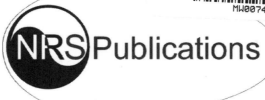

NUTRITION:
The Good, The Bad and The Politics

IS A PRODUCT OF THE
NRS PUBLICATIONS EDUCATION SE-
RIES

NUTRITION: The Good, The Bad and The Politics
ISBN 0-9756920-8-9
Copyright 2006

Nutrition: The Good, the Bad and the Politics

The START

The GOOD...

The BAD ...

And the POLITICS...

Start Here....

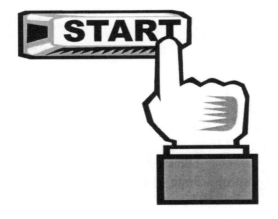

ACKNOWLEDGMENTS.

I would like to thank the following people for their direct and indirect help.

Mr Peter Daale of the Cancer Support Association of W.A. for allowing me to vent my spleen in the Cancer Wellness Newsletter where many of these short papers were published.

Dr. Myke Stanbridge for his foreword, technical help and constant inspiration for 30 years.

Mrs. Val Allen for opening new avenues of understanding for me.

Mrs. Betty Foster for keeping an eye on me.

Sheena Martin who predicted that I would do this.

Dr. Don Watts for teaching me real chemistry.

Dr. Ted Haywood for allowing lateral thinking in his ward.

Dr. David Haydon for his technical support and lateralism.

Mr. Les Spartalis for his constant support.

Ms. Mary Paul (connoisseur of ovine products) for her past help.

Mr. John Bryant for his constructive criticism.

The Staff at my clinic who have seen my work in action.

PREFACE

There are three assumptions that are fundamental in Mainstream Medicine that will always lead doctors to the wrong decisions.

Wrong assumption 1 is "Once a diagnosis has been made, this is permanent and unalterable".

Wrong assumption 2 is "Studies in the basic sciences relating to causation of illness are not applicable in clinical practice".

Wrong assumption 3 is "Only Mainstream Medicine has effective treatments".

When you give up these unhelpful mindsets, you can really start to help people.

However, I did not write this book for doctors. They have been so effectively brainwashed by pharmaceutical companies and health authorities that they can never be expected to use logic again. But health consumers have had enough. They read, they surf the net and they are not happy with the current direction of modern medicine. Doctors either have to listen and learn or they will be drowned in the eventual tide of discontent. Presently, they sleep too comfortably in their castle of ignorance. They respond like this "If all this stuff about magnesium were true, then why hasn't someone told me about it?" What they mean is, why hasn't the information been plonked on their desks. Actually they are too lazy to investigate the information for themselves. But even if it had been plonked on their desks, they wouldn't look at it. Why? Because there's no gloss, no plentiful cleavage and no free lunch to go with it.

They have another problem. Nutritional Medicine explains to the patient why things have gone wrong. Therefore it is a transparent healing modality. No mystique, no sleight of hand. It's logical and it works with processes that can be applied to many disorders. This is totally unsatisfactory for the ego driven medical profession. We can't possibly let the patient understand what we are doing for them can we now? Hence the warning on the cover. If you read this, then prepare to use logic again in medical decision-making. Otherwise you can stay locked in your bedazzled pharmaceutical comfort zone and keep dishing out the pills. Maybe the truth will be plonked on your desk one day. However, if you want to begin the search, there are over 2000 references here to get you started.

But one more thing. Doctors tend to hide behind the skirt of the "double blind randomised trial". I don't need such a trial to know that if I took the battery out of my car that it wouldn't start. Why? Because the battery is *part of the design*. I don't need to take the batteries out of 100 randomly chosen motor vehicles either. Drugs are **not** part of the design of the human body. There is no way use can use the experimental structure and ideology of double blind randomised trials to analyse nutrients properly. We are not using nutrients "therapeutically' we are using them "correctly".

Since my first book, many practitioners have attended my lectures and courses. The feedback has been very positive. All of them have left at the end of the day with a better understanding of how the human body works and a better understanding of why governments and big businesses collude to keep the population at large slightly sick. The name of the game is to extract the maximum amount of profit and tax from the herd and then kill them off slowly.

FOREWORD (to Dr Tabrizian's original book)

This book is about nutrition. Broadly, this includes what food we get to eat, what water we get to drink and what air we get to breathe. It can also include supplements to a poor diet, and in some cases, special medications. Our biological machinery must cope with all these and every other chemical, no considered a nutrient, to which we have daily exposure. Healthy bodies can cope, provided they maintain a proper balance. This includes a tranquil lifestyle with stress-free physical and mental exercise. A robust constitution, or a proven genetic line, is not able to deliver health if one's nutrition is out of balance.

Human beings have evolved with nature for millions of years. Over that time, injury and infection have been a constant threat to our life and wellbeing. Naturally, we have evolved mechanisms to cope with a vast range of internal changes caused by external agents. These may be organic and/or inorganic, entering our body in what we eat, drink and breathe, or let in via exposed skin or open wounds. Our success as a biological machine is a consequence of our ability to act upon an environmental stage that changes rapidly, but where natural adaptation to a persistent change is a very slow process. Our health relies on us keeping our finely tuned biological machine functioning smoothly. Our almost 100% adaptation to a past environment, but a fraction of 1% to the insults of the modern world, has geared us to function with only minimum harm in a biologically hostile world, not in an artificial chemically engineered world. Our successful evolution among other living things, parasites, microbes and all, is a battle for survival among the fittest. That we have survived so far is a remarkable fact due in large part to our ability to maintain a biological balance.

The external agents that can harm us are as diverse as they are numerous. They include fungi, bacteria, viruses and the more subtle mycoplasmas and prions. As well as this, we have to cope with various toxic substances from plant, animal and mineral sources. Any of these could be unknown parts of what we eat, drink or breathe, or a by-product of digestive and/or metabolic interactions. It may be a surprise to learn that all this applies to a nature unadulterated by modern human activities. No artificial chemicals, like drugs, dyestuffs, plastics, solvents, food additives, pesticides, etc. Especially, no genetic mods to life that have not first passed the long-term safety filter of evolution. In our modern world most of us take it for granted that very strict controls exist that minimise such potentially harmful external agents, but that is a myth of monstrous proportions – we need to regain control.

Regaining control over our life begins by ensuring an appropriate nutritional regime that fits our lifestyle. But this is a lot easier said than done. The majority of people need professional guidance to discover their appropriate nutritional regime. Learning how to maintain a proper nutritional balance can then help them to regain control over their wellbeing. In a global economy obsessed with quantity over quality – with its pressures to use artificial production methods to lower costs – nutrition is the big loser. Once we could depend on the nutritional values of foods – never worrying about the chemical traces they carried into our bodies, but not any more. Indeed, that a need even exists for dietary supplements and corrective medications is an indictment of the modern system. We can regain control if we understand the effects that poor nutrition has, what symptoms appear when a nutritional imbalance exists for a given lifestyle. Regaining control can be as simple as recovering nutritional balance. Dr. Tabrizian explains – steadfastly – in this book his broad experiences in general medicine and life that have led to his quantitative nutritional rebalancing approach to healing. In our long and wide-ranging association, he has demonstrated a dedication to understanding the very difficult chronic health issues. He has discovered how nutritional imbalances in our biological machinery lead to the onset of particular symptoms, and how to correct nutritional imbalances to eliminate the underlying cause of the symptoms. As will become clear on reading this book, the real connections between nutrition and health have far reaching consequences. Dr. Tabrizian's general findings go to the heart of good health and wellbeing at a time when the world is under chemical siege – from a burgeoning number of fronts, including pharmaceuticals over prescription in general and falling food, water and air quality in particular. Utilizing quantitative nutritional rebalancing is a novel approach to total health care that augments the superficial amelioration of symptoms by a simple prescription of drugs.

For good health to be a reality with shrinking health care budgets – a worldwide happening – doctors need to be able to practice 'reality' medicine. Unfortunately, the time needed to fully assess a patient appears eroded to the point where the general medical practice has become a sort of 'turnkey' operation. An operation designed for packaged health care outcomes based on identifying the drugs-set indicated to ameliorate the patient's symptoms in the shortest time at the lowest social cost. Although the ordering of tests may precede the prescription of the drugs-set, with the purpose of 'catching' abnormalities that appear consistent with the patient's symptoms, this can exacerbate the problem. For example, simple serum tests for zinc will not reveal the true biological status of zinc in a patient's body, but hair analysis will.

This goes to the philosophy of diagnosis – know thy patient's true biochemical status. Of course, the initial costs in time and tests rise, but the health care outcomes get better at a lower social cost. The practice of 'reality' medicine is the essence of this book.

While drugs are a very important part of the medical tool kit, they are not always a part of the ultimate health care solution. In many cases, a change in lifestyle and/or nutrition can be of greater benefit. Recognising this can be very difficult in chronic illnesses, where the immune system is hypersensitive to poorly understood pathogens and/or allergens. For example, mycoplasmas are agents with systemic effects that often confuse a diagnosis. The consequence can be a general treatment of symptoms by drug therapy that leaves the cause untouched – likewise with certain allergens that may be 'nutritional' elements for the majority, yet traumatic for a few, as in products containing allergenic materials. So, the chronic problem with its associated consumption of drugs will persist. In such cases, the ultimate health care solution would be to eliminate the cause of the symptoms, because then the drugs used to ameliorate the symptoms are unnecessary with benefits to patient and society. Of course, trying to wean the practitioners and their patients off unnecessary drugs is not that easy, especially under drugs marketing pressures and the modern quick fix mentality.

Nutritional Medicine: Fact & Fiction is a book that is long overdue. Dr. Tabrizian has compiled a very easy to read and digest insight into human wellbeing. It gives in a concise format the details needed to regain control over a range of health issues via balanced nutrition. The methods of quantitative nutritional rebalancing combine advanced analytic techniques with a deep understanding of how our basic biochemical machinery functions.

This direct approach to the resolution of chronic illness, and the provision of preventative medicine, has a great deal to recommend it. The results presented here have taken many years to accumulate, to understand and to put into practice in a clinically effective way. As a technology consultant, with medical training and an understanding of applied chemistry I know the principles introduced here by Dr Tabrizian are well founded. Their application long ago was a possibility, but uneconomic in the practice of general medicine due to the high costs of clinical testing. Fortunately, the technologies used to accurately determine a patient's biochemical status have now advanced sufficiently to permit general application at a reasonable cost. As a final point, the principles used arise in common sense – they have obvious simplicity at the level of patient understanding. Bringing nutritional medicine to the attention of the public, at its functional level, requires a book like this.

Myke Stanbridge Augsut 2001

INTRODUCTION.

Everything comes down to molecules. Sorry to tell you this, but it all comes down to very small particles like Magnesium, Zinc, Iron, even protons (hydrogen ions). So to those people selling their drugs, herbs, "glyconutrients" or whatever, move over for cellular nutrition. Nutritional Medicine encompasses many facets of medicine and complementary therapies. It is just one of many ways of viewing and solving medical problems.

It is really based upon applied clinical biochemistry and immunology with a bit of lateral thinking.

It looks for disturbances of cellular processes and matches them to clinical settings and symptoms using data collected from many sources.

By examining on a cellular level, paradoxically one develops holistic solutions. For example in the investigation of panic attacks, magnesium is frequently found to be lacking (as confirmed by Red Blood Cell Magnesium level). Those with low magnesium levels will often have headaches, leg cramps, unstable blood sugars, blurred vision, wheeze with exertion or have painful periods. One can reassure the patient that these symptoms are indeed related and will improve. The reassurance that the patient has 7 symptoms relating to one cause rather than 7 illnesses proves that they are not hypochondriacs (in contrast to what they may have been told previously).

The rules of nutrition:
1] There is no average person.
2] There is no average or typical cell – each cell is a specialist cell.
3] Each cell has an output that defines it.
4] Drug companies control studies and publications.
5] Doctors are threatened not to exceed the boundaries of what they were taught.

Take home message: The truth is not being told to doctors because they are manipulated too cleverly to have any insight into the extent of the misinformation shovelled to them. The proof of this is the information in this book. Most doctors are not aware of the amount of good research already undertaken in the field of molecular medicine.

I first got involved with nutritional medicine quite sceptically. After 14 years in hospital training, I ventured into General Practice. So I started a new phase of life involving both anaesthetics and general practice in a country town. It became clear after a while that there were severe deficiencies in the information available to doctors for solving all the problems that presented.

My first experience of this was with a 20 year-old Hamersley Iron worker who kept coming down with tonsillitis. I vaguely recalled from my medical school training that low zinc was associated with immune defects and so I ordered a zinc level. To my surprise and horror, it came back low. So, instead of giving antibiotics, I gave him zinc. Also to my surprise, (apart from stopping the tonsillitis) he started to sleep better, his hay fever and eczema cleared up and his asthma became easily controllable.

So I started to do more zinc levels on patients with allergies, asthma, hay fever, eczema and I kept getting abnormal results. They all got better on zinc! So I started to research zinc and found many papers on the subject, but *not* in medical journals. Looking up papers on magnesium, I found that suboptimal levels could cause anxiety, tremor, muscle cramps, headaches, insomnia and hypertension. So when patients presented with these conditions I would check the magnesium levels. Lo and behold, they came back low and/or the problems responded to magnesium.

So then I started to check things like selenium and Vitamin C. More abnormal results. I had not expected this at all. I was told that if you have a good diet that these things could not happen. What else was going on? Could there be a problem with the food we eat or in the way we absorb these nutrients from the gastrointestinal tract? So then I started surveying the patients for digestive symptoms such as bloating after meals, wind, burping, reflux. To my surprise, the deficient patients had more of the symptoms!

I then came across a pamphlet by the Society of Gastroenterologists. They said that the stomach infection caused by Helicobacter pylori affected

40% of Australians. I started checking the patients for Helicobacter and found about 60% of them had the bug. After treatment, their levels stayed up without supplements. However some patients had digestive symptoms but did not have Helicobacter. All of these patients had either low zinc, Vitamin B1 or Vitamin B6. It turns out that these nutrients are needed for the making of stomach acid. The stomach acid stimulates the pancreas to release picolinic acid, which binds zinc and allows it to be absorbed. So the circle was complete. If you don't absorb zinc, you don't make stomach acid and if you don't make stomach acid, you can't absorb zinc.

So now I had identified the commonest cause of malabsorption to be low zinc and/or Helicobacter infection.

The next question was why was the zinc low in the first place? Where does the zinc come from? There are two sources; animals and plants. As a rule, we absorb zinc better from animal flesh. We're talking about foods like beef, fish, crab, oysters, salmon and veal. From plants we're talking about cashews, sunflower seeds, nuts, lentils, chickpeas, brown rice, barley, cracked wheat. So how does the zinc get into the plants? It comes from the soil.

How much zinc is in WA soils? According to the geologists, no rocks in WA have any zinc! So the amount of zinc depends upon the level in the soil. So how do we put more zinc in the soil? We add superphosphate fertilisers. Is that the end of the story? No, because these superphosphates contain the toxic mineral cadmium in concentrations of beteween 2-130mg per kilogram (depending on the source).

The problem with cadmium is that it interferes with the plant's uptake of zinc. Worst of all, we absorb the cadmium from the bread made from such plants and the cadmium interferes with our zinc! After the zinc containing food gets to our tables, we have to eat it and absorb it (if we have enough stomach acid).

The next problem is can we store it? Stress depletes zinc levels and so do some food additives (the colouring E102 for instance). Some blood pressure medications such as diuretics and Ace-inhibitor (Ramipril, Enalapril, etc) also deplete zinc levels. So, all in all, it's not that hard to get zinc depleted. Other factors such as pregnancy, breast-feeding, the oral contraceptive and women's hormone replacement therapy also deplete zinc. So, add the 40% figure for Helicobacter and then another 20% for environmental factors related to zinc deficiency but did not have abnormal blood tests. The same with magnesium and selenium. So what was going on? I then decided to investigate Anti-nutrients. What are Anti-nutrients, see page 19. These are molecules that antagonise the good nutrients. For example lead versus iron; cadmium versus magnesium; copper versus zinc. So how could one determine if this was happening if the blood tests were normal? The answer comes down to tissue mineral analysis. What tissue? Hair. Yes, the answer came down to hair analysis. So then I started doing hair analysis and started getting some real answers. However these created even more questions as to the real effect of the environment on our health. Yes, indeed there were Anti-nutrients blocking the effect of the nutrients and the identification of these "hidden" enemies filled in the missing pieces of the nutritional puzzle.

This work linked directly with the work of Dr. John R Lee who noticed that estrogen excess or progesterone deficiency could lead to copper excess, low zinc and low magnesium. This linked to studies that showed how pesticides, plastics, petroleum products and ingested hormones from food lead to the accumulation of false estrogens which in turn cause high copper, low zinc and low magnesium. We've all had exposure to these long lasting poisons. This linked to work done on personality and mental disorders by Dr. William Walsh. It confirmed my suspicion that diagnoses like ADD were becoming epidemic as a result of these mineral imbalances.

Then the horror and the extent of the disaster was obvious. Through environmental poisons, farming malpractice, prescription drug administration and the Helicobacter epidemic (15% of the world's population), the picture was complete. We are killing ourselves, with the encouragement of the Health Insurance Commission and our government. We are all sick of it and now we want answers.

The term Nutritional Medicine often misleads doctors into thinking that the specialty primarily involves diet and lifestyle changes. Orthomolecular Medicine is probably a better description but it has a rather tarnished reputation. So we resort to the term Nutritional Medicine so as not to alienate our patients and colleagues.

Page one of any pathology textbook will tell you that by the time disease is detectable by microscopy it must have involved a structural change. The structural change must have involved an alteration in the biochemistry in a direction away from the direction that nature intended. They will say "look up a biochemistry book" to find out what this change entails. This biochemistry books fail to link the pathobiochemistry with the clinical symptoms and everybody basically passes the buck. The truth is that Nutritional Medicine links the various specialties and tries to be the middleman, the explainer of all phenomena.

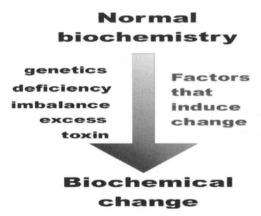

The process that drives normal biochemistry to abnormal biochemistry involves any combination of five factors. Genetics, deficiency, excess, imbalance or toxins. In order to understand these processes, there are tools required and access to the appropriate literature. Most of these tools were never taught to doctors and the source of the literature was never pointed out because it involved technical areas "outside of our business". So in order to solve certain problems, new areas of knowledge must be learned. These include Soil science, Dietetics, Tissue mineral science and Environmental science. Only after being armed with these extra tools can a full analysis be made. The problem is that many doctors do not wish to exceed the boundaries of what they were taught because their teachers in medical

Tools required

Soil science

Digestion

Dietetics

Nutrient metabolism
[biochemistry]

Tissue mineral science

Environmental
Science

Mechanism

deficiency

imbalance

excess

toxin

school or post graduate training programs would threaten them if they did. Consequently potentially useful pieces of information presented to them were probably discarded. This is an example of how medicine deals with information. Let's say you got a puzzle for your birthday. You look at the box cover quickly and say, "It's a beach scene". You start sifting through the pieces. You find an air conditioner. What is *this* doing here? Obviously packed in the wrong box- chuck it out. Next you find a Ferrari. What is *this* doing here? Obviously packed in the wrong box- chuck it out. Next a 747. What is this doing here? Obviously packed in the wrong box- chuck it out. Finally, you finish the puzzle and there are pieces missing! Well, the beach scene was near the Gold Coast. The aircon was on top of the beach house. The Ferrari was a reflection in a pair of expensive sunglasses. The 747 was in the edge of the picture because the flight path comes over the beach. This is how orthodox medicine deals with information outside the square. Nutritional medicine NEVER throws away a piece.

The problem is that the pieces come from a variety of scientific disciplines, each with their own nomenclature and histories. This creates a problem for linear thinkers. Everything is connected to everything! For the narrow minded brainwashed medical profession, this type of mindset is intolerable and unfortunately it involves *unlearning* some things. It involves questioning the objectivity of some key concepts in medicine and in fact it involves key concepts at the very bottom of the Aristotelian based knowledge pyramid, of which we are so proud. Could our hallowed teachers have been wrong? Could they have been *really* wrong? Could *their* teachers have been wrong too?

Moreover, who controls the curriculum of a medical school? Who controls not only what is included, but also what is excluded from such curricula? At this point, the issues become political. Unfortunately many issues in nutritional medicine *are* political, especially about toxins in the environment. Many nutritional medicine doctors harbour antiestablishment sentiment, because they see the truth behind the illness that confronts them every day. The truth ignored by the majority of the profession. People who tell the truth have never been popular in history. The world turns predominately because the majority of the affluent create a reality and stick to it by consensus. Working in nutritional medicine is very much like the X-files of medicine. Thousands of anecdotes adding up to a huge conspiracy. The conspiracy to perpetuate chronic illness. And behind that, the vested interests in that outcome.

One good example of this refers to the biochemistry of serotonin. The pathway is below . It includes the co-factors (never emphasized in medical schools of course). We say to the patients that they have a "chemical imbalance" and that they need chemicals to fix this. We never ask, "Why can't this patient make serotonin?" If the biochemistry has been worked out for 20 years, then why are we encouraged to use SSRI's instead of investigating such patients?

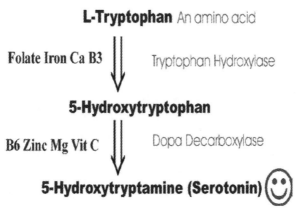

L-Tryptophan An amino acid

Folate Iron Ca B3 ⇓ Tryptophan Hydroxylase

5-Hydroxytryptophan

B6 Zinc Mg Vit C ⇓ Dopa Decarboxylase

5-Hydroxytryptamine (Serotonin) ☺

Moreover, supplements containing tryptophan and hydroxy-tryptophan are either unavailable or Schedule 4 items. Put the power to prescribe them in the hands of those least likely to use it! This is where the politics enter the equation.

NUTRIENTS AND ANTI-NUTRIENTS: THE IMPORTANCE OF BALANCE.

A theme which readers may have picked up from my articles relates to the concept of balance within biological systems. This is a feature of eastern medicine, which is generally not incorporated into western science, perhaps with the exception of physics. Balance can be described as "when two opposing components balance a biological system". In other words, these can be naturally opposing components like zinc and copper or a nutrient and it counteracting anti-nutrient such as zinc and cadmium. A list below shows examples of such nutrient anti-nutrient combinations.

ANTI-NUTRIENTS

Copper blocks Zinc, Magnesium, Molybdenum, Cobalt, Manganese, Iron, Boron, Vit B1, Vit C, Vit E, Folic Acid
Lead blocks Iron, Calcium, Molybdenum, Manganese, Chromium, Sulphur, Cobalt
Mercury blocks Zinc, Selenium, Iron, Sulphur, Cobalt
Cadmium blocks Zinc, Magnesium, Selenium, Sulphur
Arsenic blocks Vit E, Selenium, Sulphur
Aluminium blocks Vit E, Vit C, Vit B1, Zinc, Selenium, Sodium, Potassium, Phosphorus
Antimony blocks Zinc, Selenium

In this situation, minerals are somewhat easier to understand because we could mentally imagine one mineral blocking another's function with an enzyme. What is poorly understood is that Anti-nutrients can cause havoc within cells without being labelled as toxic i.e. below "toxic" levels. The definitions of toxicity are primarily defined by industry, not medicine. These industries wish to define toxicity by the least sensitive method of detection. Tissue mineral analysis (hair analysis) is the most sensitive method of detection of heavy metals; hence industry will not use this tool. This spills over into the medical profession, who cannot understand why hair analysis is so useful for the improvement

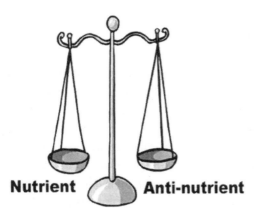

Nutrient **Anti-nutrient**

of health.

The point is this: you cannot understand the level of a nutrient unless you measure its opposing component. For instance, a normal ferritin in the presence of lead, will still give symptoms of iron deficiency. A normal red cell zinc in the presence of excess copper will still give the symptoms of zinc deficiency. A normal red cell magnesium in the presence of cadmium will still give symptoms of magnesium deficiency. Just measuring the blood levels and making assumptions about the opposing component will not always work. In fact it may lead to unnecessary and prolonged supplementation, with the eventual increasing of dose to control symptoms. If the copper is rising, then you need more Vitamin C over time to prevent say bleeding gums.

Mineral balance is not just a simple set of scales; it involves three or four dimensional axes. For instance, copper, zinc, magnesium and molybdenum need to be balanced for correct energy cycles. Abnormalities of these four minerals are the main problem in chronic fatigue syndrome. Another balance is between magnesium, sodium, potassium and calcium. The balance of these minerals determines nervous system function. When one overlaps the two sets, with magnesium in the centre, we see that alterations in one group eventually lead to a change in the other group. These balances cannot be determined by blood test. Only a tissue sample will provide this type of information. More importantly the solution requires understanding why the imbalance occurred and at which point, did disruption occur.

My final point is this: an analysis of why these groups get out of balance is paramount in finding long-term solution. Secondly, those who prescribe nutrients without an appreciation of Anti-nutrients and balance do not understand the whole process of illness. They are simply symptom prescribing.

REFERENCES:

1] Abe T., el al. High hair and urinary mercury levels of fish eaters in the non-polluted environment of Papua New Guinea. Arch Environ Health. 50:367-373, 1995

2] Abraham J.E., Svare C.W. & Frank C.W. The effect of dental amalgam restorations on blood mercury levels. J Dent Res. 63:71-73, 1984.

3] Alexander. The uptake of lead by children in differing environments. Environ Hlth Prospectus. 1974.

4] Aller A.J. the clinical significance of beryllium. J Trace Elements and Electrolytes in Health and Dis. 4,1, 1990.

5] Altmann P., et al. Disturbance of cerebral function by aluminium in haemodialysis patients with overt aluminium toxicity. Lancet. Jul, 1989.

6] Ames B.N. Dietary carcinogens and anticarcinogens. Science. 221:1256-1264, 1983.

7] Annest J.I., et al. Chronological trend in blood lead levels between 1976 and 1980. N.E.J.M. 308, 23, 1983.

8] Anthony H., et al. Environmental Medicine in Practice. Southhampton: BSAENM Publications. 204-208, 1997.

9] Aposhian H.V. DMSA and DMPS-water soluble antidotes for heavy metal poisoning. Ann Rev Pharmacol Toxicol. 23:193-215, 1983.

10] Aschner M., et al. Interactions of methylmercury with rat primary astrocyte cultures: inhibition of rubidium and glutamate uptake and induction of swelling. Brain res. 530:235-250, 1990.

11] Ashby J., et al. Studies on the genotoxicity of beryllium sulphate in vitro and in vivo. Mutation Res. 240,3, 1990.

12] Atchison W.D. & Hare M.F. Mechanisms of methylmercury-induced neurotoxicity. FASEB J. 8:622-629, 1994.

13] Baaumslag N., et al. trace metal content of maternal and neonate hair. Zinc, copper, iron and lead. Arch Environ. Hlth. 29, 1974.

14] Baker E.L., et al. A nationwide survey of heavy metal absorption in children living near primary copper, lead and zinc smelter. Am J Epidemiology. 206,4, 1977.

15] Bapu C., Rao P. & Sood P.P. Restoration of methylmercury inhibited adenosine triphosphatases during vitamin and monothiol therapy. J Environ Path toxicol Oncol. 17:75-80, 1998.

16] Barregard L., Sallsten G. & Jarvholm B. People with high mercury uptake from their own dental amalgam fillings. Occup Envrion med. 52:124-128, 1995.

17] Barth G., Ed. The Lewis and Clark Expedition, Selections from the Journals Arranged by Topic. New York: Bedford St. Martins. 158-162, 1998.

18] Batuman V., et al. Contribution of lead to hypertension with renal impairment. N.E.J.M. 309,1, 1983.

19] Beattie J.H. & Peace H.S. The influence of low-boron diet and boron supplementation on bone, major mineral and sex steroid metabolism in postmenopausal women. Brit J Nutr. 69,3, 1993.

20] Bhat R.K., et al. trace elements in hair and environmental exposure. Sci Total environ. 22(2):169-178, 1982

21] Bigazzi P.E. Lessons from animal models: the scope of mercury-induced autoimmunity. Clin Immunol Immunopathol. 65:81-84, 1992.

22] Birchall J.D. & Chappell J.S. Aluminium, chemical physiology and Alzheimer's disease. Lancet. Oct, 1988.

23] Blakley B.R., Sisodia C.S. & Mukkur T.K. The effect of methylmercury, tetraethyl lead, and sodium arsenite on the humoral immunity response in mice. Toxicol Appl Pharmacol. 52:245-254, 1980.

24] Blumer W. & Reich T. leaded gasoline – a cause of cancer. Environmental International. 3:456-471, 1980.

25] Bonhomme C., et al. Mercury poisoning by vacuum-cleaner aerosol. Lancet. 347:115, 1996.

26] Boogaard P.J., et al. Effects of exposure to elemental mercury on nervous system and the kidneys in workers producing natural gas. Arch Environ Health. 5:108-115, 1996.

27] Boyce B.F., et al. Hypercalcaemic osteomalacia due to aluminium toxicity. Lancet. Nov, 1982.

28] Boyd N.D., et al. Mercury from dental "silver" tooth fillings impairs sheep kidney function. Am J Physiol. 261:R1010-R1014, 1991

29] Capel I.D., et al. Assessment of zinc status by the zinc tolerance test in various groups of patients. Clin Biochem. 15(2):257-260, 1982

30] Cavalleri A. & Gobba F. Reversible color vision loss in occupational exposure to metallic mercury. Environ Res. 77:173-177, 1998.

31] Chang L.W. Neurotoxic effects of mercury. A review. Environ Res. 14:329-373, 1977.

32] Cheraskin E. & Ringsdorf W.M. The distribution of lead in human hair. J of Med Assoc of Alabama. April, 1979.

33] Cheraskin E. & Ringsdorf W.M. Prevalence of possible lead toxicity as determined by hair analysis. J Orthomol Psych. 8,2. Am J Ind Med. 2,1,5-14, 1981.

34] Cianciola M.E., et al. Epidemiologic assessment of measures used to indicate low-level exposure to mercury vapor. J Toxicol Environ Health. 52:19-33, 1997.

35] Cimino J.A. & Demopoulos H.B. Introduction: Determinants of cancer relevant to prevention, in the war on cancer. J Environ, Path. & Toxi.3:1-10, 1980.

36] Clarke N.E., Clarke C.N. & Mosher R.E. The "in vivo" dissolution of metastatic calcium: An approach to athero-sclerosis. Am J Med Sci. 229:142-149, 1955.

37] Clarke A.N. & Wilson D.J. Preparation of hair for lead analysis. Arch Environ Hlth. 28, 1974.

38] Clarkson T.W., Amin-Zaki L. & Al-Tikriti S.K. An outbreak of methylmercury poisoning due to consumption of contaminated grain. Fed Proc. 35:2395-2399, 1976.

39] Clarkson T.W., et al. Mercury. In: Clarkson T.W., Friber L., Nordberg G.F., Sager P.R., eds. Biological Monitoring of Toxic Metals. New York: Plenum Press; 199-246, 1988.

40] Coccini t., et al. Low-level exposure to methylmercury modifies muscarinic cholinergic receptor binding characteristics in rat brain and lymphocytes: physiologic implication and new opportunities in biological monitoring. Environ Health Perspect. 108:29-33, 2000.

41] Collipp P.J., et al. Hair zinc levels in infants. Clin Pediatr. 22(7):512-513, 1983.

42] Cooper G.P. & Manalis R.S. Influence of heavy metals on synaptic transmission: a review. Neurotoxicology. 4:69-83, 1983.

43] Cornett C.R., Markesbery W.R. & Ehmann W.D. Imbalances of trace elements related to oxidative damage in Alzheimer's disease brain. Neurotoxicology. 19:339-346, 1998.

44] Crapper-McLaughlin D.R. Aluminium toxicity in senile dementia: Implications for treatment. Read before Fall Conference, American Academy of Medical Preventics, Las Vegas, NV, Nov 8, 1981.

45] Cranton E.M., et al. Standardization and interpretation of human hair for elemental concentrations. J Holistic Med. 4:10-20, 1982.

46] Crinnion W.J. Unpublished research. Healing Naturally. Kirkland, WA. 1999

47] David O., et al. Lead and hyperactivity, behavioural response to chelation: A pilot study. Am J Psychiatry. 133:1155-1158,1976

48] De Souza Queiroz M.L., et al. Abnormal antioxidant system in erthrocytes of mercury exposed workers. Human & Exp Toxicol. 17:225-230, 1998

49] Del Maestro R.F. An approach to free radicals in medicine and biology. Acta Physiol Scand. 492(suppl):153-168, 1980.

50] Diamond G. & Zalups R.K. Understanding renal toxicity of heavy metals. Toxicol Pathol. 26:92-103, 1998.

51] Dieter M.P., et al. Immunological and biochemical responses in mice treated with mercuric chloride. Toxicol Appl Pharmacol. 68:218-228, 1983.

52] Dirks M.J., et al. Mercury excretion and intravenous ascorbic acid. ArchEnviron Health. 49:49-52, 1994.

53] Dix Y. Metabolism of polycyclic aromatic hydrocarbon derivatives to ultimate carcinogens during lipid peroxidation. Science. 221:77, 1983.

54] Dormandy T.L. Free radical reaction in biological systems. Ann R Coll Surg Engl. 62:188-194, 1980.

55] Dormandy T.L. free radical oxidation and antioxidants. Lancet i:647-650, 1978.

56] Druet P., et al. Immune type glomerulonephritis induced by HgC12 in Brown Norway Rat. Ann Immunol (Inst Pasteur). 129C:777-792, 1978

57] Durham H.D., Minotti S. & Caporicci E. Sensitivity of platelet microtubles to disassembly by methylmercury. J. Toxicol Enviro Health 48:57-69, 1997

58] Ely J.T., et al. Urine mercury in micromercurialism: a bimodal distribution and its diagnostic implications. Unpublished.

59] Ely D.L., et al. Aerometric and hair trace metal content in learning-disabled children. Environ Res. 25(2):325-339, 1981.

60] Giaziano J.H. Role of 2.3-dimercaptosuccininc acid in the treatment of heavy metal poisoning. Med Toxicol. 1:155-162, 1986.

61] Grazino J.H. & Blum C. Lead exposure from lead crystal. Lancet. 337, 1991.

62] Gunderson E.L. FDA Total Diet Study, April 1982 – April 1986. Dietary intake of pesticides, selected elements and other chemicals. Distributed by : Association of Official Analytical Chemists. Arlington, VA.

63] Hahn L.J., et al. Dental "silver" tooth fillings: a source of mercury exposure revealed by whole-body image scan and tissue analysis. FASEB J. 3:2641-2646, 1989.

64] Hahn L.J., et al. Whole body imaging of the distribution of mercury released from dental fillings into monkey tissue. FASEB J. 4:3256-3260, 1990.

65] Halbach S., et al. Compartmental transfer of mercury released form amalgam. Hum Exp Toxicol. 16:667-672, 1997.

66] Halbach S., et al. Systemic transfer of mercury from amalgam fillings before and after cessation of emission. Environ Res. 77:115-123, 1998.

67] Hansen J.C., Christensen L.B. & Tarp U. Hair lead concentration in children with minimal cerebral dysfunction. Danish Med Bull. 27:259-262, 1980.

68] Harada M., et al. The present mercury contents of scalp hair and clinical symptoms in inhabitants of the Minamata area. Environ Res. 77:160-164, 1998.

69] Harnly M., et al. Biological monitoring for mercury within a community with soil and fish contamination. Environ Health Perspect. 105:424-429, 1997.

70] Harrison W., Yurachek J. & Bensen C. The determination of trace elements in human hair by atomic absorption spectroscopy. Clin Chim Acta. 23(1):83-91, 1969.

71] Herrstrom P., et al. Dental amalgam, low-dose exposure to mercury and urinary proteins in young Swedish men. Arch environ Health. 50:103-110, 1995.

72] Hibberd A.R., Howard M.A. & Hunnisett A.G. Mercury from dental amalgam fillings: studies on oral chelating agents for assessing and reducing mercury burdens in humans. J Nutr Environ Med. 8:219-231, 1998.

73] Homma-Takeda S., et al. Selective induction of apoptosis of renal tubular cells caused by inorganic mercury in vivo. Environ Toxicol Pharmacol. 7:179-187, 1999

74] Huel G., Boudene C. & Ibraham M.A. Cadmium and lead content of maternal and newborn hair: Relationship to parity, birth weight and hypertension. Arch Environ Health. 35(5):221-227, 1981.

75] Hunt C.D., Shuler T.R. & Mullen L.M. Concentration of boron and other elements in human foods and personal-care products. J Am Diet Assoc. 91,5, 1991.

76] Hurry V.J. & Gibson R.S. The zinc, copper and manganese status of children with malabsorption syndromes and in-born errors of metabolism. Biol Trace Element Res. 4:157-173, 1982

77] InSug O., et al. mercuric compounds inhibit human monocyte function by reactive oxygen species, development of mitochondrial membrane permeability transition and loss of reductive reserve. Toxicology. 124:211-224, 1997.

78] Jenkins D.W. Toxic Trace Metals in Mammalian Hair and Nails. US Environmental Protection Agency publication No. (EPA)-600/4-79-049. Environmental Monitoring Systems Laboratory. 1979.

79] Jenkins D.W. Biological monitoring of toxic trace metals Vol.1. Biological monitoring and surveillance. EPA 600/3-80-089, 1980. Clin Chem. 36,3, 1990.

80] Jones R.J. The continuing hazard of lead in drinking water. Lancet. Sept 16,

1989.

81] Kanematsu N., et al. Mutagenicity of cadmium, platinum and rhodium compounds in cultures mammalian cells. Gifu Shika Zasshi. 17,2, 1990.

82] Kin N., et al. The effect of in ovo boron supplementation on bone mineralization of the vitamin D-deficient chicken embryo. Biol Trace Element Res. 31,1, 1991.

83] Kissel K.P. Teens fall ill after taking, playing with mercury. The Seattle Times: January 15, 1998.

84] Klevay L. Hair as a biopsy material-assessment of copper nutriture. Am J. Clin Nutr. 23(8):1194-1202, 1970.

85] Kolata G. new suspect in bacterial resistance: amalgam. The New York Times: April 24, 1993.

86] Kopito L., et al. Chronic plumbism in children. Diagnosed by hair analysis. J.A.M.A. 209,2, 1969.

87] Langworth S., Elinder C.G. & Sundqvist K.G. Minor effects of low exposure to inorganic mercury on the human immune system. Scan J Work Environ Health. 19:405-413, 1993.

88] Lebel J., Mergler D. & Lucotte M. Evidence of early nervous system dysfunction in Amazonian populations exposed to low-levels of methylmercury. Neurotoxicology. 17:157-167, 1996.

89] Levine S.A. & Reinhardt J.H. Biochemical-pathology initiated by free radicals, oxidant chemicals and therapeutic drugs in the etiology of chemical hypersensitivity disease. J Orthomol Psychiatr. 12(3):166-183, 1983.

90] Lichtenberg H. Symptoms before and after proper amalgam removal in relation to serum-globulin reaction to metals. J Orthomolec Med. 11:195-204, 1996.

91] Lieb J. & Hershman d. Isaac Newton: mercury poisoning or manic depression. Lancet. 1479-1480, 1983.

92] Magour S., Maser H. & Grein H. the effect of mercury and methylmercury on brain microsomal Na+, K+ ATPase after partial delipidisation with Lubrol. Pharmacol Toxicol. 60:184-186, 1987.

93] Maloney S.R., Phillips C.A. & Mills A. Mercury in the hair of crematoria workers. Lancet. 352:1602, 1998.

94] Marlow M., et al. Increased lead burdens and trace mineral status in mentally retarded children. J Spec Educ. 16:87-99, 1982.

95] Marlowe M. et al. lead and mercury levels in emotionally disturbed children. J Orthomol Psychiatr. 12(4):260-267, 1983.

96] Marlowe M. & Mood C. Hair aluminium concentration and non-adaptive classroom behaviour. J of Advancement in Med. 1,3, 1998.

97] Matte T.D., et al. Acute high-dose lead exposure from beverage contaminated by traditional Mexican pottery. Lancet. 344, 8929, 1994.

98] Matthews A.D. Mercury content of commercially important fish of the Seychelles and hair mercury levels of a selected part of the population. Environ Res. 30:305-312, 1983.

99] Medeiros D.M. & Borgman R.F. Blood pressure in young adults as associated with dietary habits, body conformation and hair element concentrations. Nutr Res. 2:455-466, 1982.

100] Medeiros D.M. Pellum L.K. & Brown B.J. The association of selected hair minerals and anthropometric factors with blood pressure in a normotensive adult population. Nutr Research. 3:51-60, 1983.

101] Medeiros D.M. & Pellum L.K. Elevation of cadmium, lead and zinc in the hair of adult black female hypertensives. Bull Environ Toxicol. 32, 1984.

102] Miettinen J.K. Absorption and elimination of dietary mercury (2+) ion and methylmercury in man. In: Miller MW, Clarkson T.W., eds. Mercury Mercurials and Mercaptans. Proceedings 4th International Conference on Environmental Toxicology. New York: Plenum Press; 1973

103] Miller O.M., Lund B.O. & Woods J.S. Reactivity of Hg(II) with superoxide: evidence for the catalytic dismutation of superoxide by Hg(II). J Biochem Toxicol. 6:293-298, 1991.

104] Miura K., et al. The involvement of microtubular disruption in methylmercury-induced apoptosis in neuronal and nonneuronal cell lines. Toxicol Appl Pharmacol. 160:279-288, 1999.

105] Moser P.B., Krebs N.K. & Blyler E. Zinc hair concentrations and estimated zinc intakes of functionally delayed normal sized and small-for-age children. Nutr Research. 2:585-590, 1982.

106] Musa-Alzudbaidi L., et al. Hair selenium content during infancy and childhood. Eur J Pediatr. 139:295-296, 1982.

107] Nakatsuru S., et al. Effect of mercurials on lymphocyte functions n vitro. Toxicology. 36:297-305, 1985.

108] Narang A.P.S., et al. Arsenic levels in opium eaters in India. Trace Elements inMed. 4,4, 1987.

109] Ngim C.H., et al. Chronic neurobehavioural effects of elemental mercury in dentists. Dr J Indust Med. 49:782-790, 1992

110] Niculescu T., et al. Relationship between the lead concentration in hair and occupational exposure. Brit J Industrial med. 40,67, 1983

111] Ninomiya T., et al. Expansion of methylmercury poisoning outside of Minamata: an epidemiological study on chronic methylmercury poisoning utside Minamata. Environ Res. 70:47-50, 1995.

112] Nolan K.R. Copper toxicity syndrome. J Orthomol Psychiatr. 12(4):270-282, 1983.

113] Nordlind K. Inhibition of lymphoid-cell DNA synthesis by metal allergens at various concentrations. Effect on short-term cultured non-adherent cell compared to non-separated cells. Int Arch Allergy Appl Immunol. 70:191-192, 1983.

114] Nriagu J.O. Lead and Lead Poisoning in Antiquity. Wiley N.Y. 1983.

115] Orloff K.G., et al. Human exposure to elemental mercury in a contaminated residential building. Arch Environ Health. 52:169-172, 1997.

116] Ortega H.G., et al. Neuroimmunological effects of exposure to methylmercury forms in the Sprague-Dawley rat. Activation of the hypothalamic-pituitary-adrenal axis and lymphocyte responsiveness. Toxicol Indust Health. 13:57-66, 1997.

117] Oskarsson A., et al. Total and inorganic mercury in breast milk and blood in relation to fish consumption and amalgam filling in lactating women. Arch Environ Health. 51:234-241, 1996.

118] Oudar P., Caillard L. & Fillon G. In vitro effects of organic and inorganic mercury on the serotonergic system. Pharmacol Toxicol. 65:245-248, 1989.

119] Patterson J.E., Weissberg B. & Dennison P.J. Mercury in human breath from dental amalgam. Bull Environ Contam Toxicol. 34:459-468, 1985.

120] Pearl D.P., et al. Intraneuronal aluminium accumulation in Amyotrophic Lateral Sclerosis and Parkinsonism-Dementia of Guam. Science. 217, 1982.

121] Pendergrass J.C., et al. Mercury vapour inhalation inhibits binding of GTP to tubulin in rat brain: similarity to a molecular lesion in Alzheimer's disease brain. Neurotoxicity. 18:315-324, 1997.

122] Pendergrass J.C. & Haley B.E. Mercury-EDTA complex specifically blocks brain beta-tubulin-GTP interactions: similarity to observations in Alzheimer's disease. In: Friberg L.T., Scrauzer G.N., eds. Status Quo and perspectives of Amalgam and other Dental Materials. Stuttgar: Georg Thieme Verlag,98-105, 1995.

123] Peters H.A. Trace minerals, chelating agents and the por-phyrias. Fed Proc. 20(3)(Part II)(suppl 10):227-234. 1961.

124] Peters H.A., et al. Arsenic, chromium and copper poisoning from burning treated wood. N Engl J Med. 308(22):1360-1361, 1983.

125] Peters H.A., et al. Seasonal arsenic exposure from burning treated wood. J.A.M.A. 11;25,18,2393-2396, 1984.

126] Petro R., et al. Can dietary beta-carotene materially reduce human cancer rates? Nature. 290:201, 1981.

127] Rajanna B. & Hobson M. Influence of mercury on uptake of dopamine and morepinephrine by rat brain synaptosomes. Toxicol Lett. 27:7-14, 1985.

128] Rajanna B., et al. Effects of cadmium and mercury on Na+, K+, ATPases and the uptake of 3H-dopamine in rat brain synaptosomes. Arch Int Physiol Biochem. 98:291-296, 1990.

129] Redhe O. & Pleva J. Recovry from Amyotrophic Lateral Sclerosis and from allergy after removal of dental amalgam filling. Int J Risk Safety Med. 4:299-236, 1994.

130] Rees E.L. Aluminium poisoning of Papua New Guinea natives as shown by hair testing. J Orthomol Psychiatr. 12(4):312-313, 1983.

131] Salonen J.T., et al. Intake of mercury from fish, lipid peroxidation, and the risk of myocardial infarction and coronary, cardiovascular, and any death in eastern Finnish men. Circulation. 91:645-655, 1995.

132] Schroeder H.A. & Perry H.M. Jr. Antihypertensive effects of metal binding agents. J Lab Clin Med. 45:416, 1955.

133] Seven M.J. & Johnson L.A. (eds). Metal Binding in Medicine: Proceedings of a Symposium Sponsored by Hahnemann Medical College and Hospital, Philadelphia. Philadelphia, J.B. Lippincott Co., 1960.

134] Sharp D.S. & Smith A.H. Elevated blood pressure in treated hypertensives with low-level lead accumulation. Arch environ Hlth. 44,1, 1989.

135] Shenker B.J., Guo T.L. & Shapiro I.M. Low-level methymercury exposure causes human T-Cells to undergo apoptosis: evidence of mitochondrial dysfunction. Enviro Res. 77:149-159, 1998.

136] Siblerud R.L. The relationship between mercury from dental amalgam and mental health. Am J Psychotherapy. 43:575-587, 1989.

137] Sitprija V., et al. Metabolic problems in northeastern Thailand: possible role of vanadium. Mineral and Electrolyte Metabol. 19,1, 1993.

138] Skerfving, S. Mercury in women exposed to methylmercury through fish consumption, and in their newborn babies and breast milk. Bull environ Contam toxicol. 41:475-482, 1988.

139] Stopford W. & Goldwater L.J. Methylmercury in the environment: a review of current understanding. Environ Health Perspect, 12:115-118, 1975.

140] Stortebecker P. Mercury Poisoning from Dental Amalgam, A Hazard to Human Brian. Stockholm: Stortebecker Foundation for Research. 24, 1985.

141] Szylman P., et al. Potassium-wasting nephropathy in an outbreak of chronic organic mercurial intoxication. Am J Nephrol. 15:514-520, 1995.

142] Thatcher R.W., et al. Effects of low levels of cadmium and lead on cognitive functioning in children. Arch Environ Health. 37(3):159-166, 1982.

143] Thimaya S. & Ganapathy S.N. Selenium in human hair in relation to age, diet, pathological condition and serum levels. Sci Total environ. 24:41-49, 1982.

144] Thompson C.M., et al. Regional brain trace-element studies in Alzheimer's disease. Neurotoxicology. 9:1-8, 1988.

145] Ting K.S., et al. Chelate stability of sodium dimercaptosuccinate on the intoxication from many metals. Chinese Med J. 64:1072-1075, 1965.

146] Tollefson L. & Cordle F. methylmercury in fish: a review of residue levels, fish consumption and regulatory action in the United States. Environ Health Perspect. 68:203-208, 1986.

147] Trepka M.J., et al. Factors affecting internal mercury burdens among East Germany children. Arch environ health. 52:134-138, 1997.

148] Vanderhoff J.A., et al. Hair and plasma zinc levels following exclusion of biliopancreatic secretions from functioning gastrointestinal tract in humans. Dig Dis Sci. 28(4):300-305, 1983.

149] Vimy M.J. & Lorsheider F.L. Intra-oral air mercury released from dental amalgams. J Dent Res. 64:1069-1071, 1985.

150] Vimy M.F. & Lorsheider F.L. Serial measurements of intra-oral air mercury: estimation of daily dose from dental amalgams. J Dent res. 64:1072-1075, 1985.

151] Walker P.R., LeBlanc J. & Sikorska M. Effects of aluminium and other cations on the structure of brain and liver chromatin. Biochem. 28,9, 1989

WHY HAIR ANALYSIS IS SO USEFUL.

Tissue mineral analysis can be done on any body tissue, but hair is a non-invasive way to sample. Also, the reference ranges have been determined mostly for this type of sample. This technology uses mass spectrometry and it is reliable. Contrary to what many doctors and dieticians think, hair analysis is a very scientific method of detecting tissue disturbances. But, as with any test, the person who interprets it is a significant determiner of its usefulness.

In a hair analysis, most of the nutrient minerals are measured. These are calcium, magnesium, sodium, potassium, copper, zinc, iron, selenium, chromium, manganese, molybdenum, phosphorus, cobalt and boron. The test tells whether the levels are low, normal or high, but more importantly, it tells whether they are *in balance* or not. The hair analysis also detects heavy metals such as lead, mercury and cadmium. In this setting, it is much more sensitive than a blood test. If you detect lead in the blood, there is already liver damage. If detect cadmium in the blood, there is already kidney damage. Is this the time that you want to find out about this sort of problem? No, you want to know as *early* as possible.

The reason for this discrepancy is that the blood is just a transport system. *If all the minerals were stored in the blood, we would be dead.* Most intracellular mineral stores have the same feature, in that deficiencies don't show up in a blood test. Most doctors should know this, but they choose to believe the blood test rather than the patient. Unfortunately, this type of medicine is encouraged by the regulators of the Medicare system.

Heavy metals are sequestered (or stored) into the tissues to protect the blood. Hence the tissue levels offer a better insight if analysed, not the blood. Patient's problems are in their tissues, not the blood. The only diseases of blood are things like anaemia and leukaemia! Patients have problem with hearts, muscle, brains, joints, livers, stomachs NOT their blood. A tissue sample, NOT a blood test is the method of addressing these problems.

In terms of the nutrients, the body tries to keep everything in balance. The common pairs are calcium-magnesium; sodium-potassium; copper-zinc, copper-molybdenum, cobalt-potassium and chromium-vanadium as examples. Many illnesses result from imbalance between these pairs. The commonest abnormalities arise from imbalances between copper, zinc and molybdenum. This imbalance has at its root the Estrogen hormones or chemicals which have as estrogens (pesticides, petroleum products, plastics and hormones in food). Obviously, these will not show up on a blood test, so don't expect your doctor to look for them or even to understand a hair analysis report. Most of medical school teaching was about sodium, potassium and calcium.

I was very skeptical about hair analysis the first time a patient suggested it. Coming from a "hard" medical training (Physician Medicine and Anaesthetics) I had never heard of such tests and certainly never been taught in medical school about the value of tissue samples for any application other than histopathology. So when my patient showed me his test 5 years ago I responded with "I can't see this test being of any use in my practice". He then pulled out a book (by David L Watts) and said "but there's a book!" Being a bit of a bookworm, he had me hooked and I reluctantly borrowed the book for 2 weeks. I was surprised by the amount of references and the diversity of the information. I started talking more to my farmer friends and farmer patients about soil and plant analysis and realized there could be some valuable information in such a test if it was applied clinically.

Do we take the mineral levels at face value?

Minerals with charges like sodium, potassium, calcium, magnesium, iron, zinc, copper, manganese, molybdenum and chromium are very easy to study because deficiencies of them give "tell-tale" symptoms. There are hundreds of studies in humans and thousands of studies in animals about the function of these. Therefore making a list of specific symptoms for each of these could be used in a questionnaire and correlated to any testing (blood, urine, hair). For hair analysis, in some situations the symptoms do match the levels, but in many situations they do not. In the case of magnesium and zinc, normal (and high) levels can still give rise to symptoms as well as the more obvious low levels. So is it only low levels that really mean anything or is there a problem with the interpretation of these too? We sometimes see on hair analysis say, zero level of potassium or molybdenum. Can we then assume that the level equates to the whole body? Clearly not, because some of these levels (if extrapolated) would be incompatible with life! However, the same pattern is probably happening somewhere in the body and this needs a practitioner to assess. A test is not a diagnosis.

Mineral Control Mechanisms are like Aircon Systems

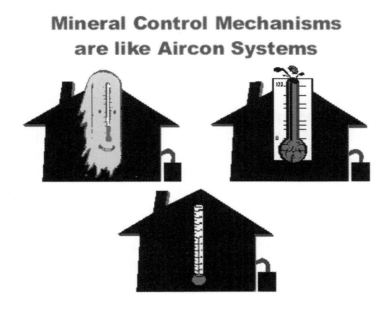

Why do mineral levels move out of range?
I believe it is more fruitful to examine why minerals vary from the reference ranges. Imagine a room in a building that is monitored by a central air-conditioning system. If you went into that room and it was cold, it wouldn't really matter if it were 3 degrees or 4 degrees. There is something wrong with the control mechanism that sets and adjusts the temperature. Same with the minerals. Variations from the reference ranges could also be due to incorrectly set management systems. The mineral level that is out of range is a message that the system is damaged or perhaps being influenced by a toxic compound. There are plenty of examples of this. A viral illness will cause a rise in temperature above the normal range. Caffeine may cause a rise in heart rate above the normal range. Therefore evaluation of the nutrient elements should take into account everything that we know about the patient (including past toxin exposure and the toxic elements). A computer that generates a report

31

may be programmed to take into account the effect of heavy metals, but generally it cannot. It sees the information "cold" and without history or context. Xenoestrogens such as DDT (which cannot be seen on a hair analysis) typically cause copper levels to rise on hair analysis to over 7 p.p.m. That is why clinical interpretation will always be more relevant and more powerful. The practitioner provides history and context.

Toxic elements like arsenic, cadmium, lead and aluminium affect the nutrient mineral levels by pushing some minerals higher than the reference range. Is the level of toxic element on hair analysis proportional to the amount in the body? No, definitely not. Sometimes you do not see that magnitude of the toxic load until you provoke the system to push out some of these toxins. Intravenous chelation practitioners use provocation studies to confirm heavy metals, but we see the same thing on sequential Hair analysis.

Mercury affects the hair analysis differently by blocking transmembrane channels that allow nutrients into the cells. Mercury causes lower levels on hair samples especially potassium, but may also cause cobalt to rise substantially. Now imagine the combined effect of say cadmium and mercury, which might give rise to the combination of say high calcium, magnesium, cobalt and boron, but low potassium. The computer would say" cut out dairy (to reduce the calcium and hence the magnesium)" and "The high cobalt and boron may not be causing problems at this time but should be further investigated". This would be Path 1 for the practitioner and probably wouldn't give long-term results. Path 2 would be to point out that even "minor" levels of mercury and cadmium can cause this profile, and a trial of heavy metal detox with follow up hair analysis in 6 months would be useful. Well, after 5,000 plus samples of going down Path 2, I have to say that following the assumptions that I've mentioned above work better than following the computer!

At the end of the day, a test is not a diagnosis; it is just the beginning of another investigation. In addition, a test is only as useful the person interpreting it. So for those people contemplating doing a hair analysis, my advice is "Find someone who can interpret it in terms of your specific problem". Even practitioners should seek an opinion from a colleague.

In summary, the hair analysis not only tells you what is wrong, it tells you how to fix it!

WHY DIGESTION IS SO IMPORTANT.

Topologically, the human body is like a torus. That is the "inside" of us (digestive tract) is actually the outside. This poses the problem of security against things that may hurt us. In the years of past it were just bacteria, viruses and fungi, and luckily our stomach acid and the immune system did the trick. These days we have preservatives, food colourings, heavy metals and other nasties to deal with. So what's the problem? With a physiology basically thousands of years old, we are struggling to cope with the ingested dangers of the 21st Century. So we need to promote the natural defence system that includes the stomach and the liver.

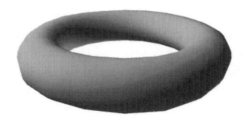

Fig 1 A torus.

So many people have symptoms such as reflux, heartburn, bloating after meals and they do not realise that these are symptoms of a failing defence system. These are the symptoms of reduced stomach acid and they are the start of many impending disasters about to befall the people who have them. Just reducing stomach acid will impair the ability to absorb Iron, Calcium and Magnesium (Page 148). Bad enough you may say, but these people also will have trouble with the digestion of the salicylates (natural aspirins). These foods include citrus, tomatoes, pineapple, kiwi fruit, strawberries, stone fruit, capsicum, chilli, mushrooms and onions. These plants accumulate natural aspirins as a defence mechanism to avoid being eaten before ripening. The only species who take them off the tree fully laden with salicylates are humans; and they do this for money and to take short cuts with nutrition. Salicylate intolerance was a rare thing 50 years ago, but now it is almost as endemic as helicobacter. Which brings us the next piece of our digestive puzzle. Helicobacter was discovered when investigators were trying to find out why some people got ulcers when on anti-inflammatory drugs. It turns out that helicobacter made them more likely to get an ulcer in the stomach. Well guess what relatives the anti-inflammatory drugs have? Aspirins (salicylates). So, those people with salicylate intolerance may well have Helicobacter brewing in their stomachs.

Helicobacter is a chronic stomach infection of worldwide epidemic proportions. It gained notoriety when it was discovered that it could cause stomach ulcers. When this information came out, everyone said "But nothing can live in the stomach; it's too acidic". Well, the truth of the matter is that we were all told that the stomach killed anything nasty as part our defence system, and so hearing the Helicobacter was the exception was rather odd. We were told that this bug is so perverse that it loves acid, and that is why we must suppress acid. The obvious (and completely overlooked) corollary hypothesis is that helicobacter could only survive if the acid was low and the commonest reason for this would be zinc deficiency. Zinc is required for the enzyme Carbonic Anhydrase which make the proton (hydrogen ion). What happens if your zinc is chronically low? You get low stomach acid and reduced defence against infections! You might say that this would suggest that zinc could be useful in the treatment of Helicobacter infections, and yes, there are some studies, which have used zinc for Helicobacter eradication.

This is not the only anomaly. Helicobacter supposedly causes gastritis. Most tissues when inflamed do not function properly, and yet the gastroenterologist claim that stomach acid must be high. Of all the medical examples above, you can see that indeed gastritis is special condition according to the medical specialists in this field of digestion. Really?

There is one more anomaly. Helicobacter is supposed to cause ulcers. Apparently, forty percent of Australians have helicobacter. Quite clearly then, most people with helicobacter do not develop ulcers. What factors predispose those to getting the ulcers? Probably low zinc.

Now, many of my patients turn up with the diagnosis of "Candida". The two commonest reasons for this overgrowth of this yeast is low stomach acid and lack of acidophilus in the intestine. Try this experiment. Put some pieces of melon in the fridge for a couple of weeks. What you will find is a heavy growth of a white fungus. This is Candida albicans. Stomach acid is supposed to kill fungi, right? Then these fungi should be killed if there is adequate digestive power in the stomach. So the best treatment is not just a low Candida diet, not just antifungals, but put back the defence system! Give them Zinc Vitamin B1, Vitamin B6 or digestive enzymes supplements or just plain Betaine hydrochloride (which converts to stomach acid). As for the acidophilus. The name says it all. Philos means to love, for example paedophile. These bacteria need an acid environment to survive, so low stomach acid creates an environment hostile to these organisms in the intestine. They also like molybdenum and zinc, and you know how much of these we get in our diet! A good intestinal environment will protect from food poisoning, travellers diarrhoea, and antibiotic induced thrush and probably from bowel cancer. One of the functions of molybdenum is to detoxify aldehydes, sulphites and carcinogens such as nitrosamines in the diet. Hence, the association of gastric tract cancers with low molybdenum. This was demonstrated in China about 30 years ago.

The widespread problems with digestion are causing major illness but in indirect ways. The inactivation of the topical defence system, the impaired absorption of important nutrients like Zinc and Selenium and the increased incidence of food intolerances (as opposed to food allergies) are powerful driving forces towards ill health. Fix the gut and the rest falls into place.

Just to reinforce why stomach acid is so important in the chain of digestion, the diagram on page 148 depicts the connection between the production of gastric acid and the absorption of Zinc and other minerals. The take home message is this. If you don't make acid, you don't absorb zinc, and if you don't absorb zinc, you don't make stomach acid.

List of foods with a very high content of salicylates:-
Fruit: Sultanas (dried), prunes, raisins (dried), currants (dried), raspberry, redcurrant, grape, loganberry, blackcurrant, youngberry, cherry, orange, blueberry, plum, pineapple, boysenberry, guava, apricot, blackberry, cranberry, date, strawberry, rock melon, tomatoes and tomato products (pastes, sauce, puree).
Vegetables: gherkin, endive, champignon, radish, olives, capsicum,

zucchini, chicory, hot pepper, chili, snow peas/unshelled peas.
Nuts: Almonds, water chestnuts.
Spices & Sauces: Cumin, chicory, cayenne, sage, vinegar (cider),
aniseed, mace, curry, paprika, thyme, Worcester Sauce, dill, turmeric,
Vegemite, Marmite, rosemary, oregano, garam marsala, mixed herbs,
mint, cumin canella, tarragon, mustard, Five Spice, pickles.
Drinks: Tea - all brands, alfalfa, peppermint. Cereal coffee -Nature's
Cuppa, any with chicory content Alcohol - liqueurs, port, wine, rum,
and cider
Other - MSG, Chinese food, Parmesan cheese, aspirin, Disprin,
tartrazine (food colouring 102), benzoates (food additives 210-211),
Licorice, peppermints, honey, mints/Minties

Digestion references

1] Barrie S.A., et al. Comparative absorption of zinc picolinate, zinc
citrate and zinc gluconate in humans. Agents and Actions. 5:1-6, 1986
2] Birdsall T. C. Zinc picolinate: Absorption and supplementation. Alt
Med Rev. 1:26-30, 1996
3] Bulbena EG. Zinc compounds, a new treatment in peptic ulcer.
Drugs under Experimental and Clinical Research.15(2):83-89 1989
4] Cater, R. E. 2nd. Helicobacter pylori as the major causal factor in
chronic hypochlorhydria. Med Hypotheses. 39:367-374, 1992.
5] Cave, D. R., et al. Effect of a Campylobacter pylori protein on acid
secretion by parietal cells. Lancet. 2:187-189, 1989.
6] Cho, C. H., et al. Zinc deficiency: its role in gastric secretion and
stress-induced gastric ulceration in rats. Pharmacol Biochem Behav.
26:293-297, 1987.
7] El-Omar,.E. M., et al. Divergent effects of H. pylori on acid
secretion. Gut. 37(Supplement 2):A6, 1995.
8] Frommer D.J. The healing of gastric ulcers by zinc sulphate. Med J
Austr. 2:793, 1975
9] Gaby, A. R. Helicobacter pylori eradication: are there alternatives
to antibiotics? Alternative Medicine Review. 6(4):355-366, 2001.
10] Giannella, R. A., et al. Influence of gastric acidity on bacterial and
parasitic enteric infections. Ann Int Med. 78:271-276, 1973.
11] Graham, D. Y., et al. Iatrogenic Campylobacter pylori infection is

a cause of epidemic achlorhydria. Am J Gastroenterol . 83:974-980, 1988.

12] Grossman, M. I., et al. Basal and histalog-stimulated gastric secretion in control subjects and in patients with peptic ulcer or gastric cancer. Gastroenterology. 45:15-26, 1963

13] Halter, F., et al. Long-term effects of Helicobacter pylori infection on acid and pepsin secretion. Yale J Biol Med. 69:99-104, 1996.

14] Hunt, J. N., et al. Relation between gastric secretion of acid and urinary excretion of calcium after oral supplements of calcium. Dig Dis Sci. 28:417-421, 1983

15] Kelly, G. S. Hydrochloric acid: physiological functions and clinical implications. Alternative Medicine Review. 2(2):116-127, 1997.

16] Kitchen, J. Hypochlorhydria: a review, part 1. Townsend Letter for Doctors and Patients. October 2001.

17] Murray et al Harper's Biochemistry 22nd Ed p 577 and p 581 1990

18] Murray, M. J., et al. A gastric factor promoting iron absorption. Lancet. 1:614, 1968

19] Sturniolo, G. C., et al. Inhibition of gastric acid secretion reduces zinc absorption in man. J Am Coll Nutr. 10(4):372-375, 1991.

20] O'Connor, H. J., et al. Vitamin C in the human stomach: relation to gastric pH, gastroduodenal disease, and possible sources. Gut. 30:436-442, 1989.

21] Prousky, J. E. Is vitamin B3 dependency a causal factor in the development of hypochlorhydria and achlorhydria? Journal of Orthomolecular Medicine. 16(4): 225-237, 2001.

22] Reed, P. I. Vitamin C, Helicobacter pylori infection and gastric carcinogenesis. Int J Vitamin Nutr Res. 69(3):220-227, 1999.

23] Solomons N.W. Competitive interaction of iron and zinc in the diet: consequences for human nutrition. J Nutr. 116:927-935, 1986

24] Sterniolo G.C., et al. Inhibition of gastric acid secretion reduces zinc absorption in man. J Am Coll Nutr. 10:372-375, 1991

25] Wapnir R.A. Zinc Deficiency, Malnutrition and the Gastrointestinal Tract. J. Nutr. 130:1388S-1392S, 2000

The Good …..

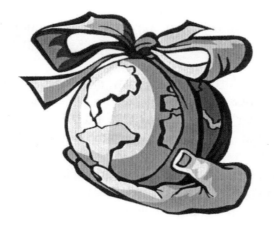

ZINC, MY KINGDOM FOR SOME ZINC.

Zinc is important for so many enzyme systems ranging from liver function to DNA synthesis, serotonin production (mood chemical), sex hormone production, insulin production, stabilisation of mast cells (these cause itching when they release histamine); immune function and preventing free radical build up. Most of the cancer patients I see have low zinc levels. Zinc deficiency is associated with diabetes, raised cholesterols, heart disease, anorexia, allergies, recurrent infections, delayed wound healing, arthritis, hair loss, pimples, eczema, infertility, depression, insomnia, learning disorders, and hyperactivity in children.

A mid-summer's night zinc deficiency

Zinc sits between copper and gallium and above cadmium and mercury on the periodic table. Unfortunately it's all bad news when it comes to this mineral. A detailed list of foods that contain zinc will show just how unplentiful it is compared with iron or calcium and to compound the problem there is the variation of zinc levels in soils where such products are grown. Zinc is the cornerstone of many nutritional deficiencies because it is required for making stomach acid. Now, despite what you hear from the medical profession, stomach acid is a **good** thing to have. Humans have had lots of stomach acid for thousands of years until recently. Now we are finding that hypochlorhydria (low stomach acid) is associated with many medical problems. Low stomach acid starts a chain of events, which eventually disable correct nutrition.

The body absorbs zinc by producing an acid called picolinic acid (which is made by the liver and kidney). This is released by the pancreas during meal times and binds zinc (along with several other trace elements) to facilitate its absorption. Problems occur because the amount of this acid is reduced if stomach acid is low. This leads to an eventual spiralling drop in zinc levels, which is insidious. The irony is that if you can't produce stomach acid your pancreas won't help you absorb zinc and if you can't absorb zinc, you can't make stomach acid.

The next problem is what does a plant include in its structure if it can't get enough zinc? Plants can grow in zinc and selenium deficient soils without apparent change in appearance. Unfortunately, trace element substitution can occur, which will fill up zinc's "spot" with some other mineral. There is concern that superphosphates contain cadmium (15-21mg per kg as a contaminant) and that cadmium will substitute for zinc. Cadmium is a toxic heavy metal.

Now the really bad news. It is possible that not only could one consume foods that are low in zinc, and be able to absorb them, but also worst of all they may contain a toxic heavy metal such as cadmium or mercury or other minerals such as copper. Now you see the problem with zinc's position in the periodic table (location, location, location!). Moreover, if the body accumulates copper as a result, this will further inhibit the absorption of zinc. Cadmium competes for absorption with zinc also. Cadmium has been implicated in the genesis of prostate cancer and atherosclerosis.

What about losses of zinc? Zinc is secreted into body fluids as an antiseptic. That's why low levels are associated with sore throats, lung infections, gastroenteritis, ulcers, urinary tract infections and thrush. Diuretics (things that make you go to the toilet) lower zinc levels. This includes the ACE inhibitors (Captopril, Enalapril etc.), Lasix (and other diuretics), coffee, tea, alcohol and the food additive Tartrazine (additive 102, which is just about everything yellow, green or orange in this country). Some people sweat zinc as zinc chloride. This explains why levels may be lower in summer (hence the comment about midsummer deficiency).

Then there's the problem of zinc storage. The syndrome of estrogen dominance (where there is an apparent lack of progesterone or an inappropriately high estrogen level) accounts for the high prevalence of zinc deficiency.
A pound of flesh yields much zinc.

Yes, animal flesh contains plentiful, easily absorbed zinc. So what are the common manifestations of zinc deficiency? Zinc falls during the day, and so low levels are often encountered in the late afternoon. Hypoglycaemia (low blood sugars) usually develops 2-2 hours after a meal, so the first hypo's begin about 3-4pm when the patient looks for a sugar fix. The next spot is about 10:30 – 11pm. Those with low zinc tend to need to eat frequently. It may cause poor concentration or mental apathy. Low zincs are associated with sleep disturbance. If the body runs low on zinc, the first symptoms may be a disrupted sleep pattern, or circadian rhythm disturbance. These people have poor sleep patterns.

Then, there's the problem of allergies, eczema/dermatitis, hay fever, and asthma. Zinc deficiency is associated with depression and disrupted sleep cycles, because you need it to make serotonin (your happy chemical) and melatonin (your sleep chemical). See the figure below to see where zinc fits into the picture.

When could such a deficiency start- at birth?

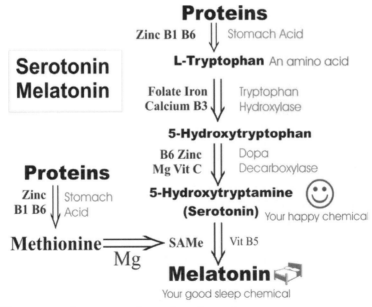

Fig. 1. How to make serotonin and melatonin

The seven ages of man. What it is to have a life without zinc.
Let's take the example of mother and baby with zinc deficiency. Mother

41

has become depleted in zinc during pregnancy and maybe breastfeeding. Her low zinc has produced problems with her brain not making the happy chemical serotonin (post natal depression). She is also low in melatonin (your sleep chemical), which is the next step down from serotonin. Baby is low in zinc and develops hypoglycaemia. Baby needs extra frequent feeds and is either a reflux baby or a colicky baby (low stomach acid leads to poor digestion). Baby also can't sleep properly (low melatonin).

Some manifest as allergies such as eczema or hay fever. Ironically, the parents may start to exclude dairy products in an effort to reduce "dairy induced mucus" symptoms, but dairy products are the main source of zinc for a child.

Next, come the frequent colds, sore throats and ear infections especially during times of growth spurts (increased DNA synthesis for growing puts pressure on zinc stores) or the skin will flare up from eczema, thrush or warts (viruses don't like zinc). If the eczema gets infected, they can't mount an effective immune reaction and so secondary infection (Staph or fungus) will complicate the issue and confuse the doctor who uses cortisone creams, because while they suppress the eczema and fungal infection, but they will aggravate any bacterial infection. Zinc deficiency may manifest in the lung and cause "asthma". These children are usually fussy eaters. They lose the sense of smell and so are reliant upon taste (salt, sweet, sour or bitter). In the case of vegetables, they tend to like peas or carrots (because they can taste the sweetness) but avoid other vegetables with innate bitterness that would normally be masked by the aroma (smell) of the plant. These children also have low stomach acid, which might make them sensitive to acidic foods such as grapes, citrus and tomatoes. These foods will either give them a headache (mummy, my head's sore) abdominal pains (mummy, my tummy's sore), skin problems (mummy, I'm itchy) and poor sleep (mummy, can I sleep in your bed?). They will either be hyperactive or moody, and suffer the hypoglycaemia effects with features such as pre-dinner tantrums and temper outbursts. They often have a persistently runny nose, but react strangely to antihistamine medications.

Later they may develop anorexia/bulimia, acne or teenage depression. If they are infected with the glandular fever virus, they will not recover quickly and have a high chance of developing chronic fatigue syndrome. If they have a baby, then the cycle starts all over again. Later, in life they will have a higher chance of diabetes, raised cholesterol, arthritis, depression and cancer. Alas poor Yorick.

Zinc, zinc, where art thou zinc?

A work of warning, don't expect your doctor to believe that zinc deficiency exists. They were taught that people on a good diet could never become zinc deficient. What they weren't taught is that we have a problem with soil depletion; digestive problems or excessive losses which can lead to clinical zinc deficiency, but it won't show up in the serum zinc level. However it may show up in the RED CELL ZINC level or in hair analysis. Zinc is an intracellular molecule. It exhibits the pattern of deficiencies typical of these, in that one can become deficient without if showing up in a blood test. An editorial in the British Medical Journal suggested that the best way to diagnose zinc deficiency was to give a trial of zinc!

References:

1] Abbassi A.A., et al. Experimental zinc deficiency in man. Effect on testicular function. J Lab Clin Med. 96(3):544, 1980

2] Aliaga A. Psoriasis: clinical trial of an aerosol for topical use formulated with zinc pyrithione at 0.2% and sodium methyl ethyl sulfate at 0.1%. Hospital General, Valencia.1982

3] Al-Nakib W., et al. Prophylaxis and treatment of rhinovirus colds with zinc gluconate lozenges. J Antimicrob Chemother. 20(6):893-901, 1987

4] Amer M., et al. Serum zinc in acne vulgaris. Int J Dermatol. 21(8):481-482, 1982

5] Ananda S., et al. Duration of symptoms and plasma cytokine levels in patients with the common cold treated with zinc acetate. Annals of Internal Medicine. 133(4):245-252, 2000

6] Anderson R.A., Roussel A-M, Zouari N. et al. Potential antioxidant effects of zinc and chromium supplement in people with type II diabetes mellitus. J Am Coll Nutr. 20(3):212-218, 2001

7] Apisariyakulm A., et al. Zinc monoglycerolate is effective against oral herpetic sores. Med J Aust. 152(1):54, 1990

8] Arnold et al. Does hair zinc predict amphetamine improvement of ADD/hyperactivity? Int J Neuroscience. 50:103-107, 1990

9] Bakan R. The role of zinc in anorexia nervosa: Etiology and treatment. Medical Hypotheses. 5:731-736, 1979

10] Bakan R., et al. Dietary Zinc Intake of Vegetarian and Nonvegetarian Patients with Anorexia Nervosa. Int. J. Eat. Disord. 13:229-233, 1993

11] Balogh Z., et al. Plasma zinc and its relationship to clinical symptoms and drug treatment in rheumatoid arthritis. Ann Rheum Dis. 39(4):329032, 1980

12] Barbarino F., et al. Effects of zinc-aspartate and zinc-glycinate in healthy rats and on reserpine-induced gastric lesions. Biol Trace Elem Res. 16(3):253-267, 1988

13] Barrie S.A., et al. Comparative absorption of zinc picolinate, zinc citrate and zinc gluconate in humans. Agents and Actions. 5:1-6, 1986

14] Baum M.K., et al. Zinc status in human immunodeficiency virus infection. Journal of Nutrition. 130(5):1421S-1423S, 2000

15] Beach, R.S., et al. Altered thymic structure and mitogen responsiveness in postnatally zinc-deprived mice. Dev Comp Immunol. 3:725-738, 1979

16] Bekaroglu M., et al. Relationships between serum free fatty acids and zinc, and attention deficit hyperactivity disorder: a research note. J Child Psychol Psychiatry. 37(2):225-227, 1996

17] Bellanti J. A., et al. ADHD: Causes and Possible Solutions Conference. Arlington, VA, USA. Nov 4-7, 1999

18] Bhutta A., et al. Prevention of diarrhea and pneumonia by zinc supplementation in children in developing countries: pooled analysis of randomized controlled trials. Zinc Investigators' Collaborative Group. J Pediatr. 135(6):689-697, 1999

19] Blechman S., et al. Zinc: low levels restrict aerobic capacity. Muscular Development. 36(12):53, 1999

20] Birmingham C.L., et al. Controlled trial of Zinc Supplementation in Anorexia Nervosa. Int. J. Eat. Disord. 15:251-255, 1994

21] Birdsall T. C. Zinc picolinate: Absorption and supplementation. Alt Med Rev. 1:26-30, 1996

22] Bradshaw A.D. Populations of Agrostis tenuis Resistant to Lead and Zinc Poisoning. Phytopath. Z. 12:, HF. 1:1-112, 1939

23] Brandao-Neto J., et al. Zinc acutely and temporarily inhibits adrenal cortisol secretion in humans. A preliminary report. Biol. Trace Elem. Res. 24:83-89, 1990

24] Bresink I., et al. Zinc changes AMPA receptor properties: results of binding studies and patch clamp recordings. Neuropharmacology. 35(4):503-509, 1996

25] Brewer G.J., Johnson V.D., Dick R.D. et al. Treatment of Wilson's disease with zinc. XVII: Treatment during pregnancy. Hepatology 31, 364-370, 2000

26] Brody I. Topical treatment of recurrent herpes simplex and post-herpetic erythema multiforme with low concentrations of zinc sulphate solution. British Journal of Dermatology. 104:191, 1981

27] Browning J.D., et al. Reduces Food Intake in Zinc Deficient Rats is normalized by Megestrol Acetate but not by Insulin-like growth factor-1. J. Nutr. 128:136-142, 1998

28] Bryce-Smith D. & Simpson R.I. Case of Anorexia Nervosa responding to Zinc Sulphate. Lancet. 2:350, 1984

44

29] Bryce-Smith D. Prenatal zinc deficiency. Nursing Times. 1985

30] Buamah P.K., et al. Maternal zinc status: a determination of central nervous system malformation. Br J Obstet Gynaecol. 91(8):788-790, 1984

31] Bulbena EG. Zinc compounds, a new treatment in peptic ulcer. Drugs under Experimental and Clinical Research.15(2):83-89 1989

32] Bush I.M., et al. Zinc and the prostate. Presented at the annual meeting of the American Medical Association. Chicago, 1974

33] Calhoun N.R., et al. The effects of zinc on ectopic bone formation. Oral Surg. 39(5):698-706, 1975

34] Caruthers R. Oral zinc in cutaneous healing. Drugs. 6:164. 1973

35] Cass Smith W.P. & Harvey H.L. Zinc Deficiency of Flax. J. Dep. Agric. W. Aust. 25:136-42, 1948

36] Castillo-Duran C., et al. Controlled trial of Zinc Supplementation during recovery from Malnutrition: Effects on Growth and immune Function. Am. J. Clin. Nutr. 45:602-608, 1987

37] Chan S., et al. The role of copper, molybdenum, selenium, and zinc in nutrition and health. Clin Lab Med. 18(4):673-685, 1998

38] Chauser A. Zinc, Insulin and Diabetes. J of American College of Nutrition. 17(2):109-115, 1998

39] Chen M-D, Lin P-Y. Zinc-induced hyperleptinaemia relates to the amelioration of sucrose-induced obesity with zinc repletion. Obesity Res. 8(7), 525-529, 2000

40] Chester C.G.C. & Robinson G.N. The Role of Zinc in Plant Metabolism. Biol. Rev. 26:239-52, 1951

41] Chiricolo M., et al. Enhanced DNA repair in lymphocytes of Down syndrome patients: The influence of zinc nutritional supplementation. Mutat Res Dnaging Genet Instab Aging (Netherlands). 295(3):105-111, 1993

42] Christian P., et al. Zinc supplementation might potentiate the effect of vitamin A in restoring night vision in pregnant Nepalese women. American Journal of Clinical Nutrition. 73(6):1045-1051, 2001

43] Chuong C.J. & Dawson E.B. Zinc and copper levels in premenstrual syndrome. Fert. Steril. Aug 62:2, 313-20 1994

44] Cohen C. Zinc sulphate and bed sores. Br Med J. 2:561,1968

45] Collip P.J., et al. Zinc deficiency: improvement in growth and growth hormone levels with oral zinc therapy. Ann Nutr Metab. 26(5):287-290, 1992

46] Cordova A., et al. Behavior of zinc and physical exercise: A special reference to immunity and fatigue. Neuroscience and Behavioral Reviews. 19(3):439-444, 1995

47] Cordova A, et al. Effect of training on zinc metabolism: changes in serum and sweat zinc concentrations in sportsmen. Ann Nutr Metab. 42(5):274-282, 1998

48] Costello L.C., et al. Novel role of zinc in the regulation of prostate citrate metabolism and its implications in prostate cancer. Prostate. 35(4):285-296, 1998

49] Cunliff W.J., et al. A double-blind trial of a zinc sulphate/zinc citrate complex and tetracycline in the treatment of acne. British Journal of Derm. 101:321-325, 1979

50] Demetree J.W., et al. The effect of zinc on sebum secretion rate. Acta

Dermatovenerol. 60(2):166-169, 1980

51] Dinsmore W.W., et al. Zinc Absorption in Anorexia Nervosa. Lancet 1:1041-1042, 1985

52] Donadini A., et al. Plasma levels of Zn, Cu and Ni in healthy controls and in psoriatic patients. Acta Vitamin Enzymol. 1:9-16, 1980

53] Dreno B., et al. Low doses of zinc gluconate for inflammatory acne. Acta Derm Venereol. 69:541-543, 1989

54] Duchateeau J., et al. Influence of oral zinc supplementation on the lymphocyte response to mitogens of normal subjects. Am J Clin Nutr. 34:88-93, 1981

55] Duchateau J., et al. Beneficial effects of oral zinc supplementation on the immune response of old people. Am J Med. 70:1001-1004, 1981

56] Duncan J., et al. Thymidine kinase and DNA polymerase activity in normal and zinc deficient developing rat embryos. Proc Soc Exp Biol Med. 159:39-43, 1978

57] Eby G.A., et al. Reduction in duration of common colds by zinc gluconate lozenges in a double-blind study. Antimicrobial Agents and Chemotherapy. 25:20, 1984

58] Eby G. Use of topical zinc to prevent recurrences of orolabial and genital herpetic infections: Review of literature and suggested protocols. Medical Hypotheses. 17(2):157-165, 1985

59] Editor Another look at Zinc. Br Medical Journal. 282:1098-99, 1981

60] Eggleton W.G. The Zinc Content of Epidermal Structures in Beri-beri. Biochem. J. 33(i): 403-6, 1939

61] Elcoate P.V., et al. The Effect of Zinc Deficiency on the Male Genital System. J. Physiol. 129:53, 1955

62] Esca S.A., et al. Kwashiorkor-like zinc deficiency syndrome in anorexia nervosa. Acta Derm Venereol. Stockholm. 59:361-364, 1979

63] Evans G.W., et al. Effect of iron, vitamin B-6 and picolinic acid on zinc absorption in the rat. Journal of Nutrition. 111(1):68-75, 1981

64] Fabris N., et al. AIDS, zinc deficiency and thymic hormone failure. Journal of the American Medical Association (Letter). 259:839-840, 1988

65] Fabris N., Mocchegiani E., Muzzoli M., and Provinciali M. Role of zinc in neuroendocrine-immune reactions during aging. In: Physiological Senescence and its Postponement. Annals of the New York Academy of Sciences, Volume 621, by Walter Pierpaoli and Nicola Fabris (editors). 314-326, 1991

66] Fahim M., et al. Zinc treatment for the reduction of hyperplasia of the prostate. Federation Proceedings. 35(3):361, 1976

67] Federico A., Lodice P., Federico P. et al. Effects of selenium and zinc supplementation on nutritional status in patients with cancer of digestive tract. Eur J Clin Nutr. 55 (4):293-7, 2001

68] Fernandes G., et al. Impairment of cell-mediated immune function by dietary Zn deficiency in mice. Proceedings of the National Academy of Sciences, USA. 76:457-461, 1979

69] Ferrigno D., et al. Serum copper and zinc content in non-small cell lung cancer: abnormalities and clinical correlates. Monaldi Arch Chest Dis (Italy), Jun. 54(3):204-

8, 1999

70] Finnerty E. F. Topical zinc in the treatment of herpes simplex. Cutis. 37(2):130-131, 1986

71] Fischer P.W.F., et al. The effect of dietary zinc on intestinal copper absorption. American Journal of Clinical Nutrition. 34(9):1670-1675, 1981

72] Fong L.Y.Y., et al. Zinc deficiency and the development of oesophageal and forestomach tumours in Sprague-Dawley rats fed precursors of N-nitroso-N-benzylmethylamine. Journal of the National Cancer Institute. 72:419-425, 1984

73] Frank J. Zinc and your skin. Australian Wellbeing. 10:69-71, 1985

74] Fraker P.J., et al. Interrelationships between zinc and immune function. Fed Proc. 45:1474-1479, 1986

75] Fraker P.J. The dynamic link between the integrity of the immune system and zinc status. Journal of Nutrition. 130 (5S Supplement). 1399S-1406S, 2000

76] Freeland-Graves J.H., et al. Effect of zinc supplementation on plasma high-density lipoprotein cholesterol and zinc. American Journal of Clinical Nutrition. 35(5):988-992, 1982

77] Frithiof L., et al. The relationship between marginal bone loss and serum zinc levels. Acta Med Scand. 207(1):67-70, 1980

78] Frommer D.J. The healing of gastric ulcers by zinc sulphate. Medical Journal of Australia. 2:793, 1975

79] GaoY., et al. Zinc enhancement of genistein's anabolic effect on bone components in elderly female rats. Gen Pharmac. 31(2):199-202, 1998

80] Garfinkel D. Is aging inevitable? The intracellular zinc deficiency hypothesis of aging. Med Hypotheses. 19(2):117-137, 1986

81] Gersdorff M., et al. [The zinc sulfate overload test in patients suffering from tinnitus associated with low serum zinc. Preliminary report]. Acta Otorhinolaryngol Belg. 41(3):498-505, 1987

82] Godfrey J.C., et al. Zinc for treating the common cold: review of all clinical trials since 1984. Alternative Therapies in Health & Medicine. 2(6):63-72, 1996

83] Golik A., et al. Effects of captopril and enalapril on zinc metabolism in Hypertension Subjects . J. of Am College of Nutrition. 17(1): 75-78, 1998

84] Gong H., et al. Optic nerve changes in zinc-deficient rats. Exp Eye Res. 72(4):363-369, 2001

85] Goransson K., et al. Oral zinc in acne vulgaris: a clinical and methodological study. Acta Derm Venereol. 58(5):443-8, 1978

86] Goto T., et al. Long-term zinc deficiency decreases taste sensitivity in rats. Journal of Nutritiion. 131(2):305-310, 2001

87] Greaves M.W., et al. Double-blind trial of zinc sulphate in the treatment of chronic venous leg ulceration. Brit Jour of Derm. 87:63251,1972

88] Hadden J.W. The treatment of zinc deficiency is an immunotherapy. International Journal of Immunopharmacology. 17(9):697-701, 1995

89] Hagino N. & Kobayashi J. Strange Osteomalacia "Itaiitai" Disease in the Jintsu River Basin, Polluted with Zinc, Lead and Cadmium I. Private Communication, 1960

90] Haglund et al. Evidence of a relationship between childhood onset type 1 diabetes and low groundwater concentration of zinc. Diabetes Care Aug. 19:8 873-5, 1996

91] Hambridge K.M., et al. Zinc nutritional status during pregnancy: a longitudinal study. Am J Clin Nutr. 37:429-42, 1983

92] Hartoma T.R., et al. Zinc, plasma androgens and male sterility. Letter to the Editor. The Lancet. 3:1125-1126, 1977

93] Hasegawa H., et al. Effects of zinc on the reactive oxygen species-generating capacity of human neutrophils and on the serum opsonic activity in vitro. Luminescence. 15(5):321-327, 2000

94] Hess F.M., et al. Zinc excretion in young women on low zinc intakes and oral contraceptive agents. J Nutr. 107, 1977

95] Heyneman C.A. Zinc deficiency and taste disorders. Ann Pharmacotherapy Feb. 30:2 186-7, 1996

96] Higashi A., et al. A prospective survey of serial zinc levels and pregnancy outcome. J Ped Gastro. 7:430-33, 1988

97] Hillstrom L., et al. Comparison of oral treatment with zinc sulfate and placebo in acne vulgaris. British Journal of Dermatology. 97:679-684, 1977

98] Hirt M., et al. Zinc nasal gel for the treatment of common cold symptoms: a double-blind, placebo-controlled trial. Ear, Nose, & Throat Journal. 79(10):778-782, 2000

99] Horning M. S., et al. Endogenous mechanisms of neuroprotection: role of zinc, copper, and carnosine. Brain Res. 852(1):56-61, 2000

100] Huang X., Cuajungco M.P.,.Atwood C.S., et al. Alzheimer's disease, beta-amyloid protein and zinc. J Nutr. 130, 1488S-1492S, 2000

101] Humphries L., et al. Zinc deficiency and eating disorders. Journal of Clinical Psychiatry. 50(12):456-459, 1989

102] Humphries L.L., et al. Anorexia Nervosa, Zinc Supplementation and weight gain. In: Anderson H, ed. Biology of Feast and Famine: Relevance to Eating Disorders, Symposium on Nutrition Research. Toronto: University of Toronto. 124-136, 1990

103] Hunt C.D., et al. Effects of dietary zinc depletion on seminal volume and zinc loss, serum testosterone concentrations, and sperm morphology in young men. Am J Clin Nutr. 56(1):148-157, 1992

104] Iitaka M. et al. Induction of apoptosis and necrosis by zinc in human thyroid cancer cell lines. J Endocrinol. 169(2):417-24, 2001

105] Jackson E.A. Are zinc acetate lozenges effective in decreasing the duration of symptoms of the common cold? J Fam Pract. 49(12):1153, 2000

106] Joseph C.E., et al. Zinc deficiency changes in the permeability of rabbit periodontium to 14 C-phenytoin and 14 C-albumin. J Periodontol. 53:251-256, 1982

107] Karayalcin S., et al. Zinc plasma levels after oral zinc tolerance test in nonalcoholic cirrhosis. Dig Dis Sci. 33:1096-1102, 1988

108] Katz R.L., et al. Zinc deficiency in anorexia nervosa. J Adolesc Health Care.

8(5):400-406, 1987

109] Kneist W., et al. Clinical double-blind trial of topical zinc sulfate for herpes labialis recidivans. Arzneimittelforschung. 45:524-526, 1995

110] Kobayashi J. & Hagino N. Strange Osteomalacia "Itaiitai" Disease in the Jinsu River Basin Polluted with Zinc, Lead and Cadmium II. Private Communication, 1960

111] Koo S.I. & Turk D.E. Effect of Zinc Deficiency on the Ultrastructure of the Pancreatic Acinar Cell and Intestinal Epithelium in the Rat. J. Nutr. 107:896-908, 1977

112] Korant B.D., et al. Zinc ions inhibit replication of rhinoviruses. Nature. 248:588-590, 1974

113] Korant B.D., et al. Inhibition by zinc of rhinovirus protein cleavage: Interaction of zinc with capsid polypeptides. J Virol. 18:298-306, 1976

114] Krieger I., et al. Tryptophan deficiency and picolinic acid: effect on zinc metabolism and clinical manifestations of pellagra. American Journal of Clinical Nutrition. 46:511-517, 1987

115] Krotkiewski M., et al. Zinc and muscle strength and endurance. Acta Physiol Scandinavia. 116(3):309-311, 1982

116] Kruis W. et al. Zinc deficiency as a problem in patients with Crohn's disease and fistula formation. Hepatogastroenterol. 32(3):133-134, 1985

117] Kugelmas M. Preliminary observation: oral zinc sulfate replacement is effective in treating muscle cramps in cirrhotic patients. J Am Coll Nutr. 19(1):13-15, 2000

118] Lally E.V., et al. An element of uncertainty: The clinical significance of zinc deficiency in rheumatoid arthritis. Int Medicine. 8(1):98-107, 1987

119] Larue J.P., et al. [Zinc in the human prostate]. Journal of Urology (Paris). 91(7):463-468, 1985

120] Lask B., et al. Zinc Deficiency and childhood-onset Anorexia Nervosa. J. Clin. Psychiatry. 54:63-66, 1993

121] Leake A., et al. Subcellular distribution of zinc in the benign and malignant human prostate: evidence for a direct zinc androgen interaction. Acta Endocrinol (Copenhagen). 105:281-288, 1984

122] Leissner K.H., et al. Concentration and content of zinc in the human prostate. Investigative Urology. 18:32-35, 1980

123] Liang J.Y., et al. Inhibitory effect of zinc on human prostatic carcinoma cell growth. Prostate. 40(3):200-207, 1999

124] Lin D.D., et al. Zinc-induced augmentation of excitatory synaptic currents and glutamate receptor responses in hippocampal CA3 neurons. J Neurophysiol. 85(3):1185-1196, 2001

125] Loneragen J.F. The Effect of Applied Phosphate on the Uptake of Zinc by Flax. Aust. J. Sci. Res. Ser. B,4:108-14, 1951

126] Macknin M.L. Zinc lozenges for the common cold. Cleveland Clin J Med. 66:27-32, 1999

127] Mantzoros C.S., et al. Zinc may regulate serum leptin concentrations in humans. J. Am. Coll. Nutr. 17:270-275, 1998

128] Marchesini G., et al. Zinc supplementation improves glucose disposal in patients with cirrhosis. Metabolism. 47:792-798, 1998

129] Marone G. et al. Physiological concentrations of zinc inhibit the release of histamine from human basophils and lung mast cells. Agents Actions. 18:103-106, 1986

130] Marshall S. Zinc gluconate and the common cold. Review of randomized controlled trials. Canadian Family Physician. 44:1037-1042, 1998

131] Mattingley P.C., et al. Zinc sulphate in rheumatoid arthritis. Annals of the Rheumatic Diseases. 41:456-457, 1982

132] Mawson C.A. & Fischer M.I. The Occurrence of Zinc in the Human Prostate Gland. Canad. J. Med. Sci. 30:336-9, 1952

133] Mawson C.A. & Fischer M.I. Zinc and Carbonic Anhydrase in Human Semen. Biochem. J. 55:696, 1953

134] McCarthy M. Zinc Lozenges shorten duration of common cold. Lancet. 348:184, 1996

135] McClain C.J., et al. Zinc-deficiency-induced retinal dysfunction in Crohn's disease. Dig Dis Sci. 28:85, 1983

136] McClain C.J., et al. Zinc deficiency in the alcoholic: A review. Alcoholism: Clin Exp. 7:5, 1983

137] McClain C.J., et al. Zinc status before and after zinc supplementation of eating disorder patients. Journal of the American College of Nutrition. 11(6):694-700, 1992

138] McLoughlin I.J., et al. Zinc in depressive disorder. Acta Psychiatrica Scandinavica. 82(6):451-453, 1990

139] Mechegiani E., et al. Zinc-dependent low thymic hormone level in type I diabetes. Diabetes. 12:932-937, 1989

140] Merialdi M., et al. Adding zinc to prenatal iron and folate tablets improves fetal neurobehavioral development. Am J Obstet Gynecol. 180(2 Partt 1):483-490, 1999

141] Merluzzi V.J., et al. Evaluation of zinc complexes on the replication of rhinovirus 2 in vitro. Res Commun Chem Pathol Pharmacol. 66(3):425-440, 1989

142] Michaelsson G., et al. Effects of oral zinc and vitamin A in acne. Archives of Dermatology. 113:31-36, 1977

143] Michaelsson G., et al. Serum zinc and retinol-binding protein in acne. British Journal of Dermatology. 96:283-286, 1977

144] Michaelsson G., et al. A double blind study of the effect of zinc and oxytetracycline in acne vulgaris. British Journal of Dermatology. 97:561-565, 1977

145] Miller M.J., et al. The Effect of Dietary Zinc Deficiency on the Reproductive System of Male Rats. Rev. Canad. de Biol. 13 No.5, 1954

146] Millikan C.R. Effect of Phosphates on the Development of Zinc Deficiency Symptoms in Flax. J. Dept. Agric. Victoria. 45: 273-8, 1947

147] Mocchegiani E., et al. The zinc-melatonin interrelationship: A working hypothesis. Ann NY Acad Sci. 719:298-307, 1994

148] Mocchegiani E., et al. Therapeutic application of zinc in human immunodeficiency virus against opportunistic infections. Journal of Nutrition. 130(5S Supplement):1424S-1431S, 2000

149] Mocchegiani E., at al. The immuno-reconstituting effect of melatonin or pineal grafting and its relation to zinc pool in aging mice. J Neuroimmunol. 53:189-201, 1994.

150] Moran J., et al. A study to assess the plaque inhibitory action of a new zinc citrate toothpaste formulation. J Clin Periodontol. 28(2):157-161, 2001

151] Mossad S.B., et al. Zinc gluconate lozenges for treating the common cold. A randomized, double-blind, placebo-controlled study. Ann Int Med. 125(2):81-88, 1996

152] Munoz N., et al. Effect of riboflavin, retinol, and zinc on the micronuclei of buccal mucosa and of esophagus: A randomized double-blind intervention study in China. J Nat Cancer Inst. 79:687-691, 1987

153] Nakamura T., et al. Kinetics of zinc status in children with IDDM. Diabetes Care. 14:553-557, 1991

154] Nason A., et al. Changes in Enzymatic Constitution in Zinc Deficient Neurospora. J. Biol. Chem. 188:397-406, 1951

155] Neil F., et al. Neurobiology of zinc-influenced eating behavior. Journal of Nutrition. 130(5 Supplement):1493S-1499S, 2000

156] Netter A., et al. Effect of zinc adminisration on plasma testosterone, dehydrotestosterone and sperm count. Archives of Andrology. 7(1):69-73, 1981

157] Newsome D.A., et al. Oral zinc in macular degeneration. Arch Ophthalmol. 106(2):192-198, 1988

158] Newsome D.A., et al. Zinc uptake by primate retinal pigment epithelium and choroid. Current Eye Research. 11(3):213-217, 1992

159] Niewoener C.B., et al. Role of zinc supplementation in type II diabetes mellitus. Am J Med. 63-68, 1988

160] Nishi Y. Zinc Status in various diseases. Hiroshima J. Med. Sci. 29:69-74, 1980

161] Nishida K., et al. [A study on a low serum zinc level in Crohn's disease]. Nippon Shok Gakkai Zasshi. 82(3):424-433, 1985

162] Nishiyama S., et al. Zinc supplementation alters thyroid hormone metabolism in disabled patients with Zinc deficiency. J Am Col Nut 13(1):62-67, 1994

163] Novick S.G., et al. How does zinc modify the common cold? Clinical observations and implications regarding mechanisms of action. Medical Hypotheses. 46(3):295-302, 1996

164] Novick S.G., et al. Zinc-induced suppression of inflammation in the respiratory tract, caused by infection with human rhinovirus and other irritants. Medical Hypotheses. 49(4):347-357, 1997

165] Ochi K., et al. [The serum zinc level in patients with tinnitus and the effect of zinc treatment]. Nippon Jibiinkoka Gakkai Kaiho. 100(9):915-919, 1997

166] Om A.S. & Chung K.W. Dietary Zinc Deficiency alters 5 alpha-reduction and Aromatization of Testosterone and Androgen and Estrogen receptors in Rat Liver. J. Nutr. 126:842-848, 1996

167] Osendarp S.J., et al. Zinc supplementation during pregnancy and effects on growth and morbidity in low birthweight infants: a randomised placebo controlled trial. Lancet. 357(9262):1080-1085, 2001

168] Pandley S.P., et al. Zinc in rheumatoid arthritis. Indian Journal of Medical Research. 81:618-620, 1985

169] Park J.S., et al. Zinc finger of replication protein A, a non-DNA binding element, regulates its DNA binding activity through redox. J Biol Chem. 274(41):29075-29080, 1999

170] Petrus E.J., et al. Randomized, double-masked, placebo-controlled clinical study of the effectiveness of zinc acetate lozenges on common cold symptoms in allergy-tested subjects. Curr Ther Res. 59:595–607, 1998

171] Pfeiffer C. Zinc and other micronutrients New canan CT Keats. 1978

172] Pidduck H.G., et al. Hyperzincuria of diabetes mellitus and possible genetic implications of this observation. Diabetes. 19:240-247, 1970

173] Pilerard-Franchimont C., et al. A double-blind controlled evaluation of the sebosuppressive activity of topical erythromycin-zinc complex. European Journal of Clinical Pharmacology. 1-2(49):57-60, 1995

174] Pohit J., et al. Zinc status of acne vulgaris patients. Journal of Applied Nutrition. 37(1):18-25, 1985

175] Pories W.J.et al. Acceleration of wound healing in man with zinc sulphate given by mouth. The Lancet. 1:1069, 1969

176] Powell S.R. The antioxidant properties of zinc. Journal of Nutrition. 130(5):1447S-1454S, 2000

177] Prasad A Trace elements in human health and disease. Vol 1 Zinc and Copper. New York Academic press.1976

178] Prasad A.S., et al. Experimental zinc deficiency in humans. Ann Intern Med. 89:483, 1978

179] Prasad A.S. Clinical, Endocrinological and Biochemical Effects of Zinc Deficiency. Clin. Endocrinol Metab. 14:567-589, 1985

180] Prasad et al. Biochemistry of Zinc. New York Plenum press. 1993

181] Prasad A.S., et al. Trace elements in head and neck cancer patients: zinc status and immunologic functions. Otolaryngol Head Neck Surg Jun. 116(6 Pt 1):624-9, 1997

182] Prasad A.S., et al. Duration of symptoms and plasma cytokine levels in patients with the common cold treated with zinc acetate: a randomized, double-blind, placebo-controlled trial. Ann Intern Med. 133(4):245-252, 2000

183] Prout T.E., et al. Zinc Metabolism in Patients with Diabetes Mellitus. Metabolism. 9:109-17. 1960

184] Rao K.V.R., et al. Effect of zinc sulfate therapy on control and lipids in type I diabetes. JAPI. 35:52, 1987

185] Rapisarda E., et al. [Effects of zinc and vitamin B 6 in experimental caries in rats.] Minerva Stomatol. 30(4):317-320, 1981

186] Record I. R., et al. Protection by zinc against UVA- and UVB-induced cellular and genomic damage in vivo and in vitro. Biol Trace Elem Res. 53:15-19, 1996

187] Reed H.S. The Relation of Zinc to Seed Production. J. Agric. Res. 64:635-44, 1942

188] Ripa S., et al. Zinc and the elderly. Minerva Med. (6):275-278, 1995

189] Rogers L.H. & Wu C.H. Zinc Uptake by Oats as Influenced by Applications of Lime and Phosphate. J. Amer. Soc. Agron. 40:563-6, 1948

190] Rogers S.A. Zinc deficiency as a model for developing chemical sensitivity. Int Clin Nutr Rev. 10(1):253-59, 1990

191] Romics I., et al. Spectrographic determination of zinc in the tissues of adenoma and carcinoma of the prostate. Int Urol Nerphol. 15(2):171-176, 1983

192] Russell R.M., et al. Zinc and the special senses. Ann Int Med. 99:227-229, 1983

193] Safai-Kutti S., et al. Zinc and anorexia nervosa. Annals of Internal Medicine. 100(2):317-318, 1984

194] Safai-Kutti S. Oral Zinc Supplementation in Anorexia Nervosa. Acta. Psychiatr. Scand. Suppl. 361:14-17, 1990

195] Saha K.C. Therapeutic value of zinc in acne. Indian J Dermatol. 23(2):25-31, 1978

196] Sakai F., et al. [Therapeutic efficacy of zinc picolinate in patients with taste disorders]. Nippon Jibiinkoka Gakkai Kaiho. 98:(7)1135-1139, 1985

197] Salvin S.B., et al. The effect of dietary zinc and prothymosin a on cellular immune responses of RF/J mice. Clin Immunol Immunopathol. 43:281-288, 1987

198] Salvin S.B., et al. Resistance and susceptibility to infection in inbred murine strains. IV. Effects of dietary zinc. Cellular Immunol. 87(2):546-552, 1984

199] Sandstrom B. et al. Absorption of zinc from soy protein meals in humans. J Nutr. 117 321-327, 1987

200] Sanstead H.H. W.O. Atwater memorial lecture. Zinc: Essentiality for Brain Development and Function. Nutr. Rev. 43:129-137, 1985

201] Sanstead H.H. Zinc in Human Nutrition: Disorders of mineral metabolism. Vol 1. Academic press N.Y. 1981

202] Saxton C.A., et al. The effect of dentifrices containing zinc citrate on plaque growth and oral zinc levels. J Clin Periodontol. 13(4):301-306, 1986

203] Sayeg Porto M.A., et al. Linear growth and zinc supplementation in children with short stature. J Pediatr Endocrinol Metab. 13(8):1121-1128, 2000

204] Sazawal S., et al. Zinc supplementation reduces the incidence of acute lower respiratory tract infections in infants and preschool children: a double-blind controlled trial. Pediatrics. 102:1-5, 1998

205] Schauss A.G., et al. Evidence of zinc deficiency in anorexia nervosa and bulimia nervosa. In: Nutrients and brain function. Essman, W. B. (editor). Basel: Karger, 151-162, 1987

206] Schauss A. & Costin C. Zinc as a Nutrient in the Treatment of Eating Disorders. Am. J. Nat. Med. 4:8-13, 1997

207] Scholmerich J., et al. Zinc and vitamin A deficiency in liver cirrhosis. Hepatogastroenterol. 30:119-125, 1983

208] Schoelmerich J., et al. Zinc and vitamin A deficiency in patients with Crohn's disease is correlated with activity but not with localization or extent of the disease. Hepatogastroenterology. 32(1):34-38, 1985

209] SchÜtte K.H. The Influence of Zinc upon the Stomata of Citrus Leaves. Unpublished. 1962

210] Scott D.A. & Fisher A.M. Insulin and Zinc Content of Bovine Pancreas. J. Clin. Invest. 17:725, 1938

211] Scott M.E., et al. Zinc deficiency impairs immune responses against parasitic nematode infections at intestinal and systemic sites. Journal of Nutrition. 130(5 Supplement): 1412S-1420S, 2000

212] Sempertegui F., et al. Effects of short-term zinc supplementation on cellular immunity, respiratory symptoms, and growth of malnourished Equadorian children. Eur J Clin Nutr. 50(1): 42-46, 1996

213] Seri S., et al. Effects of dietary tryptophan bioavailability on zinc absorption in rats. IRCS Medical Science. 12:452-453, 1984

214] Shambaugh G.E. Zinc: the neglected nutrient. Am J Otol. 10(2):156-160, 1989

215] Shankar A.H., et al. Zinc and immune function: the biological basis of altered resistance to infection. American Journal of Clinical Nutrition. 68(Supplement):447S-463S, 1998

216] Shay N.F., Mangian H.F. Neurobiology of zinc-influenced eating behaviour. J Nutr 130, 1493S1499S, 2000

217] Simkin P.A. Treatment of rheumatoid arthritis with oral zinc sulfate. Agents and Actions. (Suppl.) 8:587-595, 1981

218] Simkin P.A. Oral zinc sulphate in rheumatoid arthritis. The Lancet. 2:539, 1976

219] Singh R.B., et al. Current zinc intake and risk of diabetes and coronary artery disease and factors associated with insulin resistance in rural and urban populations of North India. J Am Coll Nutr. 17:564-570, 1998

220] Singh K.P., et al. Effect of zinc on immune functions and host resistance against infection and tumor challenge. Immunopharmacol Immunotoxicol. 14:813-840, 1992

221] Singh R.B., et al. Current zinc intake and risk of diabetes and coronary artery disease and factors associated with insulin resistance in rural and urban populations of North India. J Am Coll Nutr. 17:564-570, 1998

222] Sjogren A., et al. Magnesium, potassium and zinc deficiency in subjects with type II diabetes mellitus. Acta Med Scand. 224(5):461-466, 1988

223] Solomons N.W., et al. Zinc deficiency in Crohn's disease. Digestion. 16:87, 1977

224] Song M.K., et al. Effects of Bovine Prostate Powder on Zinc, Glucose and Insulin Metabolism in Old Patients with Non-insulin-dependent Diabetes Mellitus. Metabolism. 47:39-43, 1998

225] Sparkman D. Zinc: lower risk of heart disease, diabetes. Muscular Development. 36(6):44, 1999

226] Staker E.V. Progress Report on the Control of Zinc Toxicity in Peat Soils. Soil

Sci. Amer. Proc. 7:387-92, 1943

227] Sterling M. New zinc resarch reveals more applications. Nutrition Science News. July 2001

228] Svenson K.L., et al. Reduced zinc in peripheral blood cells from patients with inflammatory connective tissue diseases. Inflammation. 9(2):189-199, 1985

229] Swanson C.A. & King J.C. Zinc and pregnancy outcome. AM J Clin Nutr. 46(5): 763-71, 1987

230] Takeda A., et al. Zinc homeostasis in the brain of adult rats fed zinc-deficient diet. J Neurosci Res. 63(5):447-452, 2001

231] Takihara H., et al. Zinc sulfate therapy for infertile males with or without variococelectomy. Urology. 29(6):638-641, 1987

232] Tang, X-h., et al. Zinc has an insulin-like effect on glucose transport mediated by phosphoinositol-3-kinase and akt in 3t3-11 fibroblasts and adipocytes. Journal of Nutrition. 131(5):1414-1420, 2001

233] Terhune M.W., et al. Decreased RNA polymerase activity in mammalian zinc deficiency. Science. 177:68-69, 1972

234] Terwolbeck K., et al. Zinc in lymphocytes-the assessment of zinc status in patients with crohn's disease. Journal of Trace Element, Electrolytes, Health and Disease. 6(2):117-121, 1992

235] Tikkiwal M., et al. Effect of zinc administration on seminal zinc and fertility of oligospermic males. Indian J Physiol Pharmacol. 31(1):30-34, 1987

236] Toke G.B.& Dhamne B.K. A study of serum copper, serum zinc and Cu/Zn ratio as diagnostic and prognostic index in cases of head, neck and face tumors. Indian J Pathol Microbiol Apr. 33(2):171-4, 1990

237] Tuormaa T.E. Adverse effect of zinc deficiency: A review from the literature. J Orthomol Med. 10(3):149-162, 1995

238] Tvedt K.E., et al, Intracellular distribution of calcium and zinc in normal, hyperplastic, and neoplastic human prostate: x-ray microanalysis of freeze-dried cryosections. Prostate. 15:41-51, 1989

239] Van Binsbergen C.J., et al. Nutritional Status in Anorexia Nervosa: Clinical Chemistry, vitamins, iron and zinc. Eur. J. Clin. Nutr. 42:929-937, 1988

240] Van Campen D.R. Zinc interference with copper absorption in rats. Journal of Nutrition. 91:473, 1967

241] Vasquez A. Zinc treatment for reduction of hyperplasia of prostate. Townsend Letter for Doctors & Patients. 100,1996

242] Vega Robledo G.B., et al. Effect of zinc on Entamoeba histolytica pathogenicity. Parasitol Res. 85:487-492, 1999

243] Verm K.C., et al. Oral zinc sulphate therapy in acne vulgaris: A double-blind trial. Acta Dermatovener. 60:337-340, 1980

244] Voelker R. Zinc reduces pneumonia. Journal of the American Medical Association. 283(2), 2000

245] Wallace E.C. Diabetic epidemic. Energy Times. 9(4):24-28, 1999

246] Walsh C.T., et al. Zinc health effects and research priorities for the 1990's. Environ Health Perspect. 102:5-46, 1994

247] Wapnir R.A. Zinc Deficiency, Malnutrition and the Gastrointestinal Tract. J. Nutr. 130:1388S-1392S, 2000

248] Ward N., et al. The influence of the chemical additive tartrazine on the zinc status of hyperactive children, a double blind placebo controlled study. J Nut Med. 1: 51-57, 1990

249] Watts D. The Nutritional relationships of Zinc. J Ortho Med. 2: 99-108, 1989

250] Wear J.I. Effect of Soil pH and Calcium on the Uptake of Zinc by Plants. Soil Sci. 81:311-15, 1956

251] Weimar V., et al. Zinc sulphate in acne vulgaris. Arch Dermatol. 114(12):1776-1778, 1978

252] Wilkinson E.A.J., et al. Does oral zinc aid the healing of chronic leg ulcers? A systematic literature review. Arch Dermatology. 134(12):1556-1560, 1998

253] Wood J.G. & Silby P.M. Carbonic Anhydrase Activity in Plants in Relation to Zinc Content. Aust. J. Sci. Res. B, 5:244-55, 1952

254] Wood R.J. Assessment of Marginal Zinc Status in Humans. J. Nutr. 130:1350S-1354S, 2000

255] Wray D.W. A double blind trial of systemic zinc sulfate in recurrent aphthous stomatitis. Oral Surg. 53(5):469, 1982

256] Wright J.V. Treatment of benign prostate hypertrophy with zinc. Townsend Letter for Doctors & Patients. 82, April 1996

257] Yamaguchi H., et al. Anorexia Nervosa responding to Zinc Supplementation: a case report. Gastroenterol Jpn. 27:554-558, 1992

Hypertension and Cadmium
Glauser, S., et al: Blood-Cadmium levels in normotensive and untreated hypertensive humans. The Lancet. 1:717-718. 1976

Enlarged Prostate and Cadmium
Habib, F.K., et al: Metal-androgen interrelationships in carcinoma and hyperplasia of the human prostate. J. End. 71(1):133-141. 1976

SO DOCTOR, I APPEAR TO HAVE AROPAX DEFICIENCY. WHAT ABOUT MAGNESIUM?

I recently had a conversation with a GP who had never heard of Magnesium being used for PMT headaches. It was the old "I never learned that in Medical school, so it can't be true" syndrome. My advice is this: you can either bite the bullet and learn something new or you can just retreat back in ignorance, but eventually the truth will bite you in the gluteals.

Go easy on your doctor. If they become hostile when you mention magnesium, then they probably didn't understand any of their undergraduate biochemistry. If they are heart specialists you're in big trouble, because they will probably treat your fluid with calcium channel blockers (Cardizem, Verapamil or Adalat) and your atrial fibrillation with digoxin, and not realise that all of these conditions could be caused by low magnesium. Never mind, you'll just have to go along with the provisional diagnosis that you have Digoxin, Adalat or Lasix deficiency and keep your mouth shut. The specialist knows best. After all, they've been thoroughly trained in this high tech stuff.

If you mention magnesium to most doctors, they'll probably get defensive and deny everything. Personally, I don't remember a single word being spoken about Magnesium in medical school. It wasn't until I started reading recent biochemistry and nutritional journals that I found out about it. It's a very small metallic ion, but it's important for over 300 enzyme systems in the body. That makes it the most important metallic cofactor. Next, comes Iron at 93 enzymes (only one is related to Haemoglobin in red blood cells) and zinc at 88 enzymes. We store about 25,000mg of magnesium in our body and only 1% of it is in the blood. So most of it is in the tissues. It demonstrates the features of most intracellular ions, in that you can become depleted *without it showing up in a blood test*. Unfortunately most doctors rely on blood tests (and believe them more than the patient!) and don't take the time to ask about symptoms such as headaches, unrefreshed sleep, leg or foot pain, palpitations, muscle twitching, blurred vision, mouth ulcers or anxiety symptoms.

Magnesium falls at night and so the first symptoms may be poor REM sleep cycles and leg cramps. Later, as levels continue to fall, tissues start failing so unpredictable, that the symptoms may be sporadic. Borderline stores mean that the person becomes dependent upon dietary intake of the mineral and hence may have good and bad days. This variation in manifestation often leads to doctors being suspicious of the validity of the reported symptoms to the point where they suggest that the problem is "all in your mind".

Failure of recognition of magnesium deficiency symptoms occurs from GP level to specialist level. For instance, despite over a hundred papers linking magnesium deficiency to headache, many neurologists are unaware of the connection and would prefer to prescribe drugs like mersyndol or even beta-blockers (which eventually reduce magnesium levels). Oh no, we can't have people treating headaches with minerals!

When confronted about the intracellular effects of calcium channel blockers, most doctors will eventually concede that these drugs could lead to an increase in the effect of magnesium (as a muscle relaxant) and hence lower the blood pressure. When I ask them if they had considered just giving magnesium, they will often reply, "Can you do that?" Well strangely enough several million people have done just that. Oh no, but we can't have people treating high blood pressure with minerals. They need *drugs*! These patients are suffering from Renitec or Tritace or Tenormin deficiency. Recently one of my patients told me that a specialist said that magnesium therapy would lead to muscle weakness. It's not physiological? It's not natural (of course Ventolin and Adalat are)? Magnesium shouldn't be in your body? We don't have mechanisms to excrete magnesium? Most of my patients have the opposite problem in that they can't absorb enough magnesium!

Magnesium is important for the production of serotonin and hence low levels may lead to depression. This is quite standard biochemistry available to anyone who cares to look it up, but again the standard treatment for depression is to correct the Aropax or Zoloft deficiency in these recalcitrant patients. They should put these drugs in the water supply!

One interesting aspect of magnesium is that tissues low in magnesium (such as skin & lung) have a higher rate of cancer but tissues high in magnesium (such as muscle and bone) have a lower rate of cancer. The connection may be related to the efficiency of energy cycles within the cells. Energy cycles help to ensure Apoptosis occurs when it should. That is, when all the functions of the cell are working properly, abnormalities in DNA should be detected by the internal cell "auditors", the Apoptosis "button" is pressed and the cell stops dividing. This concept of energy normalisation has lead to some exciting new work in cancer (page 140). The best studies so far used high dose Co-enzyme Q10 is mainly used for energy cycle problems like Chronic Fatigue. Co-enzyme Q10 needs the enzyme HMGCoA reductase to be made, so the cholesterol lowering agents will eventually deplete this important co-factor. This may explain why such therapies may lead to fatigue and depression.

So what is the take home message of all of this? Two messages. Firstly, there is no "average cell" as most doctors were taught. Remember the second rule of nutrition? Each cell is a specialist cell: A brain cell, a muscle cell, a skin cell, a heart cell. Secondly, when tissues get depleted in a nutrient they exhibit a dysfunction characteristic *of that tissue*. A heart cell will become irritable and try to change the heart rhythm. Or the heart muscle may not work effectively and lead to breathlessness or fluid retention. A brain cell may not keep the cerebral cortex stimulated enough and cause poor concentration. Or the cell might fail in making serotonin and cause low mood. Or the brain cell may not make enough melatonin and cause insomnia. A bronchiole may not relax properly and reduce flow into the lung causing wheeze and breathlessness. The pancreas may not release insulin appropriate to the blood glucose level and cause hyper or hypoglycaemia. A calf muscle may not be able to fully stretch and cause a leg cramp.

I hope you get the picture because most doctors really believe that all cells have the same metabolic pathways and do the same things (ask them how many mitochondria there are in a red blood cell?). Be ready for the "I'm the one with the medical degree" response. Hang in there though, one day your doctor might read a biochemistry textbook written within the last ten years and may finally understand you symptoms.

P.S. Magnesium is more important than calcium for making bone!

References:
1] Abbott L. et al. Magnesium deficiency in alcoholism: possible contribution to osteoporosis and cardiovascular disease in alcoholics. Alcoholism: Clinical and Experimental Research. 18(5):1076-1082, 1994

2] Abraham G.E., et al. Effect of vitamin B6 on plasma red blood cell magnesium levels in premenopausal women. Ann Clin Lab Sci. 11(4):333-336, 1981

3] Abraham G.E., Lubran MM. Serum and red cell magnesium levels in-patients with premenstrual tension. Am J Clin. Nutrition; 34(11) 2364-66, 1981

4] Abraham GE et al. A total dietary program emphasising magnesium instead of calcium. Effect on the mineral density of calcaneous bone in postmenopausal women on hormonal therapy. J Reprod Med. 35:5 503-7, 1990

5] Abraham et al. Hypothesis: Management of fibromyalgia: rationale for the use of magnesium and malic acid. J Nutr Med. 3:49-59, 1992

6] Adaniya H., et al. Effects of magnesium on polymorphic ventricular tachycardia induced by aconite. Journal of Cardiovascular Pharmacology. 24:721-729, 1994

7] Agarwal O.P. Role of magnesium in development of spontenous atherosclerosis in pigs. Indian J Exp Biol. 20(3):262-263, 1982

8] Ahlborg H., et al. Effect of potassium-magnesium aspartate on the capacity for prolonged exercise in man. Acta Physiologica Scandinavia. 74:238-245, 1968

9] Alamoudi O.S. Hypomagnesemia in chronic stable asthmatics: prevalence, correlation with severity and hospitalisation. Eur Resp. J

16:427-431, 2000

10] Al-Ghamdi, Saeed M.G., et al. Magnesium Deficiency: Pathophysiologic and Clinical Overview. American Journal of Kidney Diseases, November; 24(5): 737-752, 1994

11] Altura B.M., et al. Role of magnesium in the pathogenesis of hypertension updated: relationship to its action on cardiac, vascular smooth muscle, and endothelial cells. In: Laragh, J., Brenner, B. M. (editors). Hypertension: Pathophysiology, Diagnosis, and Management, 2nd Edition. Raven Press, New York, USA. :1213-1242, 1995

12] Altura B.M., et al. Mg, Na, and K interactions and coronary heart disease. Magnesium; 1:241-265, 1982

13] Altura B.M., et al. The role of magnesium in Etiology of strokes and cerebrovasospasm. Magnesium; 1:277-291, 1982

14] Altura B.M; Altura B.T. Magnesium ions and contraction of vascular smooth muscles: Relationship to some vascular diseases. Fed Proc; 40(12):2672-9, 1981

15] Altura B.M; Altura B.T. Interactions of Mg and K on blood vessels: Aspects in view of hypertension. Magnesium; 3(4-5) :175-94, 1984

16] Altura B. M., et al. Magnesium deficiency and hypertension: correlation between magnesium- deficient diets and microcirculatory changes in situ. Science. 223(4642):1315-1317, 1984

17] Altura B. M., et al. New perspectives on the role of magnesium in the pathophysiology of the cardiovascular system. Magnesium. 4:226-244, 1985

18] Altura B.T., et al. Biochemistry and pathophysiology of congestive heart failure: Is there a role for magnesium? Magnesium. 5(3-4):134-143, 1986

19] Altura B.M. Ischemic heart disease and magnesium. Magnesium. 7:57-67, 1988

20] Altura B.M., et al. Cardiovascular risk factors and magnesium: relationships to atherosclerosis, ischemic heart disease and hypertension. Magnes Trace Elem. 10(2-4):182-192, 1991-92

21] Altura B.M., et al. Magnesium: Growing in Clinical Importance. Patient Care, January 15; 130-136, 1994

22] Altura B.M., et al. Role of magnesium and calcium in alcohol-induced hypertension and strokes as probed by in vivo television microscopy, digital image microscopy, optical spectroscopy, 31P-NMR, spectroscopy and a unique magnesium ion-selective electrode. Alcohol Clin Exp Res. 18(5):1057-1068, 1994

23] Anast C.S. Impaired release of parathyroid hormone in magnesium deficiency. J Clin Endocrin Metab. 42: 707, 1976

24] Anderson T.W., et al. Ischemic heart disease, water hardness and myocardial magnesium. Canadian Medical Association Journal. 113:199, 1975

25] Ascherio A., et al. Intake of potassium, magnesium, calcium, and fiber and risk of stroke among US men. Circulation. 98:1198-204, 1998

26] Ascherio A. et al. A prospective study of nutritional factors and hypertension among US men. Circ. 86:5. 1475-84, 1992

27] Atar D., et al. Effects of magnesium supplementation in a porcine model of myocardial ischemia and reperfusion. J Cardiovasc Pharmacol. 24(4):603-611, 1994

28] Attias J., et al. Oral magnesium intake reduces permanent hearing loss induced by noise exposure. Am J Otolaryngol. 15:26-32, 1994

29] Baker S. Magnesium in primary care. Magnesium and Trace Elements. 10:251-5, 1994

30] Baker J.C., et al. Dietary antioxidants and magnesium in type I asthma Case control study. Thorax. 54(2) 115-8, 1999

31] Banki C. M., et al. Cerebrospinal fluid magnesium and calcium related to amine metabolites, diagnosis, and suicide attempts. Biol Psychiatry. 20(2):163-71, 1985

32] Barbagallo M., et al. Effects of vitamin E and glutathione on glucose metabolism: role of magnesium. Hypertension. 34(4 Part 2):1002-1006, 1999

33] Bashir Y., et al. Effects of long-term oral magnesium chloride replacement in congestive heart failure secondary to coronary artery disease. Am J Cardiol. 72:1156-1162, 1993

34] Benga I., et al. Plasma and cerebrospinal fluid concentrations of magnesium in epileptic children. J Neurol Sci. 67(1):29-34, 1985

35] Beyers E. Occurrence and Correction of Micro-element and

Magnesium Deficiencies in the Deciduous Orchards and Vineyards in the Union of South Africa. Plant Analysis & Fertilizer Problems (I.R.H.O., Paris). 1956

36] Bhargava B., et al. Adjunctive magnesium infusion therapy in acute myocardial infarction. Int J Cardiol. 52(2):95-99, 1995

37] Bjorum N. Electrolytes in blood in endogenous depression. Acta Scand Psych. 48:59-68, 1972

38] Bloch H., et al. Intravenous magnesium sulfate as an adjunct in the treatment of acute asthma. Chest. 107(6):1576-1581, 1995

39] Blondell J.M. The anticarcinogenic effect of magnesium. Med Hypotheses. 6: 863-871, 1980

40] Blum M., et al. Oral contraceptive lowers serum magnesium. Harefuah. 121(10):363-364, 1991

41] Bohmer T., et al. Magnesium deficiency in chronic alcoholic patients uncovered by an intravenous loading test. Scand J Clin Lab Invest. 42:633, 1982

42] Briggs S. Magnesium - a forgotten mineral. Health & Nutrition Breakthroughs. November 1997

43] Brilla L. R., et al. Effect of magnesium supplementation on strength training in humans. J Am Coll Nutr. 11:326-329, 1992

44] Brisco A.M. & Regan, C. Effects of Magnesium on Calcium Metabolism in Man. Am J Clin Nutr. 19, 1966

45] Britton et al. Dietary magnesium, lung function, wheezing and airway hyperreactivity in a random adult population sample. Lancet. 344:357-362, 1994

46] Brodsky M.A. Magnesium, Myocardial Infarction and Arrhythmias. Journal Am Coll of Nutr, 11(5): 607/Abstract 36, 1992

47] Brodsky M.A., et al. Magnesium Therapy in New-Onset Atrial Fibrillation. The Am J of Cardiol. 15; 73:1227-1229, 1994

48] Cairns C.B., et al. Magnesium attenuates the neutrophil respiratory burst in adult asthmatic patients. Acad Emerg Med. 3(12):1093-1097, 1996

49] Cappuccio F, Markandu N, Beynon G., et al. Lack of effect of oral magnesium on high blood pressure. BMJ 1985; 291:235-238

50] Casscells W. Magnesium and Myocardial Infarction. Lancet, April 2; 343:808-809, 1994

51] Cernak I., et al. Alterations in magnesium and oxidative status during chronic emotional stress. Magnesium Research. 13(1):29-36, 2000

52] Chipperfield B., et al. Magnesium and the heart. American Heart Journal. 93:679, 1977

53] Ciarallo L et al. Intravenous magnesium therapy for moderate to severe pediatric asthma: results of a randomized, placebo-controlled trial. J Pediatr. 129(6):809-814, 1996

54] Ciarallo L et al. Higher dose intravenous magnesium therapy for children with moderate to severe acute asthma. Arch Pediatr Adolesc medicine. 154 979-983, 2000

55] Clague et al. Intravenous magnesium loading in chronic fatigue syndrome. Letter Lancet. 340:124-125, 1992

56] Classen HG et al. The clinical importance of magnesium The indications for supplementation and therapy. Fortschr Med. 108 (10): 198-200 1990

57] Clauw D. J., et al. Magnesium deficiency in the eosinophilia-myalgia syndrome. Arth Rheum. 9:1331-1334, 1994

58] Corica F, Allegra A, Di Benedetto A, et al. Effects of oral magnesium supplementation on plasma lipid concentrations of patients with non-insulin-dependent diabetes mellitus. Magnes Res. 7:43-47, 1994

59] Corica F., et al. Changes in plasma, erythrocyte, and platelet magnesium levels in normotensive and hypertensive obese subjects during oral glucose tolerance test. American Journal of Hypertension. 12(2 Part 1):128-136, 1999

60] Cohen L Infrared spectroscopy and magnesium content in bone mineral in osteoporotic women. J Med Sci. 17: 1123-5, 1981

61] Cohen L., et al. Magnesium sulphate and digitalis-toxic arrhythmias. JAMA. 249:2808-2810, 1983.

62] Cohen L, et al. Magnesium sulfate in the treatment of variant angina. Magnesium. 3:46-49, 1984

63] Cohen L., et al. Prompt termination and/or prevention of cold-pressor-stimulus-induced vasoconstriction of different vascular beds by magnesium sulfate in patients with Prinzmetal's angina. Magnesium. 5:144-149, 1986

64] Cohen N., et al. Metabolic and clinical effects of oral magnesium supplementation in furosemide-treated patients with severe congestive heart failure. Clin Cardiol. 23(6):433-436, 2000

65] Cox et al. Red Blood cell magnesium and chronic fatigue syndrome. Lancet 337:757-760, 1991

66] Curry D.L., et al. Magnesium modulation of glucose-induced insulin secretion by the perfused mouse pancreas. Endocrinology. 101:203, 1977

67] Dahle et al. The effect of oral magnesium substitution on pregnancy induced leg cramps. AM J Obstet Gynecol. 173:1 175-80, 1995

68] Davis W. H., et al. Monotherapy with magnesium increases abnormally low high density lipoprotein cholesterol: A clinical essay. Clin Ther Res. 36:341-346, 1984

69] Demirkaya et al. Efficacy of intravenous magnesium sulfate in the treatment of acute migraine attacks. Headache. 41 171-177, 2001

70] De Swart P.M., et al. The interrelationship of calcium and magnesium absorption in idiopathic hypercalciuria and renal calcium stone disease. Journal of Urology. 159(3):669-772, 1998

71] Deulofeu et al. Magnesium and chronic fatigue syndrome. Letter Lancet 338: 66, 1991

72] Deuster P.A., et al. Responses of plasma magnesium and other cations to fluid replacement during exercise. J Am Col Nutr. 12(3):286-293, 1993

73] Dipalma J.R. Magnesium replacement therapy. Am Fam Physician. 42 (1): 173-6, 1990

74] Ditmar R.,et al. The significane of magnesium in orthopaedics Magnesium in osteoporosis. Acta Chir Orthoop Traumatol Cech. 56(2): 143-59, 1989

75] Dominguez L. J., et al. Magnesium responsiveness to insulin and insulin-like growth factor I in erythrocytes from normotensive and hypertensive subjects. J Clin Endocrinol Metab. 83:4402-4407, 1998

76] Domingez et al. Bronchial reactivity and intracellular magnesium: a possible mechanism for the brochodilating effect of magnesium in asthma. Clin Sci. 95:137-142, 1998

77] Dorup I. Magnesium and potassium deficiency. Its diagnosis, occurrence and treatment in diuretic therapy and its consequences for growth, protein synthesis and growth factors. Acta Physiol Scand. 618(Supplement):1-55, 1994

78] Drach G.W. Contribution to therapeutic decisions of ratios, absolute values and other measures of calcium, magnesium, urate or oxalate balance in stone formers. Journal of Urology. 116(3):338-340, 1976

79] Dubey A., et al. Magnesium, myocardial ischaemia and arrhythmias: The role of magnesium in myocardial infarction. Drugs. 37:1-7, 1989

80] Durlach J., et al. The Control of Central Neural Hyperexicability in Magnesium Deficiency. Nutritients and Brain Function Karger Publishers. 48-71, 1987

81] Durlach J. Magnesium depletion and pathogenesis of Alzheimer's disease. Magnesium Research . 3(3):217-218, 1990

82] Durlatch J. New trends in international magnesium research. Magnesium Research. 5: 23-27, 1992

83] Dyckner T., et al. Intracellular potassium after magnesium infusion. British Medical Journal. 1:882, 1978

84] Dyckner T., et al. Aggravation of thiamine deficiency by magnesium depletion. Acta Med Scand. 218:129-131, 1985

85] Dyckner T., et al. Effect of magnesium on blood pressure. British Medical Journal. 286(6381):1847-1849, 1983

86] Eisinger J., et al. Selenium and magnesium status in fibromyalgia. Magnesium Research. 7(3-4):285-288, 1994

87] Emelianova et al. Magnesium sulfate in management of bronchial asthma. Klin Med. 47:8 55-8, 1996

88] Facchinetti F., et al. Magnesium prophylaxis of menstrual migraine: effects on intracellular magnesium. Headache, 31:5, 298-301, 1991

89] Facchinetti F., et al. Oral magnesium successfully relieves premenstrual mood changes. Obstet Gynecol.78:2,177-81, 1991

90] Feillet-Coudray et al. Exchangeable magnesium pool masses in healthy women: effects of magnesium supplementation. American Journal of Clinical Nutrition, Vol. 75, No. 1, 72-78, January 2002

91] Fernandes J. S., et al. Therapeutic effect of a magnesium salt in patients suffering from mitral valve prolapse and latent tetany. Magnesium. 4:283-289, 1985

92] Ferrara L, Iannuzzi R, Castaldo A, et al. Long-term magnesium supplementation in essential hypertension. Cardiology. 81:25-3, 1992

93] Fiaccadori E., et al. Muscle and serum magnesium in pulmonary intensive care unit patients. Crit Care Med. 16(8):751-760, 1988

94] Flink E.B. Magnesium deficiency in alcoholism. Alcoholism. 10(6):590-594, 1986

95] Fontana-Klaiber H., et al. Therapeutic effects of magnesium in dysmenorrhea. Schweiz Rundsc Med Prax 79(16): 491-4, 1990

96] Fourman P. & Morgan D.B. Chronic Magnesium Deficiency in Man. Clin Sci Nutr 26, 1973

97] Frizel D., et al. Plasma calcium and magnesium in depression. British Journal of Psychiatry. 115:1375-1377, 1969.

98] Fugii S, Takemura T, Wada M., et al. Magnesium levels in plasma, erythrocyte, and urine in patients with diabetes mellitus. Horm Metab Res. 14:161-162, 1982

99] Gallai V., et al. Red blood cell magnesium levels in migraine patients. Cephalalgia. 13:2, 94-81, 1993

100] Galland L. D., et al. Magnesium deficiency in the pathogenesis of mitral valve prolapse. Magnesium. 5:165-174, 1986

101] Gantz N.M. Magnesium and chronic fatigue. Letter Lancet. 338 66, 1991

102] Gaspar A.Z., et al. The influence of magnesium on visual field and peripheral vasospasm in glaucoma. Ophthalmologica. 209(1):11-13, 1995

103] Gatewood J. W., et al. Mental changes associated with hyperparathyroidism. Am J Psychiat. 132(2):129-132, 1975

104] Gawaz M. Antithrombotic effectiveness of magnesium. Fortschr Med. 114: 329-332, 1996

105] Glick L.J. The role of magnesium deficiency and an hypothesis concerning the pathogenesis of Alzheimer's disease. Medical Hypotheses. 31(3):211-225, 1990

106] Gorges L.F., et al. Effect of magnesium on epileptic foci. Epilepsia. 19(1):81-91, 1978

107] Goto et al. Magnesium deficiency detected by intravenous loading dose test in variant angina pectoris. Am J Cardiol. 15 65: 709-12, 1990

108] Gottlieb S. S. Importance of magnesium in congestive heart failure. Am J Cardiol. 63:39G-42G, 1989

109] Gottlieb S. S., et al. Prognostic importance of serum magnesium concentration in patients with congestive heart failure. J Am Coll Cardiol. 16:827-831, 1990

110] Gottlieb S., et al. Effects of Intravenous Magnesium Sulfate on Arrhythmias in Patients With Congestive Heart Failure. American Heart Journal, June; 125:1645-1649, 1993

111] Gueux E., et al. The effect of magnesium deficiency on glucose stimulated insulin secretion in rats. Horm Metab Res. 15:594-597, 1983

112] Gullestad L., et al. Oral magnesium supplementation improves metabolic variables and muscle strength in alcoholics. Alcohol Clin Exp Res. 16(5):986-990, 1992

113] Gums I.J. Clinical Significance of Magnesium. Intell Clin Pharm. 21:240-46, 1987

114] Haga H. Effects of dietary magnesium supplementation on diurnal variations of blood pressure and plasma sodium, potassium-ATPase activity in essential hypertension. Jpn Heart J. 33:785-800, 1992

115] Hall R. C. W., et al. Hypomagnesemia: physical and psychiatric symptoms. Journal of the American Medical Association. 224:1749-1751, 1973

116] Hallson P., et al. Magnesium reduces calcium oxalate crystal formation in human whole urine. Clin Sci. 62:17-19, 1982

117] Hampton E. M., et al. Intravenous magnesium therapy in acute myocardial infarction. Ann Pharmacother. 28:212-219, 1994

118] Hanna S & MacIntyre, I. Influence of Aldosterone on Magnesium Metabolism. Lancet. 2, 1960

119] Harari et al. Magnesium in the management of acute and chronic treatments and Deutsches Medizinisches Zentrum's (DMZ's) clinical experience at the dead sea. J Asthma. 35:525-536, 1998

120] Hartwig A Role for Magnesium in genomic stability. Mutat Res. 475 (1-2) 113-21 2001-11-21

121] Hashimoto et al. Assessment of magnesium status in patients with bronchial asthma. J Asthma. 37:489-496, 2000

122] Hattori K., et al. Intracellular magnesium deficiency and effect of oral magnesium on blood pressure and red cell sodium transport in diuretic-treated hypertensive patients. Jpn Circ J. 52(11):1249-1256, 1988

123] Haury V.G. Blood serum magnesium in bronchial asthma and its treatment by the administration of magnesium sulfate. The Journal of Laboratory and Clinical Medicine. 26:340-344, 1940

124] Hauser S.P., et al. Intravenous magnesium administration in bronchial asthma. Scweiz Med Wochenschr. 199(46) 1633-1635, 1989

125] Henderson D.G., et al. Effect of magnesium supplementation on blood pressure and electrolyte concentrations in hypertensive patients receiving long term diuretic treatment. British Medical Journal. 293(6548):664-665, 1986

126] Henrotte J.G. Type A behavior and magnesium metabolism. Magnesium. 5:201-210, 1986

127] Herzog W.R., et al. How magnesium therapy may influence clinical outcome in acute myocardial infarction: review of potential mechanisms. Coron Artery Dis. 7(5):364-370, 1996

128] Hinds et al. Normal red cell magnesium concentrations and magnesium loading tests in patients with chronic fatigue syndrome. Ann Clin Biochem. 31:459-461, 1994

129] Hill et al. Investigation of the effect of short-term change in dietary magnesium intake in asthma. Eur Respir J. 10:2225-2229, 1997

130] Howard J. M. H. Magnesium deficiency in peripheral vascular disease. Journal of Nutrition and Medicine. 1:39-49, 1990

131] Humphries S., et al. Low dietary magnesium is associated with insulin resistance in a sample of young, nondiabetic Black Americans. Am J Hypertens. 12:747-756, 1999

132] Hwang D.L., et al. Insulin increases intracellular magnesium transport in human platelets. J Endocrinol Metab. 76:549-553, 1993

133] Ichihara A. Effects of magnesium on the renin-angiotensin-aldosterone system in human subjects. J Lab Clin Med. 112(4):432-440, 1993

134] Iseri L.T. Magnesium and cardiac arrhythmias. Magnesium. 5:111-126, 1986

135] Iseri L.T., et al. Magnesium for intractable ventricular tachyarrhythmias in normomagnesemic patients. Western Journal of Medicine. 138(6):823-828, 1983

136] ISIS-4 Collaborative Group. Fourth international study of infarct survival: protocol for a large simple study of the effects of oral mononitrate, oral captopril, and of intravenous magnesium. Am J Cardiol. 68:87-100, 1991

137] Itoh K., et al. The effects of high oral magnesium supplementation on blood pressure, serum lipids and related variables in apparently healthy Japanese subjects. Br J Nutr. November; 78:5, 737-50, 1997

138] Izenwasser S.E., et al. Stimulant-like effects of magnesium on aggression in mice. Pharmacol Biochem Behav. 25(6):1195-9, 1986

139] Jing M.A., Folsom A.R., Melnick S.L., et al. Associations of serum and dietary magnesium with cardiovascular disease, hypertension, diabetes, insulin, and carotid arterial wall thickness: the ARIC study. J Clin Epidemiol. 48:927-940, 1995

140] Joffres M.R., et al. Relationship of magnesium intake and other dietary factors to blood pressure: the Honolulu heart study. Am J Clin Nutr 45:2,469-75, 1987

141] Johansson G., et al. Biochemical and clinical effects of the prophylactic treatment of renal calcium stones with magnesium hydroxide. Journal of Urology. 124(6):770-774, 1980

142] Johansson G., et al. Magnesium metabolism in renal stone disease. Invest Urol. 18(2):93-96, 1980

143] Johansson G., et al. Effects of magnesium hydroxide in renal stone disease. Journal of the American College of Nutrition. 1(2):179-185, 1982

144] Johansson G. Magnesium and renal stone disease. Acta Med. Scand. (supplement). 661:13-18, 1982

145] Johnson C. J., et al. Myocardial tissue concentrations of magnesium and potassium in men dying suddenly from ischemic heart disease. American Journal of Clinical Nutrition. 32:967, 1979

146] Johnson S., et al. The multifaceted and widespread pathology of magnesium deficiency. Medical Hypotheses. 56(2):163-170, 2001

Jooste, P. L., et al. Epileptic-type convulsions and magnesium deficiency. Aviat. Space Environ. Med. 50(7):734-735, 1979

147] Jorgensen F. S. The urinary excretion and serum concentration of calcium, magnesium, sodium and phosphate in male patients with recurring renal stone formation. Scand J Urol Nephrol. 9(3):243-248, 1975

148] Kantak K. M. Magnesium deficiency alters aggressive behavior and catecholamine function. Behav Neurosci. 102(2):304- 11, 1988.

149] Karkkainen P., et al. Alcohol intake correlated with serum trace elements. Alcohol. 23:279-282, 1988

150] Kawano Y., Matsuoka H., Takashita S., et al. Effects of magnesium supplementation in hypertensive patients: assessment by home, office, and ambulatory blood pressures. Hypertension ;32:260-265, 1998

151] Keynes et al. Nerve & Muscle. Cambridge Uni Press. 1991

152] Kh R., et al. Effect of oral magnesium supplementation on blood pressure, platelet aggregation and calcium handling in deoxycorticosterone acetate induced hypertension in rats. Journal of Hypertension. 18(7):919-926, 2000

153] Kirov G.K., et al. Magnesium, schizophrenia and manic-depressive disease. Neuropsychobiology. 23(2):79-81, 1990

154] Klevay et al. Low dietary magnesium increases supraventricular ectopy. American Journal of Clinical Nutrition. Vol. 75, No. 3, 550-554, March 2002

155] Kozielec T., et al. Assessment of magnesium levels in children with attention deficit hyperactivity disorder (ADHD). Magnesium Research. 10(2):143-148, 1997

156] Kysters K., Spieker C., Tepel M., et al. New data about the effects of oral physiological magnesium supplementation on several cardiovascular risk factors. Magnes Res. 6:355-360, 1993

157] Labeeuw M., et al. [Role of magnesium in the physiopathology and treatment of calcium renal lithiasis.] La Presse Medicale. 16(1):25-27, 1987

158] Landon et al. Role of magnesium in regulation of lung function. J Am Diet Assoc. 93:674-677, 1993

159] Leary W.P., et al. Magnesium and deaths ascribed to ischaemic heart disease in South Africa. A preliminary report. S Afr Med J. 64(20):775-776, 1983

160] Leclercqu-Meyer et al. Effect of Calicium and Magnesium on Glucagon Secretion. Endocrinol. 93, 1973

161] Lefebvre P.J., et al. Magnesium and glucose metabolism. Therapie. 49:1-7, 1994

162] Lelord G., et al. Effects of pyridoxine and magnesium on autistic symptoms - Initial observations. J Autism Dev Disorders. 11:219-230, 1981

163] Lemke M.R. Plasma magnesium decrease and altered calcium/magnesium ratio in severe dementia of the Alzheimer type. Biol Psychiatry. 37(5):341-343, 1995

164] Lichodziejewska B., et al. Clinical symptoms of mitral valve prolapse are related to hypomagnesemia and attenuated by magnesium supplementation. American Journal of Cardiology. 79(6):768-772, 1997

165] Lind L., Lithell H., Landsberg L Blood pressure response during long-term treatment with magnesium is dependent on magnesium status. Am J Hypertens. 4:674-679, 1991

166] Lindeman R. D., et al. Magnesium in Health and Disease. SP Medical and Scientific Books, Jamaica, NY. 1980:236-245

167] Linder J., et al. Calcium and Magnesium concentrations in affective disorder: Difference between plasma and serum in relation to symptoms. Acta. Psych Scand 80:527-37, 1989

168] Ma J. Associations of serum and dietary magnesium with cardiovascular disease, hypertension, diabetes ,insulin and carotid arterial wall thickness: the ARIC study Atherosclerosis Risk in Communities. J Clin Epidem 48:7 927-40, 1995

169] MacIntyre I., et al. Intracellular Magnesium Deficiency in Man. Clin Sci 20, 1961

170] Malpuech-Brugere C., et al. Early morphological and immunological alterations in the spleen during magnesium deficiency in the rat. Magnesium Research. 11(3):161-169, 1998

171] Marlow M., et al. Decreased magnesium in the hair of autistic children. J Orthomol Psychiat. 13(2):117-122, 1984

172] Martineau J., et al. Vitamin B6, magnesium, and combined vitamin B6-Mg: Therapeutic effects in childhood autism. Biol Psychiat. 20:467-478, 1978

173] Martineau J., et al. The effects of combined pyridoxine plus magnesium administration on the conditioned evoked potentials in children with autistic behavior. Curr Top Nutr Dis. 19:357-362, 1988

174] Maruer J.R. Role of environmental magnesium in cardiovascular disease. Magnesium. 1:266-276 1982 and 2:57-61, 1983

175] Marx A & Neutra R. Magnesium in drinking water and ischemic heart disease. Epidemiol Rev.19:258-272, 1997

176] Mather H. M., et al. Hypomagnesemia in diabetes. Clin Chem Acta. 95:235-242, 1979

177] Matz R. Magnesium: Deficiencies and Therapeutic Uses. Hospital Practice. April 30, 79-72, 1993

178] Mauskop A., et al. Intravenous magnesium sulfate rapidly alleviates headaches of various types. Headache. 36:154-160, 1996

179] Mauskop A. & Altura B.M. Role of magnesium in the pathogenesis and treatment of migraines. Clin Science 89(6):633-636, 1995

180] Mauskop A., et al. Role of magnesium in the pathogenesis and Treatment of migraine. Clin Neurosciences. 5:24-27, 1998

181] McCarty M.F. Magnesium taurate and fish oil for prevention of migraine. Med Hypotheses. 47: 461-466, 1996

182] McLean R.M. Magnesium and its therapeutic uses: a review. American Journal of Medicine. 96(1):63-76, 1994

183] McNair P., et al. Hypomagnesemia, a risk factor in diabetic neuropathy. Diabetes. 27:1075-1077, 1978

184] McNair P., Christensen M.S., Christiansen C., et al. Renal hypomagnesemia in human diabetes mellitus: its relation to glucose homeostasis. Eur J Clin Invest ; 12:81-85, 1982

185] Melnick I., et al. Magnesium therapy of recurrent calcium oxalate urinary calculi. I Urol. 105:119, 1978

186] Mishima et al. Platelet ionised magnesium, cyclic AMP and cyclic GMP levels in migraine and tension type headache. Headache. 37:561-564, 1997

187] Moore M.P., Redman C.W. Case-control study of severe preeclampsia of early onset. Br Med J. 287:580-83, 1983

188] Moore T.J. The role of dietary electrolytes in hypertension. J Am Coll Nutr, 8 Suppl S. 68S-80S, 1989

189] Moorkens et al. Magnesium deficit in a sample of the Belgian population presenting with chronic fatigue. Magnes Res. 10:329-337, 1997

191] Motoyama T., et al. Oral magnesium supplementation in patients with essential hypertension. Hypertension. 13(3):227-232, 1989

192] Muenzenberg et al. Mineralogic apects in the treatment of osteoporosis with magnesium. J Am Coll Nutr. 8(5): 461, 1989

193] Muir K.W., et al. Dose optimization of intravenous magnesium sulfate after acute stroke. Stroke. 29:918-923, 1998

194] Muneyvirci-Delale O., et al. Sex steroid hormones modulate serum ionized magnesium and calcium levels throughout the menstrual cycle in women. Fertil Steril. 69(5): 958-62, 1998

195] Nadler J.L., et al. Magnesium deficiency produces insulin resistance and increased thromboxane synthesis. Hypertension. 21:1024-1029, 1993

196] Nowson C & Morgan T. Magnesium supplementation in mild hypertensive patients on a moderately low sodium diet. Clin Exp Pharmacol Physiol. 16:299-302, 1989

197] O'Brien P., et al. Progesterone, Fluid and Electrolytes in Premenstrual Syndrome. Brit Med Journal. (1) 1161-1163, 1980

198] Okayama H., et al. Bronchodilating effect of intravenous magnesium sulfate in bronchial asthma. JAMA. 257(8):1076-1078, 1987

199] Olhaberry J., Reyes A., Acousta-Barrios T., et al. Pilot evaluation of the putative antihypertensive effect of magnesium. Magnes Bull. 9:181-184, 1987

200] Omu A. E., et al. Magnesium in human semen: possible role in premature ejaculation. Arch Androl. 46(1):59-66, 2001

201] Paolisso G., et al. Daily magnesium supplements improve glucose handling in elderly subjects. American Journal of Clinical Nutrition. 55:1161-1167, 1992

202] Paolisso G., et al. Improved insulin response and action by chronic magnesium administration in aged NIDDM subjects. Diabetes

Care. 12(4):265-269, 1989

203] Paolisso G., et al. Magnesium and glucose homeostasis. Diabetologia. 33(9):511-514, 1990

204] Paolisso et al. Changes in glucose turnover parameters and improvement of glucose oxiation after 4-week magnesium administrataion in elderly non-insulin dependent diabetic patients. J Clin Endocrin Metab. 78:6 1510-4, 1994

205] Paolisso et al. Hypertension, diabetes and insulin resistance: the role of intracellular magnesium. Am J Hypertens. 10:3 346-55, 1997

206] Peikert A., et al. Prophylaxis of migraine with oral magnesium: results from a prospective, multi- centre, placebo-controlled and double-blind randomized study. Cephalalgia. June, 16:4, 257-63, 1996

207] Perticone F., et al. Antiarrhythmic short-term protective magnesium treatment in ischemic dilated cardiomyopathy. J Am Coll Nutr. 9:492-499, 1990

208] Picado M., de la Sierra A., Aguilera M., et al. Increased activity of the magnesium-sodium exchanger in red blood cells for essential hypertensive patients. Hypertension; 23(part 2):987-991, 1993

209] Poenaru S., et al. Magnesium and monoaminergic neurotransmitters: Elements of human and experimental pathaphysiology. In: Magnesium in Health and Disease. Itakawa Y., and Durlach, J. London. :291-297, 1989

210] Popoviciu L., et al. Parasomnias (non-epileptic nocturnal episodic manifestations) in patients with magnesium deficiency. Romanian Journal of Neurology and Psychiatry. 28(1):19-24, 1990

211] Porta S., et al. Significant inhibition of the stress response with magnesium supplementation in fighter pilots. Magnesium- Bulletin. 16,2:54-58, 1994

212] Purvis J. R., et al. Magnesium disorders and cardiovascular disease. Clin Cardiol. 15:556-568, 1992

213] Purvis J.R., Cummings D.M., Landsman P., et al. Effect of oral magnesium supplementation on selected cardiovascular risk factors in non-insulin-dependent diabetics. Arch Fam Med. 3:503-508, 1994

214] Ralo J. Magnesium: Another metal to bone up on. Science News. 154:134, 1998

215] Ramadan et al. Low brain magnesium in migraine. Headache.

29:590-593, 1989

216] Rasmussen H. S., et al. Intravenous magnesium in acute myocardium infarction. The Lancet. 1:234-235, 1986

217] Rasmussen H. S., et al. Influence of magnesium substitution therapy on blood lipid composition in patients with ischemic heart disease. Archives of Internal Medicine. 149:1050-1053, 1989

218] Regan R. R., et al. Magnesium deprivation decreases cellular reduced glutathione and causes oxidative neuronal death in murine cortical cultures. Brain Res. 890(1):177-183, 2001

219] Resnick L. M., et al. Intracellular free magnesium in erythrocytes of esential hypertension: Relation to blood pressure and serum divalent cations. Proceedings of the National Academy of Sciences. 81:6511, 1984

220] Resnick L. Magnesium in the pathophysiology and treatment of hypertension and diabetes mellitus: where are we in 1997? Am J Hypertension. 10:368-370, 1997

221] Reynolds I. J. Intracellular calcium and magnesium, critical determinants of excitotoxicity. Prog Brain Res. 116:225-243, 1998

222] Rheinhart R.A. Clinical correlates of the molecular and cellular actions of magnesium on the cardiovascular system. Am Heart J. 121 (5): 1513-21, 1991

223] Robinson J.B.D. & Chenery E.M. Magnesium Deficiency in Coffee with Special Reference to Mulching. Emp. J. exp. Agric. 26:259-73, 1958

224] Rolla G., et al. Acute effect of intravenous magnesium sulfate on airway obstruction of asthmatic patients. Annals of Allergy. 61:388-391, 1988

225] Romano T.J. Magnesium deficiency in systemic lupus erythematosis. Journal of Nutritional & Environmental Medicine. 107-111, 1997

226] Ruddell H., et al. Effect of magnesium supplementation in patients with labile hypertension. Journal of the American College of Nutrition. 6:445, 1987

227] Rude R. K., et al. Magnesium deficiency: possible role in osteoporosis associated with gluten-sensitive enteropathy. Osteoporos Int. 6(6):453-461, 1996

228] Rude R. Low serum concentrations of 1,25-dihyroxyvitamin D in human magnesium deficiency. J Clin Endocirn Metab. 61: 933-40, 1985

229] Rude R. Magnesium Metabolism and Deficiency. Endocrin & MetabClin N America, June. 22(2): 377-395, 1993

230] Rude R. K., et al. Magnesium deficiency induced osteoporosis in the rat: uncoupling of bone formation and bone resorption. Magnesium Research. 12:257-267, 1999

231] Rudnicki M., et al. Comparison of magnesium and methyldopa for the control of blood pressure in pregnancies complicated with hypertension. Gynecol Obstet Invest. 49(4):231-235, 2000

232] Russell R. I. Magnesium requirements in patients with chronic inflammatory disease receiving intravenous nutrition. J Am Coll Nutr. 4(5):553-558, 1985

233] Ryan M. P., et al. The role of magnesium in the prevention and control of hypertension. Ann Clin Res. 16(Supplement 43):81-88, 1984

234] Saito K., Hattori K., Omatsu T., et al. Effects of oral magnesium on blood pressure and red cell sodium transport in patients receiving long-term thiazide diuretics for hypertension. Am J Hypertens. 1:71S-74S, 1988

235] Sanjuliani A. F., et al. Effects of magnesium on blood pressure and intracellular ion levels of Brazilian hypertensive patients. Int J Cardiol. 56(2):177-183, 1996

236] Saris N.E.L., et al. Magnesium: an update on physiological, clinical and analytical aspects. Clinica Chimica Acta. 294:1-26, 2000

237] Satake et al. Relation between severity of magesuim deficiency and frequency of anginal attacks in men with variant angina. J Am Coll Cardiol. 28:4 897-902, 1996

238] Schecter M., Hod H., Marks N., et al. Beneficial effect of magnesium sulfate in acute myocardial infarction. Am J Cardiol. 66:271-274, 1990

239] Schecter M., et al. The rationale of magnesium supplementation in acute myocardial infarction. A review of the literature. Arch Intern Med. 152:2189-2196, 1992

240] Schoenen, J., et al. Blood Magnesium levels in Migraine.

Cephalalgia. 11(2) 97-99, 1991
241] Seelig M.S. Interrelationship of magnesium and estrogen in cardiovascular and bone disorders, eclampsia, migraine and premenstrual syndrome. J Am Coll Nutr Aug. 12(4): 442-58, 1933
242] Seelig M. Human requirements of magnesium: factors that increase needs. In: First International Symposium on Magnesium Deficiency in Human Pathology. Springer Verlag, Paris. 1971:11
243] Seelig M., et al. Magnesium interrelationships with ischemic heart disease: A review. American Journal of Clinical Nutrition. 27:59-79, 1974
244] Seelig M.S. Magnesium Deficiency in the pathogenesis of Disease. Plenum Pub N.Y. 1980
245] Seelig M.S.,et al. Low Magnesium: A Common Denominator in Pathologic Process in Diabetes Mellitus, Cardiovascular Disease and Eclampsia. Journal of the American College of Nutrition, October; 11(5): 608/Abstr 39, 1992
246] Seifert B., et al. Magnesium a new therapeutic alternative in primary dysmenorrhoea. Zentrabl Gynakol. 111 (11): 755-60, 1989
247] Shechter M. Magnesium For Acute MI: Although the Mechanisms of its Therapeutic Effects Are Still Being Debated, The Element Seems Likely to Secure a Place in The Armamentarium Against Myocardial Infarction. Em Med, May. 135-139, 1993
248] Sherwood R.A., Rocks B.F., et al. Magnesium and the premenstrual syndrome. Ann Clin Biochem. 23:667-70, 1986
249] Singh et al. Is Verapamil a better Magnesium agonist rather than a calcium antagonist? A Hypothesis? Med Hypotheses. 24:1 1-9, 1987
250] Singh R.B. Effect of dietary magnesium supplementation in the prevention of coronary heart disease and sudden cardiac death. Magnes Trace Elements; 9:141-151, 1990
251] Singh A., et al. Biochemical indices of selected trace minerals in men: effect of stress. Am J Clin Nut. 53(1):126-131, 1991
252] Sjogren A., et al. Oral administration of magnesium hydroxide to subjects with insulin dependent diabetes mellitus. Magnesium. 121:16-20, 1988
253] Sjogren A., et al. Oral administration of magnesium hydroxide to subjects with insulin-dependent diabetes mellitus: effects on

magnesium and potassium levels and on insulin requirements.
Magnesium. 7(3):117-122, 1988

254] Sjogren A., et al. Magnesium deficiency in coronary artery
disease and cardiac arrhythmias. Journal of Internal Medicine.
226:213-222, 1989

255] Skobeloff E.M., et al. Intravenous magnesium sulfate for the
treatment of acute asthma in the emergency department. Journal of the
American Medical Association. 262(9):1210-1213, 1989

256] Smetana R., et al. Stress and magnesium metabolism in
coronary artery disease. Mag Bulletin. 13(4):125-127, 1991

257] Soldatovic D., et al. Compared effects of high oral Mg
supplements and of EDTA chelating agent on chronic lead intoxication
in rabbits. Magnesium Research. 10:127-133, 1997

258] South J. Magnesium - the underappreciated mineral of life. Part
1. Vitamin Research News. September 1997

259] Sparkman D. Magnesium helps prevent bone loss: equal to
calcium in fighting osteoporosis. All Natural Muscular Development.
36(2):34, 1999

260] Specter M.J., et al. Studies on magnesium's mechanism of action
in digitalis-induced arrhythmias. Circulation. 52:1001, 1975

261] Starobrat-Hermelin B., et al. The effects of magnesium
physiological supplementation on hyperactivity in children with
attention deficit hyperactivity disorder (ADHD). Positive response to
magnesium oral loading test. Magnes Res. 10:149-156, 1997

262] Stebbing J.B., et al. Reactive hypoglycemia and magnesium.
Mag Bull. 2:131-134, 1982

263] Stendig-Lindberg G., et al. Changes in serum magnesium
concentration after strenuous exercise. Journal of the American
College of Nutrition. 6(1):35-40, 1987

264] Stendig-Lindberg et al. Trabecular bone density in a two year
controlled trial of peroral magnesium in osteoporosis. Mag Res. 6;2
155-63, 1993

265] Sueta C.A., et al. Effect of actur magnesium administration on
the frequency of ventricular arrhythmia in patients with heart failure.
Circulation. 89(2):660-666, 1994

266] Swain R., Kaplan-Machlis B. Magnesium for the next

millennium. South Med J Nov; 92(11): 1040-7, 1999

267] Swanson D.R. Migraine and Magnesium: Eleven neglected connections. Pespect Biol Med. 31:526-557, 1988

268] Szelenyi I., et al. Effect of magnesium orotate and orotic acid on induced blood pressure elevation and cardiopathogenic changes of the myocardium in animal experiments. Dtsch Med J.; 21(22):1405-1412, 1970

269] Taubert K. Magnesium in Migraine. Results from a multicenter pilot study. Fortschr Med. 112 (24) 328-330, 1994

270] Teo K.K., et al. Effects of intravenous magnesium in suspected acute myocardial infarction: overview of randomized trials. British Medical Journal. 303:1499-1503, 1991

271] Teo K.K., et al. Role of magnesium in reducing mortality in acute myocardial infarction. A review of the evidence. Drugs. 46:347-359, 1993

272] Teragawa H. et al. The preventive effect of magnesium on coronary spasm in patients with vasospastic angina. Chest. 118(6) 1690-95 2000

273] Theodore H. et al. Magnesium and the pancreas. Am J Clin Nutr. 26, 1973

274] Tinker P.B.H. & Bull R.A. Some Effects of Variations in Soil Potassium and Magnesium on Yield Responses and Deficiency Symptoms in Oil Palms. Proc. W. African Soils and Plant Nutrition Conference. 72-90, 1957

275] Touyz R M. Magnesium supplementation as an adjuvant to synthetic calcium channel antagonists in the treatment of hypertension. Medical Hypotheses. 36:140-141, 1991

276] Touyz R., Schiffrin E. The effect of angiotensin II on platelet intracellular free magnesium and calcium ionic concentrations in essential hypertension. J Hyperten. 11:551-558, 1993

277] Turlapaty P., et al. Magnesium deficiency produces spasms of coronary arteries: Relationship to etiology of sudden death ischemic heart disease. Science. 208:199-200, 1980

278] Turnlaud J.R., et al. Vitamin B6 depletion followed by repletion with animal- or plant-source diets in calcium and magnesium metabolism in young women. The American Journal of Clinical

Nutrition 56:905-10, 1992

279] Wacker W.E. & Vallee B.L. Magnesium Metabolism. NEJM 254, 1958

280] Wallach S. Effects of magnesium on skeletal metabolism. Magnes Trace Elem. 9(1): 1-14,1990

281] Watts D.L. The Assessment of Hypertensive Tendencies from Trace Element Analysis. Chiro Econ March. 1986

282] Watts D.L. Trace Elements and Neuropsychological problems as reflected in tissue mineral analysis (TMA) patterns. J Ortho Med. 5(3) 159-166, 1990

283] Weaver K. Magnesium and its role in vascular reactivity and coagulation. Contemp Nutr. 12(3), 1987

284] Weaver K. Magnesium in Health and Disease. Spectrum Pubs. p. 833, 1980

285] Welshman S.G., et al. The relationship of the urinary cations, calcium, magnesium, sodium and potassium, in patients with renal calculi. British Journal of Urology. 47(3):237-242, 1975

286] Wester P.O., Dyckner T. Magnesium and hypertension. J Am Coll Nutr; 6(4):321-28, 1987

287] Weston P.G., et al. Magnesium sulfate as a sedative. Am J Med Sci. 165:431–33, 1923

288] Whang R., et al. Hypomagnesemia and hypokalemia in 1,000 treated ambulatory hypertensive patients. J Am Coll Nutr. 1:317-322, 1982

289] Whang R., et al. Magnesium homeostasis and clinical disorders of magnesium deficiency. Ann Pharmacother. 28:220-225, 1994

290] Whelton P., Klag M.J. Magnesium and blood pressure: Review of the epidemiologic and clinical trial experience. Am J Cardiol. 63(14):26G-30G, 1989

291] Widman L., Webster P., Stegmayr B., et al. The dose-dependent reduction in blood pressure through administration of magnesium. Am J Hypertens. 6:41-45, 1993

292] Winterkorn J.M. The influence of magnesium on visual field and peripheral vasospasm in glaucoma. Surv Ophthalmol. 40(1):83-84, 1995

293] Wirell M., Webster P., Stegmayr B. Nutritional dose of

magnesium in hypertensive patients on beta blockers lowers systolic blood pressure: a double-blind cross-over study. J Intern Med . 236:189-195, 1994

294] Wittman J., et al. Reduction of blood pressure with oral magnesium supplementation in women with mild to moderate hypertension. Am J Clin Nutr. 60:129-135, 1994

295] Wittman J.C., et al. A prospective study of nutritional factors and hypertension among US women. Circulation, Nov. 80:5, 1320-7, 1989

296] Wong E.T., Rude R.K., Singer F.R., et al. A high prevalence of hypomagnesemia in hospitalized patients. Am J Clin Pathol. 79:348-352, 1983

297] Woods K.L., et al. Intravenous magnesium sulphate in suspected acute myocardial infarction: results of the second Leicester Intravenous Magnesium Intervention Trial (LIMIT-2). The Lancet. 339:1553-1558, 1992

298] Wright J.V. Magnesium can relieve migraine (and other magnesium-related matters). AAEM Nwsletter, Winter, p.14, 1989

299] Wunderlich W. Aspects of the influence of magnesium ions on the formation of calcium oxalate. Urol Res. 9:157-160, 1981

300] Yasui M., et al. Magnesium concentration in brains from multiple sclerosis patients. Acta Neurology Scandinavia. 81(3):197-200, 1990

301] Yeh J.K., et al. Effect of physical activity on the metabolism of magnesium in the rat. Journal of the American College of Nutrition. 10(5):487-493, 1991

302] Yu-Yahiro J.A. Electrolytes and their relationship to normal and abnormal muscle function. Orthop Nurs. 13(5):38-40, 1994

303] Zehender M., et al. Antiarrhythmic effects of increasing the daily intake of magnesium and potassium in patients with frequent ventricular arrhythmias. J Am Coll Cardiol. 29:1028-1034, 1997

304] Zorbas Y.G., et al. Magnesium loading effect on magnesium deficiency in endurance-trained subjects during prolonged restriction of muscular activity. Biol Trace Elem Res. 63(2):149-166, 1998

SELENIUM IS A DIRTY WORD.

Entrée

Just lie back on the couch and relax. What is your deepest, darkest fear?

I can't…

Your darkest dream?

I…

Yes?…

I dreamt that one of my oncology patients took selenium.

And?

They improved their immune system so much that their cancer got better.

Is that so bad?

They didn't come back.

Is that so terrible?

Why, yes. They should be having chemotherapy. Chemo good, natural bad. Chemo good, natural bad.

Do you like George Orwell?

Oh yes. His books are recommended reading for the F.R.A.C.P.

Have you read 1984?

Yes.

What do you remember of it?

"The H.I.C. is watching you."

The who?

The Health Insurance Commission.

Why are they watching you?

They're worried that I'll prescribe selenium.

Is that so bad?

I'm registered to prescribe toxic drugs, not minerals.

You mean you have to prescribe toxic drugs?

Yes. Chemo good, natural bad. I even have a quota.

That's great, but what is the worst-case scenario?

My patients get better with natural therapies.

What would that mean?

That there were serious cracks in the foundation of medicine's knowledge pyramid.

Is that so frightening?

Absolutely. Then all the Naturopaths and Homeopaths and nutritional medicine practitioners, Chiropractors, clairvoyants, Podiatrists and even my mother would be right.

That's nothing. I had a dream that all of my schizophrenia patients took selenium and they became normal. Oh, look at the time! I want you to increase your Melleril to four tablets per day and see me in four weeks.

This was a true extract from a recent consultation between a local psychiatrist and a local oncologist…. Or was it?

Main Course

Selenium is an unusual element. Its conduction of electricity increases with the amount of light hitting it. It sits in the periodic table below Oxygen and Sulphur and next to Arsenic and Bromine. Both arsenic and bromine have had interesting medical applications over the years. Selenium has had a chequered history in Australia. There was a time when the authorities declared that no one in Australia could possibly be selenium deficient and therefore banned selenium supplements. Then a strange thing happened. **They changed their minds.** Rumour has it that certain doctors, when finding a patient with selenium deficiency, would send a copy of the result to the minister for health for an explanation. Now who would do such a thing? Anyway, now you can buy selenium supplements as long as the tablet does not exceed 25 micrograms in quantity. Natural sources include Wheat Germ, Whole Grain Bread, Wheat Bran, Barley, Eggs, Mushrooms, Legumes, Liver, Kidneys, Rabbit, Chicken, Brazil Nuts, Peanuts, Herring, Tuna, Shellfish, Asparagus, Cabbage, Celery, Garlic, Onions, Potatoes, Radish, Tomatoes and Brewer's Yeast.

Selenium falls in the category of a metallic antioxidant. That is, a metal that prevents oxidation (rusting) and hence free radical build up. Free radicals damage the inside structure of cells like DNA. Their build up has been implicated in many major diseases including cancer.

Interestingly, both low and high levels of antioxidants are associated with immune suppression.

Why is selenium so important, and why don't doctors know about this? I guess that if you found that significant cancer, heart disease or diabetes was associated with low selenium levels and this information got out, then you'd have somewhat of a panic on you hands, especially if you had previously issued an edict stating that selenium deficiency couldn't happen in Australia. I guess that you'd want the laboratories to use very conservative reference ranges to reduce the chance of somebody finding the problem in epidemic proportions too. Sounds far-fetched? Ever asked the laboratories where they get their reference ranges? Ask them what size population and what kind of people their zinc and selenium ranges are based upon.

Selenium deficiency is very well hidden from doctors and the general population. Any one mentioning it is immediately eyed suspiciously rather like an alien abductee would be. Selenium? Oh that conspiracy theory again! Funnily enough, all the farmers know about it (I guess they couldn't kill all of them now could they?). So does the Agriculture Department and the dieticians and the nutritionists and even some pharmacists.

Why is selenium a dirty word? Because we find it (or can't find it) in soil. Considering the low levels of selenium in our soils (a fact known to all except the medical profession), it's difficult to know what a normal serum level of selenium should be. One way to check the tissue level is to look at the conversion of T4 (the inactive thyroid hormone) to T3 (the active level of thyroid hormone). Good levels of selenium mean that the ratio is about 3:1. That is T3 should be one third of T4.

Low selenium has been associated with several major illnesses. These are heart disease, high cholesterol, arthritis, cancer, hypothyroidism, diabetes, psoriasis and even depression. The references at the end of this article show the scope of the research and are not a complete list (only 82) by any means. The majority of studies have looked at selenium and immunity especially resistance to infection and cancer. In this sense it concords with the general trend of antioxidants such as Vitamin C, beta-carotene, zinc, manganese and Vitamin E. These nutrients seem to improve immune function but high levels are associated with immunosuppression.

Selenium has a strong role in thyroid function. It is important for both thyroid hormone production and conversion of the inactive thyroid hormone (the one the doctor gives you) into the active hormone. So without selenium even Oroxine won't improve thyroid function. Selenium has been implicated in poor heart function (cardiomyopathy) and it may have this function because it is needed for Co-enzyme Q10 production (page 136). Most of the medical profession think that Co-enzyme Q10 is a new age hippie vitamin. They are not aware that Co-enzyme Q10 is step 2 of the cytochrome system, which powers every single cell in the body (except Red Blood Cells). Was that page 1 or 2 of our biochemistry book? If you don't have co-enzyme Q10 you don't get to steps 3 and 4 (which are iron based, incidentally.) This feature may explain why selenium is useful in angina. It simply helps the heart function more efficiently and hence because it needs less oxygen and can work better on a reduced blood flow such as in coronary artery disease. But I suppose we couldn't treat angina with minerals, the manufacturers of Anginine and Imdur and Nitrodisc would lose out, wouldn't they? The cardiologists would have to study biochemistry for their fellowships and then they'd find out about magnesium and zinc and potassium. The whole fabric of medicine as we know it would crumble and there would be chaos and anarchy. Drug companies would go out of business and stop funding large studies. Hospitals and universities would have less to do and instigate staff cuts. So please don't mention selenium to your doctor. The effects would be catastrophic.

The amino acid taurine facilitates the transport of selenium into the cells from the blood stream. This may explain why taurine has been used for palpitations and hypertension, because it increases cellular selenium and hence co-enzyme Q10.

86

Most problems with low selenium are due to poor soil levels, diet or absorption. Land-based sources of selenium such as alfalfa sprouts or wheat depend upon the levels of selenium in the soil where they are grown. Plants can grow on selenium poor soils without overt signs of deficiency. The best sources are from marine based products like shellfish, but cost and cholesterol levels in these foods often mean people may not include these in their diets. Interestingly, selenium is needed for cholesterol metabolism and is also found in these foods. Just as an egg has the cholesterol in the yolk balanced by the lecithin in the white, these foods are also balanced.

Malabsorption can occur for several reasons. Reduced stomach acid from low zinc, Helicobacter stomach infection, drugs (like Losec, Zoton, Somac) and/or reduced pancreatic juice production (often as result of low stomach acid) can impair selenium absorption because selenium can best be absorbed as the picolinate form (see chapter on zinc). Cadmium and selenium can compete for absorption and there is a suspicion that cadmium will substitute itself for selenium in soils treated with super phosphates. This could create a toxic product high in cadmium and low in antioxidants.

Alcohol and smoking can deplete selenium levels. Vitamin C supplements can interfere with the absorption of sodium selenite drops (one form of selenium supplement).

Dessert

So how much selenium should I take? Well, you're pretty safe with 25 micrograms per days. If you want to take more ask your doctor for a blood test or hair analysis. Oh, and don't forget your Melleril.

Selenium, the immune system and cancer:
1] Batist, G., et al. Selenium induced cytotoxicity of human leukemia cells: interaction with reduced glutathione. Cancer Research. 46(11):5482-5485, 1986.
2] Buljevac, M., et al. Serum selenium concentration in patients with liver cirrhosis and hepatocellular carcinoma. Acta Med Croatica. 1(50):11-14, 1996.

3] Burke, E. R. Selenium: low levels linked to liver cancer. Muscular Development. 36(11):34, 1999.

4] Burke, E. R. Selenium could lower risk of prostate cancer. All Natural Muscular Development. 35(12):56, 1998.

5] Burnley, P. G. J., et al. Serologic precursors of cancer: Serum micronutrients and the subsequent risk of pancreatic cancer. American Journal of Clinical Nutrition. 49:895-900, 1989

6] Broghamer, W. L., et al. Relationship between serum selenium levels and patients with carcinoma. Cancer. 37:1384, 1976.

7] Cheng, K. K., et al. Nutrition and oesophageal cancer. Cancer Causes and Control. 7:33-40, 1996.

8] Clark, L. The epidemiology of selenium and cancer. Federation Proceedings. 44:2584-2589, 1985.

9] Clark, L. C., et al. Plasma selenium and skin neoplasms: A case control study. Nutr Cancer. 6:13, 1985.

10] Clark, L. C., et al. Decreased incidence of prostate cancer with selenium supplementation: results of double-blind cancer prevention trial. Br J Urol. 81:730-734, 1998.

11] Clark, L. C., et al. Effects of selenium supplementation for cancer prevention in patients with carcinoma of the skin. A randomised controlled trial. Nutritional Prevention of Cancer Study Group. JAMA. 276:1957-1963, 1996.

12] Combs, G. F., et al. Can dietary selenium modify cancer risk? Nutr. Rev. 43:325-331, 1985.

13] Coldsitz, G. A. Selenium and cancer prevention: promising results indicate further trials required. The Journal of the American Medical Association. 276(24):1984, 1996.

14] Combs, G. F Jr., et al. Reduction of cancer mortality and incidence by selenium supplementation. Med Klin. 92(Supplement 3):42-45, 1997.

15] Contreras, V. National cancer institute spotlights nutrients: prestigious panel focuses on substances found in plants. Journal of Longevity. #48, 1999.

16] Davis, C. D., et al. The chemical form of selenium influences 3,2'-dimethyl-4- National Research Council: Diet and Health.

17] Fex, G., et al. Low plasma selenium as a risk factor for cancer death in middle-age men. Nutr Cancer. 10:221-229, 1987.

18] Hocman, G. Chemoprevention of cancer: Selenium. Int J Biochem. 20(2):123-132, 1988.

19] Ip, C. Selenium inhibition of chemical carcinogenesis. Federation Proceedings. 44:25373-2578, 1985.

20] Ip, C. Interaction of vitamin C and selenium supplementation in the modification of mammary carcinogenesis in rats. J N C I. 77:299, 1986.

21] Kandaswami, C., et al. Differential inhibition of proliferation of human squamous cell carcinoma, gliosarcoma and embryonic fibroblast-lung cells in culture by plant flavonoids. Anticancer Drugs. 3(5):525-530, 1992.

22] Kiremidjian-Schumacher, L., et al. Supplementation with selenium and human immune cell functions; II, Effect on cytotoxic lymphocytes and natural killer cells. Biol Trace Elem Res. 41:115-127, 1994.

23] Kiremidjian-Schumacher, L., et al. Selenium and immune responses. Environmental Res. 42:277-303, 1987.

24] Knekt, P., et al. Serum selenium and subsequent risk of cancer among Finnish men and women. Journal of the National Cancer Institute. 82:864-868, 1990.

25] Kobayashi, M., et al. Inhibitory effect of dietary selenium on carcinogenesis in rat glandular stomach induced by N-Methyl-N'-nitro-N-nitro. Cancer Research. 46:2266-2270, 1986.

26] Ksrnjavi, H., et al. Selenium in serum as a possible parameter for assessment of breast disease. Breast Cancer Research and Treatment. 16:57-61, 1990.

27] Menkes, M. S., et al. Serum beta-carotene, vitamins A and E, selenium and the risk of lung cancer. New England Journal of Medicine. 315:1250, 1986.

28] Mervyn, L. Thorsons Complete Guide to Vitamins and Minerals (2nd Edition). Thorsons Publishing Group, Wellingborough, England. 1989:79.

29] McConnell, K. P., et al. The relationship between dietary selenium and breast cancer. Journal of Surgical Oncology. 15(1):67-70, 1980.

30] Moss, Ralph W. Cancer Therapy: the Independent Consumer's Guide to Non-Toxic Treatment & Prevention. Equinox Press, Brooklyn, New York, USA. 1992:109-114.

31] Moss, Ralph W. Cancer Therapy: the Independent Consumer's Guide to Non-Toxic Treatment & Prevention. Equinox Press, Brooklyn, New York, USA. 1992:109-114.

32] Nelson, R. L. Is the changing patterns of colorectal cancer caused by selenium deficiency?. Dis Colon Rectum. 459-461, 1984.

33] Nelson, R. L., et al. Serum selenium and colonic neoplastic risk. Diseases of the Colon and Rectum. 38:1306-1310, 1995.

34] Rajcok, P. Selenium: the trace element for the next millennium. Mother Nature's Health Journal Biweekly Newsletter. 2(18), 1999.

35] Redman, C., et al. Involvement of polyamines in selenomethionine induced apoptosis and mitotic alterations in human tumour cells. Carcinogenesis. 18(6):1195-1202, 1997.

36] Redman, C., et al. Inhibitory effect of selenomethionine on the growth of three selected human tumour cell lines. Cancer Letters. 125(1-2):103-110, 1998.

37] Redman, C., et al. Involvement of polyamines in selenomethionine induced apoptosis and mitotic alterations in human tumour cells. Carcinogenesis. 18(6):1195-1202, 1997.

38] Roy, M. Supplementation with selenium and human immune cell functions; I, Effect on lymphocyte proliferation and interleukin 2 receptor expression. Biol Trace Elem Res. 41:103-114, 1994.

39] Salonen, J. T., et al. Association between serum selenium and the risk of cancer. American Journal of Epidemiology. 120:342, 1984.

40] Salonen, J. T., et al. Risk of cancer in relation to serum concentrations of selenium and vitamins A and E: matched case control analysis of prospective data.

British Medical Journal. 290:417-420, 1985.

41] Scheer, J. F. 12 key antioxidants: may their 'force' be with you. Better Nutrition. 61(1):58-60, 1999.

42] Schrauzer, G. N., et al. Effects of temporary selenium supplementation on the genesis of spontaneous mammary tumours in inbred female C3H/St mice. Carcinogenesis. 1:199, 1980.

43] Schrauzer, G. N. Selenium and cancer: A review. Bioinorganic Chemistry. 5:275-281, 1976.

44] Schrauzer, G. N., et al. Cancer mortality correlation studies III: Statistical associations with dietary selenium intakes. Bioinorganic Chemistry. 7:23-34, 1977.

45] Sundstrom, H., et al. Serum selenium in patients with ovarian cancer during and after therapy. Carcinogenesis. 5(6):731-734, 1984.

46] White, E. L., et al. Screening of potential cancer preventing chemicals for induction of glutathione in rat liver cells. Oncol Rep. 5(2):507-512, 1998.

47] Yoshizawa, K., et.al. Study of prediagnostic selenium level in toenails and the risk of advanced prostate cancer. J Natl Cancer Inst. 90:1219-24, 1998.

48] Yu, S. Y., et al. A preliminary report on the intervention trials of primary liver cancer in high-risk populations with nutritional supplementation of selenium in China. Biological Trace Element Research. 29:289-294, 1991.

49] Yu, S. Y., et al. Protective role of selenium against hepatitis B virus and primary liver cancer in Qidong. Biol Tr Elem Res. 56(1):117-124, 1997.

50] Yu, S-Y, et al. Intervention trial in selenium for the prevention of lung cancer among tin miners in Yunnan, China. Biological Trace Element Research. 24:105-108, 1990.

51] Yu, S. Y., et al. Protective role of selenium against hepatitis B virus and primary liver cancer in Qidong. Biol Tr Elem Res. 56(1):117-124, 1997.

Selenium and Heart disease:

52] Addis, P. B., et al. Atherogenic and anti-atherogenic factors in the human diet. Biochem Soc Symp. 61:259-271, 1995.

53] Beaglehole, R., et al. Decreased blood selenium and risk of myocardial infarction. Int J Epid. 19:918-922, 1990.

54] Kok, F. J., et al. Decreased selenium levels in acute myocardial infarction. JAMA. 261:1161-1164, 1989.

55] Korpela, H., et al. Effect of selenium supplementation after acute myocardial infarction. Res Commun Chem Pathol Pharmacol. 65:249-252, 1989.

56] Moore, J. A., et al. Selenium concentrations in plasma of patients with arteriographically defined coronary atherosclerosis. Clin Chem. 30:1171. 1984.

57] Oster, O., et al. The serum selenium concentration of patients with acute myocardial infarction. Annals of Clinical Research. 18:36, 1986.

58] Schiavon, R., et al. Selenium enhances prostacyclin production by cultured epithelial cells: Possible explanation for increased bleeding times in volunteers taking selenium as a dietary supplement. Thrombosis Research. 34:389, 1984.

59] Schone, N. W., et al. Effects of selenium deficiency on aggregation and thromboxane formation in rat platelet. Federation Proceedings. 43:477, 1984.

60] Salonen, J. T. Association between cardiovascular death and myocardial infarction and serum selenium in a matched-pair longitudinal study. The Lancet. 2:175-179, 1982.

61] Salonen, J. T. Association between cardiovascular death and myocardial infarction and serum selenium in a matched-pair longitudinal study. The Lancet. 2:175-179, 1982.

62] Stansbury, J. Sidestep heart disease. Nutrition Science News. March 1999.

63] Suadicani, P., et al. Serum selenium concentration and risk of ischemic heart disease in a prospective cohort study of 3000 males. Atherosclerosis. 96:33-42, 1992.

Selenium and Diabetes:

64] Battell, M. L., et al. Sodium selenate corrects glucose tolerance and heart function in STZ diabetic rats. Mol Cell Biochem. 179(1-2):27-34, 1998.

65] Mukherjee, B., et al. Anbazhagan S, Roy A, Ghosh R, Chatterjee M. Novel implications of the potential role of selenium on antioxidant status in streptozotocin-induced diabetic mice. Biomed Pharmacother. 52(2):89-95, 1998.

66] Pryor, K. Nutritional approaches to optimal blood glucose and insulin levels: key factors in longevity and resistance to diabetes and other degenerative diseases. Vitamin Research News. April 2000.

Selenium and arthritis:

67] Aeseth, J., et al. Trace elements in serum and urine of patients with rheumatoid arthritis. Scand J Rheumatol. 7:237-240, 1978.

68] Honkanen V., et al. Serum zinc, copper and selenium in rheumatoid arthritis. J Trace Elem Electrolytes Health Dis. 5(4):261-263, 1991.

69] Kose, K., et al. Plasma selenium levels in rheumatoid arthritis. Biological Trace Element Research. 53:51-56, 1996.

70] Munthe, E., et al. Treatment of rheumatoid arthritis with selenium and vitamin E. Scandinavian Journal of Rheumatology. 53(Suppl.):103, 1984.

71] Peretz, A., et al. Adjuvant treatment of recent onset rheumatoid arthritis by selenium supplementation: preliminary observations [letter]. Br J Rheumatol. 31(4):281-282, 1992.

72] Tarp, U., et al. Low selenium level in severe rheumatoid arthritis. Scandinavian Journal of Rheumatology. 14:97-101, 1985.

73] Tarp, U. et al. Selenium treatment in rheumatoid arthritis. Scandinavian Journal of Rheumatology. 14:364-368, 1985.

74] Tarp, U. Selenium in rheumatoid arthritis. A review. Analyst. 120(3):877-881, 1995.

Selenium in Psychiatry:

75] Benton, D., et al. Selenium supplementation improves mood in a double-blind trial. Psychopharmacology. 102(4): 549- 550, 1990.

76] Benton, D., et al. The impact of selenium supplementation on mood. Biological Psychiatry. 29(11):1092-1098, 1991.

Clausen, J., et al. Selenium in chronic neurological diseases - multiple sclerosis and

91

Batten's Disease. Biol Trace Elem Res. 15:179-203, 1988.

77] Foster, H. D. Schizophrenia and esophageal cancer: Comments on similarities in their spatial distributions. Journal of Orthomolecular Medicine. 5(3):129-134, 1990.

78] Foster, H. D. The geography of schizophrenia: Possible links with selenium and calcium deficiencies, inadequate exposure to sunlight and industrialization. Journal of Orthomolecular Medicine. 3(3):135-140, 1988.

79] Shamberger, R. J. Selenium and the antioxidant defense system. Journal of Advancement in Medicine. 5(1):7-19, 1992.

Selenium and Skin:

80] Juhlin, L., et al. Blood glutathione peroxidase levels in skin diseases: Effect of selenium and vitamin E treatment. Acta Dermat Vener (Stockholm). 62:211-214, 1982.

81] Michaelsson, G., et al. Selenium in whole blood and plasma is decreased in patients with moderate and severe psoriasis. Acta Dermatology Venereology (Stockholm). 69:29-34, 1989.

82] White A et al. Role of lipoxygenase products in the pathogenesis and therapy of psoriasis and other dermatoses. Arch. Dermatol. 119:541-547, 1983.

AN ELEMENT OF IRONY: "IRON"

The Game Show:

Announcer: And now for the frantic minute. Your time starts now. Can you be short of breath and have normal haemoglobin?
Contestant: No.
Announcer: Wrong
Announcer: Can you have iron deficiency without being anaemic?
Contestant: No
Announcer: Wrong
Announcer: Can you have normal arterial blood saturation and be iron deficient?
Contestant: No
Announcer: Wrong.
Announcer: Can you have a normal ferritin and still be iron deficient?
Contestant: No
Announcer: Wrong.
Announcer: Does Iron deficiency predispose you to influenza?
Contestant: No
Announcer: Wrong again. Does Helicobacter cause iron deficiency by reducing production of stomach acid?
Contestant: No
Announcer: Wrong.
Announcer: The core of our planet is pure iron, but is iron deficiency the commonest deficiency on this planet?
Contestant: No.
Announcer: Wrong yet again. They sure don't teach you much about iron do they?
Announcer: Is low stomach acid the commonest cause of iron deficiency?
Contestant: No.
Announcer: Wrong.
Announcer: Is iron deficiency associated with headaches?
Contestant: No.
Announcer: Wrong. (To the audience) It's very sad.

The Post Mortem after the Show.

Contestant: I didn't realize how little I knew about iron.

Coach: You really let down the profession.

Contestant: How can you have a normal ferritin and still be iron deficient?

Coach: Ferritin is the measure of body stores of iron, but Ferritin is an acute phase reactant. That means it goes up like the ESR and the white cell count when you are sick. So if you measured it during flu it might bring it up from low to normal. Quite ironic considering it predisposes one to catching flu if it is low.

Contestant: How can you be short of breath and still have normal haemoglobin?
Coach: The haemoglobin measurement (the test for anaemia done in the Full Blood Picture) is the amount of haemoglobin per deciliter of blood. If I took 2 litres of blood from you right now and measured your haemoglobin, it could be normal for a few hours, but you would be short of breath. If I punctured one of your lungs, you could be short of breath but not be anaemic. If I put a band around your heart...

Contestant: Ok, ok. What about the iron and arterial saturation?

Coach: Arterial saturation is measured by an oximeter on the finger or by taking blood from an artery. You compare the total haemoglobin (the red stuff in red blood cells that carries the iron molecule) with the amount that has oxygen attached to it. Iron deficiency doesn't affect the percent of haemoglobin saturated. If you are iron deficient and anaemic, then the reduced amount of haemoglobin you make can still be fully saturated.

Contestant: What about the low stomach acid thing? Surely Helicobacter causes iron deficiency by making you lose blood every

94

day from your ulcer.

Coach: Most patients who have iron deficiency and who have Helicobacter, never have this prove. The world population rate for Helicobacter is about 15%. The world population rate for iron deficiency is about 10-12%. Do you think it's a coincidence that the prevalence of the world's commonest infection matches so closely the world's commonest deficiency? The doctors have assumed that the patient has lost iron through their ulcer. But how can they explain the low magnesium, calcium and potassium as well? Do you lose magnesium from an ulcer?

Any organ that's infected does not function properly. The function of the stomach is to produce acid for meals. If it's infected it doesn't produce enough acid when you eat. It's a very simple principle really. If you have myocarditis (infection of the heart) you get heart failure. If you have bronchitis, you get short of breath. If you have hepatitis (infection of the liver), you get liver impairment. If you have otitis media (infection of the middle ear) you can't hear. If you have pyelonephritis (infection of the kidney) then you get impaired kidney function. If you get encephalitis (infection of the brain) then you can't think. If you get pancreatitis (infection of the pancreas) you don't make insulin. If you get synovitis (infection of the joint lining) you joints can't bend. All organs don't work when they are infected. For some reason, the Gastroenterologists feel that the stomach should be the exception.

Contestant: Thanks coach. Can I sign up for that nutritional medicine course that you did?

The Interview.

60 Minutes (Talking to the empty chair): Now, you represent the Union of Iron Molecules. What is your beef?

Iron representative: Very funny. We're upset because doctors can't recognize iron deficiency.

60 Minutes: But can't it be measure?

Iron representative: Yes but it has to be suspected first.

60 Minutes: What are the symptoms?

Iron representative: Tiredness, headaches, itchy skin, poor immunity, heavy periods…

60 Minutes: But I thought that that heavy periods caused iron deficiency.

Iron representative: Low iron can cause heavy periods too. Anyway, to continue. Anaemia, depression.

60 Minutes: But I thought that the tiredness was due to anaemia.

Iron representative: I once had a conversation with a haematologist. I asked him what iron was used for in the body. He said it was for haemoglobin. I showed him a list of 90 enzymes that iron was needed for and asked him about the other 89. "Oh they are not as important as haemoglobin" he replied. "How many red blood cells are there in the body?" I asked him. "Oh… about 30 million million (3×10^{13})" he said. "How many cells have Cytochromes?" I asked. His heart sank. He knew at that moment that I had him. "About 100 million million million (10^{20})" he reluctantly trotted out.

60 Minutes: So he completely miscalculated the importance of iron in the body?

Iron representative: Absolutely. Most doctors think that iron is used only for haemoglobin and oxygen transport. They completely neglect the fact that you can't make ATP without iron. Iron's in the Cytochromes inside the mitochondria.

60 Minutes: What's ATP?

Iron representative: It's the energy currency of each cell. Without it, the cells can't run properly.

60 Minutes: So why don't the doctors know about this?

Iron representative: They do. They just choose to ignore the biochemistry. They say that a normal haemoglobin excludes iron deficiency. They completely misunderstand that iron deficiency causes symptoms 2 to 3 years before you become anaemic. By the time you are anaemic, anyone can diagnose it!

60 Minutes: How else can it make you feel tired?

Iron representative: You need iron to convert lysine to carnitine. Carnitine is needed for transporting fatty acids into the mitochondria for energy production.

60 Minutes: What about depression?

Iron representative: You need iron to make serotonin.

60 Minutes: What about hormone imbalance?

Iron representative: You need iron to make oestrogen and testosterone.

60 Minutes: What about immunity?

Iron representative: You need iron for making peroxide.

60 Minutes: So blondes have lots of iron?

Iron representative: No smarty-pants, peroxide for killing bacteria. For example Myeloperoxidase is the enzyme that makes organisms when the white blood cell eats one. If you can't make peroxide you can't defend yourself against infection. If you don't have iron you can't make peroxide and you have an immune defect.

60 Minutes: So what would you say is the commonest cause of iron deficiency?

Iron representative: Ignorance.

60 Minutes: Say what?

Iron representative: Ignorance of the common predisposing causes.

60 Minutes: Like What?

Iron representative: Low stomach acid.

60 Minutes: What possibly could alert a doctor to this?

Iron representative: Reflux, heartburn, bloating after meals and flatulence.

60 Minutes: How could these symptoms be of use?

Iron representative: They are symptoms of low stomach acid.

60 Minutes: But I thought that everyone has excess stomach acid. How could low stomach acid cause reflux?

Iron representative: When there is low stomach acid, food ferments in the stomach instead of being digested. This fermentation distends the stomach to the point where the valve at the bottom of the gullet can't hold the pressure. Eventually the stomach contents push up into the lower gullet causing reflux. These people often have bad breath too.

60 Minutes: How come the specialists don't see this?

Iron representative: When do the patients have symptoms?

60 Minutes: After meals.

Iron representative: When do they endoscope them?

60 Minutes: Fasting from overnight.

Iron representative: Of course they won't see it then, will they?

60 Minutes: What is this condition called?

Iron representative: Hypochlorhydria.

60 Minutes: Why do the doctors think that all of us suffer from excessive acid?

Iron representative: Because the drug companies make more money by convincing the doctors that the patients need drugs to reduce stomach acid. Anybody can buy enzymes from a health food shop. But they need a script to buy proton pump inhibitors (drugs that reduce stomach acid). And each script is subsidized by the Government. Very lucrative business, stomach acid. The doctors are totally spellbound by the hype and misinformation provided to them. They get pens and notepads and other goodies to remind them that every patient must have excessive stomach acid as the cause of all dyspepsia.

60 Minutes: Are there any other nutrients affected by low stomach acid?

Iron representative: Magnesium, calcium, potassium and vitamin C.

60 Minutes: So you mean that if 40% of the population have Helicobacter, then magnesium, potassium, and vitamin C deficiency could be a lot more common than previously thought? That these

deficiencies could arise from chronic infection with Helicobacter?

Iron representative: That's exactly what I'm saying. Iron deficiency is the tip of the iceberg. If you find it, expect problems with the other nutrients too.

60 Minutes: Is it possible to have too much iron?

Iron representative: Yes it is. Too much iron can predispose you to heart attacks, colon cancer, lung cancer, diabetes and liver damage.

Interviewer: That's been very illuminating. Thank you.

Iron representative: If you think this has been illuminating, wait until you interview Neon!

References
1] Arvidsson, B., et al. Iron prophylaxis in menorrhagia. Acta Obstet Gynecol. Scandinavia. 60:157-160, 1981.
2] Bates CJ Vitamins, Iron and physical work Lancet 2:313-14 1989
3] Beutler E et al Iron therapy in chronically fatigued non-anaemic women: A double-blind study Ann Intern Med 52:378-394 1960
4] Beisel WR Single nutrients and immunity Am J Clin Nutr 35:417-68 1982
5] Dallman et al Iron deficiency and the immune response Am J Clin Nutr 46:329-334 1987
6] Dhur et al Iron status, immune capacity and resistance to infections Comparative Biochemistry and Physiology 94A:11-19 1989
7] Dillman E et al Hypothermia in iron deficiency due to altered triiodothyronine metabolism Am J Physiol 239 1980
8] Edgerton VR et al Iron deficiency anaemia and its effect on worker productivity and activity patterns Br Med J 2:1546-1549 1979
9] Fairbanks, V.F. Clinical disorders of iron metabolism 2nd Ed Grune & Stratton. 1971
10] Fielding J et al Iron deficiency without anaemia Lancet 2 1965
11] Halberg L. Search for nutritional confounding factors in the

relationship between iron deficiency and brain function. Am J Clin Nutr 50:598-606 1989

12] Hambidge KM et al Acute effects of iron therapy on zinc status during pregnancy. Obstet Gynecol 70(4): 593-6 1987

13] Heinrich, H.C. Iron deficiency without anaemia. Lancet 1968

14] Helman AD Darnton Hill I . Vitamin & iron status in new vegetarians Am J Clin Nutr 45(4): 785-9 1987

15] Herscko et al Iron and infection Br Med J 296:660-664 1988

16] Kuleschora EA Riabova NV Effect of iron deficiency of the body on the work capacity of women engaged in mental work. Ter Arkh 61(1): 92-95

17] Leiber RL Behavioural and biochemical correlates of iron deficiency J Am Diet Assoc 77:398-404 1977

18] Lewis, G. J. Do women with menorrhagia need iron? British Medical Journal. 284:1158, 1982.

19] Lozoff B Brittenham GH Behavioural aspects of iron deficiency. Proc Hematol New York 14:23-53 1986

20] MacDougall, L.G. The immune response in iron deficient children: Impaired cellular defence mechanisms with altered humoral components. J Paediatrics 86 1975

21] O'Brien et al Prenatal iron supplements impair zinc absorption in pregnant Peruvian women J Nutr 130 22251-5 2000

22] O'Keefe, S. T., et al. Iron status and restless legs syndrome in the elderly. Age and Ageing. 23(5):200-203, 1994.

23] Oppenheimer SJ Iron and infection: the clinical evidence Acta Paed Scand Sci 361:53-62 1989

Oski, F. Iron deficiency in infancy and childhood. The New England Journal of Medicine. 329:190-193, 1993.

24] Parks YA Wharton BA Iron deficiency and the brain. Acta Paed Scand Suppl 361:71-77 1984

25] Pollet E Cognitive effects of iron deficiency anaemia Lancet 1:158 1985

26] Pollet E et al Iron deficiency & behavioural development in infants and pre-school children. Am J Clin Nutr 43(4): 555-65 1989

27] Rosen, G. M., et al. Iron deficiency among incarcerated juvenile delinquents. J Adolesc Health Care

6:419-23, 1985.

28] Rushton DH et al Ferritin and fertility Letter Lancet 337: 155415 1991

29] Scrimshaw NS Functional consequences of iron deficiency in human populations J Nutr Sci Vitaminol 30:47-63 1984

30] Sherman AR Influence of iron and immunity and disease resistance Ann NY Acad Sci 587: 140-146 1990

31] Taymor, M. L., et al. The etiological role of chronic iron deficiency in production of menorrhagia. JAMA. 187:323-327, 1964. Sandstrom B et al Oral iron dietary ligands and zinc absorption J Nutr 115: 411-4 1985

32] Tucker DM et al Iron status and brain function: serum ferritin levels associated with asymmetrics of cortical electro-physiology and cognitive performance. Am J Clin Nutr 39(1):105-113 1984

33] Wallenberg HSC et al Effect of oral iron supplements during pregnancy on maternal and foetal iron status. J Perinatal Med 12(1):7-12 1984

34] Webb, T. E., et al. Behavioural status of young adolescents with iron deficiency anaemia. J. Special Ed. 8(2):153-156, 1974.

35] Youdim, M. B., et al. Putative biological mechanisms of the effect of iron deficiency on brain biochemistry and behaviour. American Journal of Clinical Nutrition. 50(3 Supplement):607-15, 1990.

MOLYBDENUM: THE UNPRONOUNCEABLE, YET PRECIOUS METAL.

When told they are molybdenum deficient, most of my patients say, "What on earth is molybdenum?" Molybdenum is a secret metal only known to farmers, vets, metallurgists and bicycle salespersons. Ironically it turns out to be pivotal mineral in the copper-zinc balance. Even more unbelievable is that the WA copper-zinc-molybdenum problem has been known about for 75 years. I guess it takes time for this sort of thing to filter down to the medical profession.

The average human body contains about 9,000mg of Molybdenum. Molybdenum is an antioxidant and is important in the defence against cancer and carcinogens. It has a defence role within the gastrointestinal tract by detoxifying compounds that cause cancer.

Molybdenum is important for kidney function and helps excrete heavy metals like mercury and lead. Molybdenum is often found with iron in for cell energy cycles. The brain and nervous system rely on molybdenum to keep the peace. This is why molybdenum deficiency causes anxiety and irritability. Molybdenum is necessary for the metabolism of dietary fats. It has been used in many forms of arthritis with success. It is necessary for the formation of tooth enamel and hence helps prevent tooth decay. It is needed for the following enzymes Xanthine Oxidase, Aldehyde Oxidase, Nitrate Reductase and Sulphite oxidase. Molybdenum helps Aldehyde Oxidase break down formaldehyde and many other aldehydes, which, we absorb from the clothes we wear, furniture we own, chipboard, carpets, glues, perfumes, etc. These are inhaled and need to be eliminated, but aldehydes can also be produced internally by bacteria, parasites, fungi, yeast, etc.

Molybdenum has been shown to prevent breast and gastrointestinal cancers. Molybdenum protects the body from the carcinogenic effects of dietary nitrosamines (due to its incorporation into the Nitrate Reductase enzyme that prevents the conversion of Nitrates to Nitrosamines within the Stomach).

Molybdenum has been used in the treatment of Wilson's disease because it facilitates the excretion of excess Copper. Hence it is extremely useful in treating copper excess. Male impotence has benefited from Molybdenum supplementation. Molybdenum is blocked by lead and copper excess. Excess molybdenum can lead to gout (need 15,000mg per day to cause this).

The most important function of molybdenum is to keep copper in check. You see Mother Nature is aware of copper's Jekyll and Hyde personality. She knows that when copper becomes too plentiful that it ceases to be a nutrient and starts becoming a nuisance! So she built in a moderator to control this tendency: Molybdenum. Now we have three problems in WA. Firstly, molybdenum is very scarce and needs to be added to fertilisers. The second problem is that fluoride inhibits the absorption of molybdenum. The third problem is that when molybdenum is low, copper absorption is much higher than expected. That means the "conservative" calculations of the total absorption of copper through water that are published by the Water Authority underestimates actual copper absorption under these circumstances. So "safe" levels of copper in water are no longer safe in the presence of Molybdenum deficiency.

Sources are Wheat Germ, Oats, Brown Rice, Cottage Cheese, Eggs, Lentils, Green Peas, Split Peas, Fish, Kidneys, Spinach, Cauliflower and Brewer's Yeast.

The recommended daily allowance (RDA) of Molybdenum (for adults) is 75 - 250 mcg per day.
The therapeutic uses of molybdenum are Asthma, recurrent tinea or thrush, cancers of the gastrointestinal system, Copper excess, Mercury toxicity, Anxiety, Arthritis, and dental caries (tooth decay).
References:
1] Berg, J. W., et al. Epidemiology of gastrointestinal cancer. Proc Natl Cancer Congr. 7:459-463, 1973.
2] Brewer, G. J. Treatment of Wilson's disease with ammonium tetrathiomolybdate; Initial therapy in 17 neurologically affected patients. Archives of Neurology. 51:545-554, 1994.

3] Brewer, G. J. Practical recommendations and new therapies for Wilson's disease. Drugs. 50:240-249, 1995.

4] Erdmann R & Jones M: Minerals: the Metabolic Miracle Workers. Century. London, UK. 110-111 1988

5] Fleisher MA Mercury detoxification Townsend Letter for Doctors and Patients 214 May 64-71 2001

6] Komada, K., et al. Effects of dietary molybdenum on esophageal carcinogenesis in rats induced by N-methyl-N-benzylnitrosamine. Cancer Res. 50:2418-2422, 1990.

7] Losee, FL et al. A study of the mineral environment of caries-resistant navy recruits. Caries Res 3:23-31, 1969.

8] Luo, X. M., et al. Molybdenum and oesophageal cancer in China. Federation Proceedings. Federation of the American Society for Experimental Biology. 46:928, 1981.

9] Luo, X. M., et al. Inhibitory effects of molybdenum on esophageal and forestomach carcinogenesis in rats. J Natl. Cancer Inst. 71:75-80, 1983.

10] Moss, M. A. Effects of Molybdenum on Pain and General Health: A Pilot Study Journal of Nutritional & Environmental Medicine. 5(1):56-61, 1995.

11] Nakadaira H et al Distribution of selenium and molybdenum and cancer mortality in Niigata, Japan. Arch Envir Health Sep 50:5 374-80 1995

12] Papaioannou R et al: Sulfite sensitivity unrecognised threat: Is molybdenum the cause? J Ortho Mol Psyhc 13 (2) 105-110 1984

13] Sardessi VM Molybdenum: an essential trace element. Nur Clin Pract Dec 8:6 277-81 1993

14] Turnlund JR et al Molybdenum absorption, excretion and retention studies with stable isotopes in young men at five intakes of dietary molybdenum Am J Clin Nutr Oct 62:4 790-6 1995

15] Wei, H. J., et al. Effect of molybdenum and tungsten on mammary carcinogenesis in Sprague-Dawley (SD) rats Chung Hua Liu Tsa Chih. 9:204-207, 1987.

16] Yang, C. S. Research on esophageal cancer in China: a review. Cancer Research. 40:2633-2644, 1980.

MANGANESE THE ENIGMA.

Manganese is an underrated nutrient mineral. It is one of the three transitional elements I treat with great respect. The other two are iron and copper. This is because these three minerals have narrow therapeutic ranges. Their absence or blockade causes problems and certainly high levels (or retention) of these minerals will also cause problems. Manganese's relationship with iron, cobalt and magnesium will affect cognitive function. Interestingly, three of these minerals appear as consecutive elements in the transition series of the periodic table. Total body manganese is about 20 mg with high levels in kidneys, liver and bone. It is excreted in the bile, like copper.

Brain function and manganese.

Studies identifying problems with both low and high levels of manganese confirm the importance of this mineral with respect to the nervous system. Low levels are associated with epilepsy, poor memory, muscle twitching, dizziness and Schizophrenia. High levels are associated with severe brain dysfunction with some writers even blaming high manganese levels for "mad cow disease". In particular, Manganese excess can cause aggressiveness, apathy dementia, hallucinations, Schizophrenia and speech impairment.

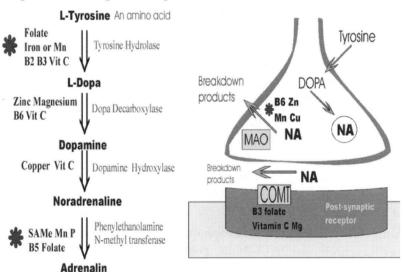

One of the reasons for these symptoms is due to the role of Manganese in the adrenergic neurotransmitter pathways. In the conversion of tyrosine to adrenaline, Manganese turns up twice as shown by the asterixes (see above).

In the terminal bulb of a noradrenergic neuron (see figure above) Manganese is important for the efficient breakdown of noradrenaline.

The balance of the neurotransmitters Dopa and Noradrenaline is important in the prevention of hallucinations and Schizophrenia. It turns out that Manganese, Copper, Vitamin B3 and Vitamin C must all be in balance for this system to function normally.

Manganese and allergy.

Manganese deficiency can cause skin rashes and eczema. This may be due to its importance in the breakdown of histamine. In fact the balance of copper, zinc, molybdenum and manganese significantly affects histamine metabolism (see pathways below).

Histamine Metabolism

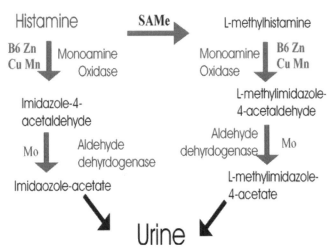

Manganese and glucose regulation.

Manganese turns up in the glycolytic pathway in an enzyme called enolase, where it can substitute for magnesium. Some authors suggest that manganese may actually be more important in glycolysis than previously thought. Manganese is also important for the production of insulin, and it is worthwhile checking blood levels for deficiency in Diabetes.

Manganese and energy.
In addition to its role in glycolysis, manganese is important for the production of Coenzyme Q10.
In mitochondrial Superoxide Dismutase (SOD), manganese and copper must be in balance. Imbalances will affect the way SOD handles free radicals. Copper overload drives the enzyme to a pro-oxidant state, while Copper deficiency will create an anti-oxidant state.

Cu:Mn ratio on oxidation state
of Superoxide dismutase

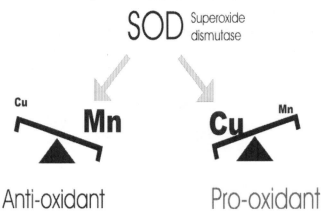

Manganese and bone/cartilage production.
Numerous studies link manganese deficiency to joint and bone problems. This due to a combination of important functions including cartilage repair, joint lubrication and bone production.

Manganese and cholesterol.
Manganese is important for the correct breakdown of LDL by the liver. Patients with high cholesterol may well turn out to be manganese deficient.

There is no RDA for manganese, but intakes of 2 to 15 mg would be appropriate in areas where refined foods abound.

Manganese References:

1] Amdur M.O., et al. The need for manganese in bone development by the rat. Proc Soc Exp Biol Med. 59:254-55, 1945

2] Aston B.A. Manganese & Man. J. Orthomol. Psych. 9,4, 1980

3] Baly D., et al. Effect of manganese deficiency on insulin binding, glucose transport & metabolism in rat adipocytes. J Nutr. 120:1075-1079, 1990

4] Banta et al Elevated manganese levels associated with dementia and extrapyramidal signs. Neurology 27:213-216 1977

5] Bentley O.G. & Philips P.H. The Effect of Low Manganese Rations upon Dairy Cattle. J. Dairy Sci. 34:396-403, 1951

6] Bolas B.D. & Portsmouth G.B. Effect os CO2 on the Availability of Manganese in Soil Producing Manganese Deficiency. Nature. 162:737, 1948

7] Burger O.J. & Hauge S.M. Relation of Manganese to the Carotene and Vitamin Contents of Growing Crop Plants. Soil Sci. 72:303-13, 1951

8] Carl E.G., et al. Association of low blood manganese concentrations with epilepsy. Neurology. 336:1584-1587, 1986

9] Caskey C.D. & Norris L.C. Further Studies on the Role of Manganese in Poultry Nutrition. Poult. Sci. 17:433, 1938

10] Chandra S.V. Neurological Consequences of Manganese Imbalance. Neurobiology of The Trace Elements,Vol.2. Dreosti, I.E., Smith R.M., Eds. Humana Press. N.J. 1983

11] Cotzias G.C. Manganese in Health and Disease. Physiol. Rev. 38:503-31, 1958

12] Cotzias G.C., et al. Slow turnover of manganese in active rheumatoid arthritis 7 acceleration by prednisone. J Clin Invest. 47:992, 1968

13] Cranton E.M. Update on hair element analysis in clinical medicine. J Holistic Med. 7(2):120-134, 1985

14] Davis et al Longitudinal changes of manganese-dependent superoxide dismutase and other indexes of manganese and iron status in women Am J Clin Nutr 55:747-752 1992

15] Davidsson et al Manganese retention in man: a method fro estimating manganese absorption in man. Am J Clin Nutr 49:170-179 1989

16] Dexter D.T., et al. Increased nigral iron content & alterations in other metal ions occuring in brain in Parkinson's disease. J. Neurochem. 52(6):1830-6, 1989

17] Doisy C.A.Jr. Micronutrient Cntrol on Biosynthesis of Clotting Proteins & Cholesterol. Trace substances in environmental health, VI. Hemphill, D.D., et al : Eds. Univ. Mo. Press. Columbia, Mo. 1973

18] Donaldson J., McGregor D., et al. Manganese neurotoxicity: a model for free radical medicated neurodegeneration. Can.J.Physiology & Pharmacol. 60:1398-1405, 1982

19] Donaldson J. & Barbeau A. Possible clues to the etiology of human brain disorders. in S.Gabay et al, Eds. Metal Ions in Neurology & Psychiatry. N.Y.

Alan R. Liss, 259-85, 1985

20] Dupont C.L. & Tanaka Y. Blood manganese levels in children with convulsive disorder. Biochem Med. 33(2):246-55, 1985

21] Failla M.L. Hormonal regulation of manganese. Manganese in Metabolism & enzyme function. Schrammk V.L.,Wedler F.C.,Eds. Academic Press. N.Y., 1986

22] Florence T.M. & Stauber J.L. Neurotoxicity of manganese. Letter. Lancet. 1:363, 1988

23] Freeland-Graves J.H. Manganese: An essential nutrient for humans. Nutrition Today. Nov./Dec. 13-19, 1988

24] Freeland-Graves J.H. & Lin P-H. Plasma uptake of manganese as affected by oral loads of manganese, calcium, milk, phosphorus, copper, & zinc. J Am Coll Nutr. 10(1):38-43, 1991

25] Gallup W.D. & Norris L.C. The Effect of a Deficiency of Manganese in the Diet of the Hen. Poult. Sci. 18:83-88, 1939

26] Greger JL Dietary standards for manganese: overlap between nutritional and toxicological studies. J Nutr 128:368S-371S 1998.

27] Guillard O., et al. Manganese concentration in the hair of greying ("salt & pepper" men reconsidered. Clin Chem. 31(7):1251, 1985

28] Hill R.M., et al. Manganese Deficiency in Rats with Relation to Ataxia and Loss of Equilibrium. J. Nutr. 53:359-371, 1950

29] Hunnisett A., et al. A new functional test of manganese status. J Nutr Med. 1:209-15, 1990

30] Hurley L.S., et al. Influence of manganese on susceptibility of rats to convulsions. Am J Physiol. 204:493-496, 1963

31] Hurley L.S. & Keen C.L. Manganese. In E. Underwood & W. Mertz, Eds. Trace Elements in Human Health & Animal Nutrition. N.Y., Academic Press. 185-223, 1987

32] Keen C.L., et al. Whole blood manganese as an indicator of body manganese. N Engl J Med. 308:1230, 1983

33] Keen C.L. & Zidenberg-Cherr S. Manganese. In: Present Knowledge in Nutrition (6th Edition). Brown M.L. (editor). International Life Sciences Institute, Washington DC, USA. 279-286, 1990

34] Keen C.L. & Lonnerdal B. Manganese Toxicity in Man & Experimental Animals. Manganese in Metabolism & enzyme Function. Schramm, V.L., Wedler F.C., Eds. Academic Press. N.Y. 1986

35] Keller J.N., et al. Mitochondrial manganese superoxide dismutase prevents neural apoptosis & reduces ischemic brain injury: supression of peroxynitrite production, lipid peroxidation, & mitochondrial dysfunction. J. Neurosci Jan. 18:2,687-97, 1998

36] Kies C., et al. Manganese availability for humans, effect of selected dietary factors.Nutritional Bioavailability of Manganese. Kies C., Ed Am Chem Soc Wash, D.C. 1987

37] Leach R.M.,Jr. Metabolism & Function of Manganese. Trace elements in Human Health & Disease. Vol.III. Prasea, A.S.,Ed. Academic Press, N.Y.,1976

38] Leach R.M., Jr., et al. Studies on the role of manganese in bone formation. II. Effect upon chondroitin sulfate synthesis in chick epiphyseal cartilage. Arch Biochem Biophys. 133:22-28, 1969

39] Leach R.M., Jr. Mn (II) and glycosyltransferases essential for skeletal development. In: Manganese in Metabolism and Enzyme Function. Schramm B.L & Wedler F.W. (editors). Academic Press, New York, NY, USA. 981-91, 1986

40] Lindegard B. Aluminium & Alzheimer's disease. Letter. Lancet. 1:267-68, 1989

41] Liu A.C., et al. Influence of manganese deficiency on the characteristics of proteoglycans of avain epiphyseal growth plate cartilage. Poultry Science. 73:663-669, 1994

42] Löhnis M.P. Manganese Toxicity in Field and Market Garden Crops. Plant and Soil. 3:193-221, 1951

43] Matsuda A., et al. Quantifying manganese in lymphocytes to assess manganese nutritional status. Clin Chem. 35(9):1939-41, 1989

44] Meissner D. [Manganese and arteriosclerosis.] Z Gesamte Inn Med. 41(4):114-115, 1986

45] Mena I. Manganese. In F Bronner,J.W. Coburn, Eds. Disorders of Mineral Metabolism. I . Trace Minerals. N.Y., Academic Press, 233-70, 1981

46] Mena I., et al. Chronic manganese poisoning. Clinical picture & manganese turnover. Neurology. 17:128-36, 1967

47] Miller E.J. Chemistry, structure & function of collagen. In L Manaker, Ed.
Biologic Basis of Wound Healing. N.Y., Harper & Row. 164-9, 1975

48] Nickolova, V et al Effect of Manganese on essential trace element metabolism. Tissue concentrations and excretion of manganese, iron, copper cobalt and zinc. Trace Elem Med 10:141-147 1993

49] Papavasilou P.S., et al. Seizure disorders and trace metals: Manganese tissue levels in treated epileptics. Neurology . 29:1466, 1979

50] Pasquier C., et al. Manganese containing superoxide dismutase deficiency in polymorphonuclear lymphocytes in rheumatoid arthritis. Inflammation. 8:27-32, 1984

51] Pfeiffer,C & Bacchi,D Copper,zinc, manganese, niacin and pyridoxine in the schizophrenias. J Appl Nutr 27(223):9-39 1975

52] Pfeiffer C.C. & LaMola S. Zinc & manganese in the schizophrenias. J Orthomol. Psychiatry. 12:215-34, 1983

53] Plumlee M.P., et al. The Effects of Manganese Deficiency upon the Growth, Development and Reproduction of Swine. J. Animal Sci. 15:352-67, 1956

54] Raloff J. Reasons for boning up on manganese. Science News. Sept. 199, 1986

55] Reginster et al Trace elements and postmenopauseal osteoporosis: a preliminary study of decreased serum manganese Med Sci Res 16:337-338 1988

56] Rosa G.D., et al. Regulation of superoxide dismutase activity by dietary manganese. Journal of Nutrition. 110(4):795-804, 1980

57] Rossander-Hulten L., et al. Competitive inhibition of iron absorption by manganese & zinc in humans. Am J Clin Nutr. 54:152-6, 1991

58] Rubinstein A.H. Manganese-induced hypoglycemia. The Lancet. 2:1348-1351, 1962

59] Rubenstein A.H., et al. Hypoglycemia induced by manganese. Nature. 194:188-9, 1962

60] Sampson P. Low manganese levels may trigger epilepsy. Journal of the American Medical Association. 238:1805, 1977

61] Sanchez-Morito N., et al. Magnesium-manganese interactions caused by magnesium deficiency in rats. J. Am Coll Nutr. 18(5),475-480, 1999

62] Schuler P., et al. Manganese Poisoning: Environmental and Medical Study at a Chilean Mine. Indus. Med. & Surg. 26:167-73, 1957

63] Shils M.E. & McCollum E.V. Further Studies on the Symptoms of Manganese Deficiency in the Rat and Mouse. J. Nutr. 26:1-19, 1943

64] Smialowicz R.J., et al. Manganese chloride enhances natural cell-mediated immune effector cell function: Effects on macrophages. Immunopharmacol. 9:1-11, 1985

65] Somers I.J. & Shive J.W. The Iron-Manganese Relation in Plant Metabolism. Plant Physiol. 17: 582-602, 1942

66] Strause L. & Saltmar P. Role of manganese in bone metabolism. Nutritional Bioavailability of Manganese. Kies C., Ed. Am. Chem. Soc. Wash., D.C. 1987

67] Sziraki I., et al. Implications for atypical antioxidative properties of manganese in iron-induced brain lipid peroxidation and copper-dependent low density lipoprotein conjugation. Neurotoxicology. 20(2-3):455-466, 1999

68] Tanaka Y. Low manganese level may trigger epilepsy. JAMA. 238:1805,

1977
69] Thome J., et al. Increased concentrations of manganese superoxide dismutase in serum of alcohol dependent patients. Alaohol alcohol. Jan. 32:1,65-9, 1997

70] Thompson S.G. The Cure of Deficiencies of Iron and Manganese. Ann. Report East Malling Research Station for 1944, 119-23, 1945

71] Thomson A.B.R., et al. Interrelation of intestinal transport system for manganese and iron. J Labs Clin Med. 73:6422, 1971

72] Van Koetsveld E.E. The Manganese and Copper Contents of Hair as an indication of the feeding condition of cattle regarding Manganese & Copper. Tijdschr. Dieregeneesk. 83:229, 1958

73] Watts D.L. The nutritional relationships of manganese. J. Orthomol. Med. 5(4):219-22, 1990

74] Watts D.L. The nutritional relationships of magnesium. J. Orthomol. Med. 3(4):197-201, 1988

75] Weiner W.J., et al. Effects of chlorpromazine on central nervous system concentrations of manganese, iron, & copper. Life Sci. 20, 1971

76] Weiner W.J. et al. Regional brain manganese levels in an animal model of tardive dyskinesia. in W.E. Fann et al, Eds. Tardive dyskinesia: Research & Treatment. N.Y.,SP Medical & Scientific Books,159-163, 1980

77] Weldie G.W. & Pound G.S. Manganese Nutrition of N. Tabacum L. in Relation to the Multiplication of Tobacco Mosaic Virus. Virology. 5:92-109, 1958

78] Wilgus H.S., et al. Factors affecting manganese utilization in the chicken. Journal of Nutrition. 18:35, 1939

79] Wimhurst J.M., et al. Comparison of the ability of Mg and Mn to activate the key enzymes of glycolysis. FEBS Letters. 27:321-326, 1972

80] Yase Y. Environmental contribution of the amyotrophic lateral sclerosis process. in G. Serratrice et al, Eds. Neuromuscular Diseases. N.Y., Raven Press, 335-39, 1984

81] Yase Y. The pathogenesis of amyotrophic lateral sclerosis. Lancet. 2:292-96, 1972

82] Zayed J., et al. Environmental factors in the etiology of Parkinson's disease. Can J Neurol Sci. 17(3):286-91, 1990

ARE YOU COPPING TOO MUCH COPPER?

In all the time I have been looking at minerals, I have not found many patients with copper deficiency. However, I have found hundreds of people with excessive copper. What sort of problems did these people have? They fell into 4 categories. Hormone imbalance, chronic fatigue, depression or cancer. Wow, you may say, how could a high copper cause all those problems? Let's begin with the sources of copper. Bee Pollen, Buckwheat, Oats, Wheat Bran, Wheat Germ, Butter, Eggs, Apples, Apricot Kernels, Bananas, Olives, Oranges, Peaches, Prunes, Raisins, Mushrooms, Burdock, Chickweed, Cocoa, Dandelion Greens, Echinacea, Eyebright, Goldenseal Parsley, Barley, Lentils, Soya Beans, Split Peas, Chicken Liver, Pork, Almonds, Brazil Nuts, Cashew Nuts, Chestnuts, Hazelnuts, Macadamia Nuts, Peanuts, Pecan Nuts, Pistachio Nuts, Coconut, Walnuts, Pine Nuts, Sunflower Oil, Chocolate, Molasses, Tomato Puree, Crab, Lobster, Oysters, Salmon, Kelp, Sunflower Seeds, Avocado, Green Beans, Beetroot, Broccoli, Fennel, Garlic, Radish, Brewer's Yeast.

Other unseen sources include vegetables sprayed with copper antifungals. But by far the most significant source would be tap water. Generally, the mains supply is low in copper, but copper piping does leach some copper into the water that comes out of the tap. It is not directly the fault of the Water Authority, but they do investigate all complaints of "blue water". The problem with copper is that our mechanism of absorption is supposed to be from copper chelates in our food. This gives a slow, predictable assimilation over several hours. With ionic copper (from tap water) we start absorbing copper from the gullet and stomach. The bioavailability of this form is higher and absorption is more rapid.

The distribution of copper in the body by tissue is as follows: Bones (44%), Muscles (25%), Liver (10%), Brain (9%), Blood (6%), Kidneys (3%), Heart (2%) and Lungs (1%).

Copper has several functions. It is needed for neurotransmitter production (L-Dopa, Dopamine and Noradrenaline); Cytochrome C oxidase: and the enzyme that breaks down Vitamin C. It is important for lactase (the enzyme you need for digesting milk); and it is needed to make collagen and elastin (the fibres that give strength and elasticity to tissues). Normally, we have several substances that protect us against the absorption of copper. These are zinc, Vitamin C, manganese and molybdenum. If copper tends to accumulate then we have cysteine, glutamine, histidine and threonine to chelate (bind to) and remove it from the body. If it accumulates in the tissues, then DHEA helps to prevent copper induced lipid peroxidation (fat breakdown that releases free radicals).

What about the work of Dr. John R Lee linking estrogens to copper excess? Copper accumulation has been linked to both prescribed estrogens (HRT and the pill) and ingested Xenoestrogens (false estrogen or estrogen mimickers). Where do false estrogens come from? There are 4 main sources. The first are pesticides like DDT, Dieldrin and their descendants. These behave as estrogens in the body and are accumulated permanently. The second group are petroleum products. Two hours in city traffic per week will incur enough of these to have an estrogenic effect. The next group are the plastics such as PVC's, BPA's, plastic wraps, plastic drink bottles, microwave containers, motor car seats and trims. We all have exposure to these. The last group are the hormones. There are two main categories. Prescribed hormones and those that come in the food chain. The food chain group has two main subtypes. These come from the poultry industry and antibiotics. Seventy five percent of the antibiotics used in Australia are not prescribed by Doctors. They are used by farmers to enhance the growth rate of animals grown for commerce.

So, when we add up all the internal and external estrogens, this can create confusion for the body. One of the effects is the accumulation of copper. In fact a high copper to zinc ratio found in hair analysis is very suggestive that there are false estrogens in the patient.

Copper overload interferes with zinc, magnesium, vitamin C, folic acid, vitamin B1 and vitamin E. For example one can have adequate zinc levels, but appear to be zinc deficient because of the high copper level. I have one patient who said that after intravenous vitamin C, there was no vitamin C detectable in her urine. She turned out to have a very high copper level, which caused the instantaneous oxidation of the vitamin C in her body. So a combination of low zinc, low molybdenum, low vitamin C in the diet coupled with Xenoestrogens and copper piping could cause a serious escalation of tissue copper levels.

There are two quite disturbing implications of this finding. The first is that many of the patients that present to doctors may be suffering from a manifestation of copper excess. The second is that because copper interferes with tissue function, this will not show up on any blood test, X-ray, ultrasound etc.

An interesting phenomenon occurs when copper is high, the patient has cravings for foods that have high *copper to zinc ratios* such as mushrooms, lobster, crab, pecans, hazelnuts, sunflower seeds, chocolate, dried peaches, canned prawns, walnuts, cod, almonds, brazil nuts, sesame seeds, French fries, brewer's yeast, oysters and liver.

So what can go wrong when to copper accumulates? Imagine a body where zinc and magnesium didn't work and none of your vitamin C lasted more than a few minutes. This is the summary of the effects of copper excess. Previous chapters have discussed the functions of zinc, magnesium and Vitamin C, so refer back to these for more detailed information. The most affected systems are immunity, hormones, joints and brain function. High copper predisposes people to viral, fungal and yeast infections. Vitamin C can help to remove copper from the body and hence may explain some of its immunostimulant activity.

Imagine such a person getting glandular fever. The chances of developing depression and anxiety would be extremely high. The likelihood would be that this person would be female and would give birth to a zinc deficient child who would eventually accumulate copper themselves. This combination of low zinc-high copper could manifest as the fashionable diagnosis of ADD/ADHD. What would that child crave? French fries and chocolate.

Does this sound like an epidemic to anyone? How many paediatricians or psychiatrists perform hair analysis? How many are likely to pick up this abnormality? Would the governmental agencies want parents to find out about this? Would the pharmaceutical companies like parents to find out about this? If copper excess can lead to cancer, would pharmaceutical companies that make chemotherapy want people to know about this? Hair analysis has been used extensively in the USA to investigate criminal behaviour and delinquency. Guess what types of abnormalities seem to crop up regularly? Yes, you guessed it; excessive metal accumulation or nutrient metal imbalance.

So, your next question would be, how would you get rid of this excessive copper? Firstly, reduce your intake: get a water filter. Secondly, a combination of zinc, vitamin C and molybdenum plus the amino acids cysteine, glutamine, histidine and threonine will do the trick. Try to reduce your intake of Xenoestrogens too!

Copper References:
1] Aggett P.J., Fairweather-Tait. Adaptation to High and Low Copper Intakes: Its relevance to Estimated Safe and adequate daily dietary intakes. Am J Clin Nut.67:1061S-63, 1998
2] Allcroft R. & Uvarov O. Parenteral Administration of Copper Compounds to Cattle with Special Reference to Copper Glycine (Copper Amino-acetate). Vet. Rec. 71: 797-810, 1959
3] Aminoff M.J. Pharmacologic management of Parkinsonism and other movement disorders. In: Katzung, B. G. (editor), Basic & Clinical Pharmacology (sixth edition). Prentice-Hall International, London. 419-431,1995
4] Arnon D.I. & Stout P.R. The Essentiality of Certain Elements in Minute Quantity for Plants, with Special Reference to Copper. Plant Physiol. 14: 371-5, 1939
5] Barber R.S. et al. Further Studies on Antibiotic and Copper Supplements for Fattening Pigs. Brit. J. Nutr. 11: 70-79, 1957
6] Baumslag N., et al. Trace metal Content of maternal and neonate hair. Arch Environ Health. 29, 1974
7] Baxter J.H. & Wyk J.S. Van A Bone Disorder Associated with Copper Deficiency. Bull. Johns Hopk. Hosp. 93: 1-23, 1953
8] Bennets H.W., et al. Studies on Copper Deficiency in Cattle: the Fatal Termination (Falling Disease). Aust. Vet. J. 18: 50-63, 1942
9] Beshgetoor L. & Hambridge M. Clinical conditions altering copper

117

metabolism in humans. Am J Clin Nutr. 67: 1017S-21S, 1998

10] Boccuzzi G., et al. Protective effect of dehydroepiandrosterone against copper-induced lipid peroxidation in the rat. Free Radical Biology & Medicine. 22(7): 1289-1294, 1997

11] Bremner I. Manifestations of Copper excess. Am J Clin Nutr. 67 1069S-73, 1998

12] Bremner K.C. & Keath R.K. The Effect of Copper Deficiency on Trichostrongylosis in Dairy Calves. Aust. Vet. J. 35: 389-95, 1959

13] Brewer G. J. Treatment of Wilson's disease with ammonium tetrathiomolybdate; Initial therapy in 17 neurologically affected patients. Archives of Neurology. 51:545-554, 1994

14] Brewer et al. Treatment of metastatic cancer with tetrathiomolybdate, an anticopper, antiangiogenic agent. Phase I study. Clin Cancer Res. 6(1): 1-10, 2000

15] Cartwright G.E. Copper metabolism in Human Subjects. Copper Metabolism, Eds. McElroy W.D. & Glass B. (Johns Hopkins Press, Baltimore) 1950

16] Cartiwright G.E., et al. Studies on Copper Metabolism. XVII. Further Observations on the Anemia of Copper Deficiency of Swine. Blood. 9: 143-53, 1956

17] Cartiwright G.E., et al. The Role of Copper in Erythropoiesis. Biosynthesis of Hemoglobin. Conference on Hemoglobin. Part II, May 1957 (Division of Med. Sci., Nat. Res. Council, U.S.A.) 1958

18] Cartwright et al. Copper metabolism in normal subjects. J Clin Nut. 14, 1964

19] Casdorph R., Walker M. Toxic Metal Syndrome: How Metal poisoning can affect your brain. Avery Press. 1995

20] Cervantes C., Gutierrez-Corona F. Copper resistance mechanisms in bacteria and fungi. FEMS Microbiol Rev. 14:121–37, 1994

21] Chandra R.H., Newberne A.M. Nutrition Immunity and Infections. Plenum Press. 1977

22] Chuong et al. Zinc and copper levels in premenstrual syndrome. Fertility & Sterility. 62 313-20, 1994

23] Cunningham I.J. & Hogan K.G. The Influence of Diet on the Copper and Molybdenum Contents of Hair, Hoof and Wool. N.Z.J. Agric. Res. 1: 841-6, 1958

24] Dabrowska E., Jablonska-Kaszewska I., Lukasiak J., et al. Serum iron and copper and their relations to hepatocellular carcinoma in porphyria cutanea tarda and hemochromatosis patients—case report. Biofactors. (Netherlands) 11(1-2) p131-4, 2000

25] Dameron et al. Mechanisms for protection against copper toxicity. AM J Clin Nut. 67 1091S-1097S, 1998

26] Daniels A.L., Wright O.E. Iron and copper retention in Young Children. J of Nutrition. 8, 1934

27] Davis G.K. The Influcence of Copper on the Metabolism of Phosphorus and Molybdenum. A Symposium on Copper Metabolism, Ed. McElroy W.D. & Glass B. (Johns Hopkins Press, Baltimore) 1950

28] Deeming S.B., Weber C.W. Hair analysis of Trace Minerals in Human Subjects as Influenced by Age, Sex, and Oral Contraceptive Use. Am J of Clin Nutrition. 23, 1970

29] Dick A.T. Studies on the Assimilation and Storage of Copper in Crossbred Sheep. Aust. J. Agric. Res. 5: 511-44, 1954

30] Dutt B. & Mills C.F. Reproductive Failure in Rats Due to Copper Deficiency. J. Comp. Path. 70: 120-5, 1960

31] Eck P. Insight into copper elimination. Ph oenix AZ Eck Institute reference sheet. 1991

32] Eck P. Introduction to copper toxicity. Phoenix AZ Eck Institute reference sheet. 1989

33] Epstein et al. Hair copper in primary biliary cirrhosis. Am J Clin Nutr. 33: 965-967

34] Fearn J.T. & Habel J.D. Parenteral Copper Therapy for Sheep in South Australia. Aust. Vet. J. 37: 224-6, 1961

35] Ferrigno D., Buccheri G., Camilla T. Serum copper and zinc content in non-small cell lung cancer: abnormalities and clinical correlates. Monaldi Arch Chest Dis (Italy), Jun. 54(3) p204-8, 1999

36] Finley E. B., et al. Influence of ascorbic acid supplementation on copper status in young adult men. American Journal of Clinical Nutrition. 47:96-101, 1988

37] Finley et al. Influences of ascorbic acid supplementtion on copper status in young adult men. Am J Clin Nut. 37, 1983

38] Fitzgerald D. Safety guidelines for copper in water. Am J Clin Nut. 67 1098S-1120S, 1998

39] Flesch P. The Role of Copper in Mammalian Pigmentation. Proc. Soc. Exp. Biol. 70: 79-83, 1949

40] Friedrich J. Stop the pain: natural remedies for migraines. Nutrition Science News. June, 1999

41] Gallagher C.H. The Pathology and Biochemistry of Copper Deficiency. Aust. Vet. J. 33: 311-17, 1957

42] Gallagher C.H., et al. The Biochemistry of Copper Deficiency. I. The Enzymological Disturbances, Blood Chemistry and Excretion of Amino

Acids. Proc. Roy Soc.,Series B. 145: 134-50, 1956

43] Gallagher C.H. et al. The Biochemistry of Copper Deficiency. II Synthetic Processes. Proc. Roy. Soc., Series B. 145: 195-205, 1956

44] Greaves J.E. & Anderson A. Influence of Soil and Variety on the Copper Content of Grains. J. Nutr. 11: 111-17, 1936

45] Gubler C.G., et al. Studies on Copper Metabolism. XX. Enzyme Activities and Iron Metabolism in Copper and Iron Deficiencies. J. Biol. Chem. 224: 533, 1957

46] Harrison D. P. Copper as a factor in the dietary precipitation of migraine. Headache. 26(5): 248-250, 1986.

47] Howell J.S. The Effect of Copper Acetate in p-Diethylaminoazobenzene Carcinogenesis in the Rat. Brit. J. Cancer. 12: 594-608, 1958

48] Howell J., McC. & Davison A.N. Copper and Cytochrome Oxidase in Swayback. Biochem. J. 72: 365-8, 1959

49] Jacob et al. Hair as a biopsy material. V. Hair metal as an index of hepatic metal in rats: copper and zinc. Am J Clin Nutr. 31: 477-480

50] Joshi N.V. & Joshi S.G. Effect of Copper Sulphate on Rice in Bombay State. Science & Culture (India) 18: 9607, 1952 (Chemical Abstracts. 47: 4538)

51] Karcioglu et al. Zinc and copper in Medicine. Springfield Charles C Thomas Pub. 1980

52] Klevey L.M. Hair as a biopsy material II. Assesment of copper nutriture. Am J Clin Nutr. 23, 1970

53] Klevay L.M. The role of copper and zinc in cholesterol metabolism. Advances in Nutritional research Draper Plenum Pub. 1971

54] Knobeloch L., Schubert C., Hayes, Clark J., Fitzgerald C., Fraundorff A. Gastrointestinal upsets and new copper plumbing-is there a connection? W.M.J. Jan. 97:1, 49-53, 1998

55] Koch M. Laugh with health. Mastertech Publishing. 1996

56] Kivirikko K., et al. Abnormalities in copper metabolism and disturbances in the synthesis of collagen and elastin. Med Biol. 60:45-48, 1982

57] Levenson C. Mechanisms of copper conservation in organs. Am J Clin Nut. 67 978S-981S, 1998

58] Lizotte L. The woman with too much copper. Total health. 19: 49, 1997

59] Lucas R.E. The Effect of Copper Fertilization on Carotene, Ascorbic Acid, Protein & Copper Contents of Plants Grown on Organic Soils. Soil Sci. 65: 461-9, 1948

60] Malter R. Copper toxicity: Psychological implications for children, adolescences and adults. Hoffman estates A Malter institute for natural development reference sheet. 1984

61] Marinov B, Tsachev K, Doganov N, et al. [The copper concentration in the blood serum of women with ovarian tumors (a preliminary report)]Akush Ginekol (Sofiia) (Bulgaria). 39(2) p36-7, 2000

62] Marston H.R. Cobalt, Copper and Molybdenum in the Nutrition of Plants and Animals. Physiol. Rev. 32: 66-121, 1952

63] Martin J.M. Overdosing on copper? Alive. 62:43-44, 1985

64] Mason K.E. A conspectus of research on copper metabolism and requirements of man. J Nutr. 109, 1979

65] Matrone G. Interrelationships of Iron and Copper in the Nutrition and Metabolism of Animals. Fed. Proc. 19: 659-65, 1960

66] McKenzie J.M. Alteration of the zinc anc copper concentration of hair. Am J Clin Nutr. 31: 470-476

67] Linder M.C.& Hazegh-Azam M. Copper biochemistry and molecular biology. Am J Clin Nutr.63: 797S-811S

68] Milde D., Novak O., Stu ka V., et al. Serum levels of selenium, manganese, copper, and iron in colorectal cancer patients. Biol Trace Elem Res (United States), Feb.79(2) p107-14, 2001

69] Mills C.F. Comparative Studies of Copper, Molybdenum and Sulphur Metabolism in the Ruminant and the Rat. Proc. Nutr. Soc. 19: 162-9, 1960

70] Morgan D.E., et al. The Effect of Copper Glycine Injections on the Live Weight Gains of Sucking Beef Calves. Anim. Prod. 4: 303-7, 1962

71] Nakakoshi T. Copper and hepatocellular carcinoma. Radiology (United States), Jan. 214(1) p304-6, 2000

72] Narasaka S. Studies in the Biochemistry of Copper. XX. Thyroid as a Factor in the Regulation of Blood Copper Level. Jap. J. Med. Sci. 4: 33-36, 1938

73] Neelakantan V. & Mehta B.V. Copper Status of Soils in Western India. Soil Sci. 91: 251-6, 1961

74] Nolan K.R. Copper toxicity syndrome. J Orthomol Psych. 12:270-282, 1983

75] O'Dell B.L. Biochemistry of Copper. The Medical Clinics of North America 60. Saunders Press. 1960

76] Osiecki Henry The Nutrient Bible. Bio Concepts Publishing. 1998

77] Owen C.A. Copper deficiency and toxicity: Acquired and inherited in plants, animals and man. Park Ridge NJ Noyes Pub. 1981

78] Pfeiffer C. Mental and Elemental Nutrients. Keats New Canaan. 1975

79] Pirrie R. Serum Copper and its Relationship to Serum Iron in Patients with Neoplastic Disease. J Clin. Path. 5: 190-3, 1952

80] Polukhina I.N.& Masljanaja H.K. Influence of Nitrogen and Copper on the Anatomical Structure of Oat Stems in Relation to the Resistance of Oats on Peat Soils. (English translation), Izv. Timir. Sol. Shokh Akad., No.1, 205-8, 1961

81] Pratt W.B. Elevated hair copper in idiopathic scoliosis and of normal individuals. Clin Chem. 24 ,1978

82] Ramaswamy M.S. Copper in Ceylon Teas. Tea Quart. 31: 76-80, 1960

83] Reavley Nicola The New encyclopaedia of Vitamins, Minerals, Supplements and Herbs. Bookman Press. 1998

84] Robertson H.A. & Broome A.W.J. Factors Influencing the Blood Copper Level of Sheep: the Effect of change in Basal Metabolic Activity. J. Sci. Fd. Agric. (Supp. Issue), 8, s. 82-s. 87, 1957

85] Roelofsen H., Wolters H., Van Luyn M.J., et al. Copper-induced apical trafficking of ATP7B in polarized hepatoma cells provides a mechanism for biliary copper excretion. Gastroenterology (United States), Sep. 119(3) : 782-93, 2000

86] Sandstead H H. Copper bioavailability and requirements. American Journal of Clinical Nutrition. 35:809-814, 1982

87] Schultze M.O. The Effect of Deficiencies in Copper and Iron on the Cytochrome Oxidase of Rat Tissues. J. Biol. Chem. 129: 729-37, 1939

88] Shore D., et al. CSF copper concentrations in chronic schizophrenia. American Journal of Psychiatry. 140:754-757, 1983

89] Sidhu K. S., et al. Need to revise the national drinking water regulation for copper. Regul Toxicol Pharmacol. 22(1): 95-100, 1995

90] Solioz M. et al Copper pumping ATPases: common concepts in bacteria and man. FEBS Lett. 346:44–7, 1994

91] Stine J.B., et al. Copper and Cheddar Flavour. Dairy World, Chicago. 32: 10-14, 1953 (Chemical Abstracts, 48,900)

92] Sugimoto Y., et al Cations inhibit specifically type 1 5 alpha-reductase found in human skin. J Invest Dermatol. 104(5): 775-778, 1995

93] Takamiya K. Anti-tumour Activities of Copper Chelates. Nature. 185: 190-1, 1960

94] Timberlake C.F. Complex Formation between Copper and some Organic Acids, Phenols and Phenolic Acids Occurring in Fruit. J. Chem. Soc. 2795-8, 1959

95] Turnlund et al. Copper absorption, excretion and retention by young men consuming low dietary copper determined by using stable isotope 65Cu. AM J Clin Nut. 67: 1219-1225, 1998

96] Van Campen D.R. Zinc interference with copper absorption in rats. Journal of Nutrition. 91:473, 1967

97] Van den Berg G.J., et al. Dietary ascorbic acid lowers the concentration of soluble copper in the small intestinal lumen of rats. Br J Nutr. 71(5): 701-707, 1994

98] Van Koetsveld E.E. The Manganese and Copper contents of hair as an indication of the feeding condition of cattle regarding manganese and copper. Tijdschr. Dieregeneesk. 83: 229, 1958

99] Vir et al. Serum and hair concentrations of copper during pregnancy. Am J Clin Nutr. 34: 2382-2388, 1981

100] Walsh W. Zinc deficiency, metal metabolism and behavioural disorders. A report of the health Research Institute March. 1996

101] Watts D. Trace Elements and other Essential Nutrients. Writer's Block. 1997

102] Watts D.L. Nutritional relationships of copper. J Orthomol Med. 4:99-108, 1989

103] Werbach M. Nutritional Influences on Illness. Third Line Press. 1996

C- I TOLD YOU SO!

The first time I ever heard of intravenous vitamin C injections I had visions of some kind of witchcraft being performed. After reviewing the extensive literature on it I understood why so many conditions might improve with such therapies, even if the therapists themselves couldn't explain why it worked!

Every retired chemist, doctor, naturopath, next-door neighbour, friend of your second cousin etc., is an armchair expert on Vitamin C, so I'll try not to bore those people. I'll try to mention information that you might not have read about in Women's Weekly or Omni.

The most surprising facts about Vitamin C aren't in the studies on cancer or the immune system, but the biochemistry of how the body uses it. Apart from its function in the defence against cancer, bacterial infections, fungal infections and viral infections, Vitamin C is important in asthma, sinusitis and mental illnesses. The highest Vitamin C concentration in any tissue is found in the adrenal gland. Why would the adrenal gland store so much of? It turns out that you need Vitamin C to make cortisol and adrenalin. Surprise surprise, that means you need more Vitamin C when you are under stress. That means that the recommended daily allowance of 60 mg might not be flexible enough for people with different environmental stresses. Now isn't it interesting that something so logical might cast doubt about the appropriateness of such tables (remember the first rule of nutrition)? That means that a serum Vitamin C level might underestimate the storage of the adrenal gland and the ability to make these hormones under pressure. This means that you could have symptoms of Vitamin C deficiency such as tiredness, low blood pressure or fainting well before you got scurvy.

The next interesting fact is that the tissue second highest in Vitamin C concentration is the brain. Now what would the brain need all that Vitamin C for? Wear and tear, collagen repair? No, to make dopamine and serotonin and melatonin. Some studies suggest that it may bind to the same sites as the antipsychotics such as Stelazine and chlorpromazine and act as a natural antipsychotic. Vitamin C keeps your sanity intact and your collagen intact too. So low levels of vitamin C could lead to insomnia, depression and lethargy. These studies suggest that low brain Vitamin C levels are associated with schizophrenia.

Wow, this sounds like a wonder drug. What about its function to chelate heavy metals and remove them? What about the fact that immune cells need it for killing bacteria?

A surprising function of Vitamin C is to activate several hormones in the blood. Many hormones are made as "pro" hormones, like yoghurt tubs with peel back foil lids. The enzyme PAM (Peptidyl-Amidating Mono-oxygenase) needs vitamin C to "peel back the foil" so the body can get to the yoghurt. See the diagram below for the range of these hormones. It's a pretty impressive list.

Sites of PAM (where Vitamin C used)

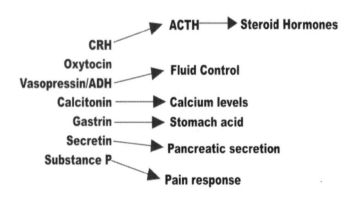

PAM = Peptidyl-amidating Mono Oxygenase

Another important use of vitamin C is to make carnitine. Start with lysine (the amino acid) and add iron and vitamin C to make carnitine. Why is this so important? All our skeletal muscles run on fatty acids to fuel them. Carnitine acts like a shovel to get these fatty acids in to the mitochondria (powerhouses in the cells). No vitamin C, and muscles don't work properly. They become weak and painful.

This is all very interesting you might say, but in Australia vitamin C deficiency must be a rare thing and not worthwhile checking for. We all eat heaps of Vitamin C containing foods everyday. Do we really? Lets take oranges. How much Vitamin C? It's an antioxidant. It's there to protect the seeds from oxidation long after the flesh has fallen away. When does this happen? During the last three days of ripening the salicylates (natural aspirins) leave the fruit while the antioxidants increase. The fruit ripens and falls off the tree in a natural, caring, free-range kind of way. Then, the fruit is quickly eaten by a passer-by, who gets all of the goodness.

Is this how all oranges are farmed today? You might have guessed that this is not what happens in the real world of commerce. So maybe our sacred sources might not be so.
Good after all? "Oh but that's nonsense – I eat lots of broccoli". There's 58mg in half a cup of boiled broccoli; 174mg in 1 cup of red capsicum; 48mg in a half cup of boiled brussel sprouts. Even a fully laden orange has only 68mg. Does anyone really believe that in today's world, 60mg is the recommended daily allowance for Vitamin C? It should be more like 600mg! Do we believe that modern day farming techniques concentrate and preserve all the antioxidants in the fruit or vegetables?

Are we exposed to more stress than our ancestors? Are we exposed to more viruses in our lifetimes than our ancestors? Are we exposed to more heavy metals than our ancestors (except perhaps the Romans who used lead plumbing and boiled their wine in lead pots to add sweetness)? Are we exposed to more chemicals than our ancestors were? Are we getting more antioxidants in our food than our ancestors did (zinc, selenium, Vitamin C)? Could there be some really major problem here? Could this contribute to the epidemics of cancer, heart disease? Does the Health Department really care? Do the Pharmaceutical companies really care? Does the Health Insurance Commission want doctors to measure things like zinc, selenium and Vitamin C? Does it want the public to know the full truth about the real number of deficiencies such as Vitamin C? You be the judge.

PS - Sources include: Acerola cherry, guava, capsicum, blackcurrants, kale leaves, parsley, collard leaves, kale, orange peel, turnip greens, dock, broccoli, brussel sprouts, mustard greens, watercress, cauliflower, jujube, strawberry, lemon, orange, spinach, lychee, currants, lime, grapefruit, kumquat, turnip, cantaloupe, asparagus, radish, tangerine, fennel, granadilla, okra, fresh beans, peas, melon, loganberry, tomato, blackberry, sweet potato, mung bean sprouts, lettuce, pineapple, leek, parsnip, quince, garlic, avocado.

References:

Vitamin C, Asthma, Bronchitis and Sinusitis

1] Anderson, R., et al. Ascorbic acid in bronchial asthma. South African Medical Journal. 63:649-652, 1983.

2] Bielory, L., et al. Asthma and Vitamin C. Annals Allergy. 73:89-96, 1994.

3] Brown, L. A., et al. Ascorbate deficiency and oxidative stress in the alveolar type II cell. American Journal of Physiology. 273(4 Part 1):L782-L788, 1997.

4] Haas, Elson M. Staying Healthy with Nutrition. Celestial Arts, Berkeley, California, USA. 1992:144.

5] Hatch, G. E. Decreased preference for foods containing vitamin C and decreased concentrations of vitamin C in blood plasma are also associated with asthma. American Journal of Clinical Nutrition. 61:625S-630S, 1995.

6] Sridhar, M. K. Nutrition and lung health. British Medical Journal. 310:75-76, 1995.

7] Mohnsenin, V., et al. Ascorbic acid exerts its effect on asthmatics through prostaglandin metabolism. American Thoracic Society 125, 1982.

8] Mohnsenin, V., et al. Effect of ascorbic acid on response to methylcholine challenge in asthmatic subjects. American Review of Respiratory Disease. 127:143-147, 1983.

ancestors? Are we exposed to more heavy metals than our ancestors (except perhaps the Romans who used lead 9]

Olusi, S. O., et al. Plasma and white blood cell ascorbic acid concentrations in patients with bronchial asthma. Clinica Chemica Acta. 92:161-166, 1979.

10] Wolfson, D. Solving sinusitis. Nutrition Science News. April 2000.

Vitamin C and Psychiatry

11] Beauclair, L., et al., An adjunctive role for ascorbic acid in the treatment of schizophrenia. Clin. Psych Pharmacol. 7:282-3; 1987.

12] Cheraskin, Emanuel, MD, et al., The Vitamin C Connection. Harper & Row, NY, 1983.

13] Gold, Mark S., MD, et al., The Good News About Depression. Villard Books, NY, 1987.

14] Kanofsky, I.D., et al., Ascorbate: An adjunctive treatment for schizophrenia. J. Am. Coll. Nutr, 8(5):425,1989.

15] Milner G., Ascorbic acid in chronic psychiatric patients: A controlled trial. Br. J, Psychiatry 109:294-9, 1963.

16] Pfeiffer, Carl C, Mental and Elemental Nutrients. Keats, New Canaan, CN, 1975

17] Quillin, Patrick PhD, RD, Healing Nutrients. Contemporary Books, Chicago, 1987.

18] Rebec, GE,, et al. Ascorbic acid and the behavioural response to haloperidol: Implications for the action of antipsychotic drugs. Science, 227:438-40: 1985

19] Suboticanec, K Vitamin C status in schizophrenia. Bibl. Nutr. Dieta 38: 173-81, 1986.

20] Suboticanec K et al. Vitamin C and schizophrenia. Acta Med Iugosl, 38(5):299-308,1984.

21] Suboticanec K, et al., Plasma levels and urinary C excretion in schizophrenic patients. Hum. Nutr. Clin. 40C;421-28, 1986

22] Tolbert, L.C., et al., Effect of ascorbic acid on neurochemical, behavioural, and physiological symptoms mediated by catecholamines. Life Sci., 25:2189- 95; 1979.

23] Tolbert, L.C., et al., Ascorbate affects conversion of tyrosine to dopamine in mouse brain. Abst., Trans. Am. Sot. Neurochem. 1979.

24] VanderKamp H., A biochemical abnormality in schizophrenics involving ascorbic acid. Intl. J of Neuropsychiatry. , 2(3):204-6, 1966

Vitamin C and Antioxidant Effects

25] Rose, R. C. Ascorbic acid protection against free radicals. In: Third Conference on Vitamin C. 1987. Annals of the New York Academy of Sciences. Volume 498, 1987.

26] Vayda, W. Prevention of aging: How to keep your cells younger, longer. Australian Wellbeing. 9:33-42, 1985.

Vitamin C and Immunity

27] Anderson, R., Oosthuizen, R., Theron, A. & Van Rensburg. The effects of increasing weekly doses of ascorbate on certain cellular and humoral immune functions in normal volunteers. American Journal of Clinical Nutrition. 33:71, 1980.

28] Anderson, R. Assessment of oral ascorbate in three children with chronic granulomatous disease and defective neutrophil motility over a two-year period. Clinical and Experimental Immunology. 43:180-188, 1981.

29] Bates, C. J. Vitamin C intake and susceptibility to the common cold - invited commentaries. British Journal of Nutrition. 78(5):857-859, 1997.

30] Boxer, L. A., et al. Correction of leukocyte function in Chediak-Higashi syndrome by ascorbate. New England J of Medicine 295:1041-1045, 1976.

31] Boxer, L. A., et al. Enhancement of chemotactic response and microtubule assembly in human leukocytes by ascorbic acid. Journal of Cellular Physiology. 100:119-126, 1979.

32] Carr, A. B., et al. Vitamin C and the common cold: Using identical twins as controls. Medical Journal of Australia. 2:411-412, 1981.

33] Carr, A. B., et al. Vitamin C and the common cold: A second MZ cotwin control study. Acta Geneticae

34] Dalton, W. L. Massive doses of vitamin C in the treatment of viral disease. J Indiana State Med Assoc. 55:1151-1154, 1962.

35] Dahl, H., et al. The effect of ascorbic acid on production of human interferon and the antiviral activity in vitro. Acta Pathologica et Microbiologica Scandinavia. 84(5):280-284, 1976

36] Destro, R. L., et al. An appraisal of vitamin C in adjunct therapy of bacterial and viral meningitis. Clin Ped. 16:936, 1977.

37] Frei, B., et al. Ascorbate is an outstanding antioxidant in human blood plasma. Proceedings of the National Academy of Sciences USA. 86:6377-6381, 1989.

38] Gerber, W. F., et al. Effect of ascorbic acid, sodium salicylate, and caffeine on the serum interferon level in response to viral infection. Pharmacology. 13:228, 1975.

39] Goodman, K. J., et al. Nutritional factors and Helicobacter pylori infection in Colombian children. J Pediatr Gastroenterol Nutr. 25(5):507-515, 1997

40] Haas, Elson M. Staying Healthy with Nutrition. Celestial Arts, Berkeley, California, USA. 1992:144.

41] Hemila, H. Does vitamin C alleviate the symptoms of the common cold? - A review of current evidence. Scand J Infect Dis. 26(1):1-6, 1994.

42] Hemila, H. Vitamin C and the common cold: A retrospective analysis of Chalmer's review. J Am Coll Nutr. 14(2):116-123, 1995.

43] Hemila, H. Vitamin C and the common cold. Br J Nutr. 67:3-16, 1992.

44] Hemila, H. Vitamin C and common cold incidence: A review of studies with subjects under heavy physical stress. International Journal of Sports Medicine. 17(5):379-383, 1996.

45] Holden, M., et al. In vitro action of synthetic crystalline vitamin C (ascorbic acid) on herpes virus. Journal of Immunology. 31:455-462, 1936.

46] Holden, M., et al. Further experiments on inactivation of herpes by vitamin C (l-ascorbic acid). Journal of Immunology. 33:251-257, 1936.

47] Horrobin, D. F., et al. The nutritional regulation of T lymphocyte function. Medical Hypotheses. 5:969-985, 1979.

48] Hovi, T., et al. Topical treatment of recurrent mucocutaneous herpes with ascorbic acid-containing solution. Antiviral Research. 27:263-270, 1995.

49] Jungeblut, C. W. Inactivation of poliomyelitis virus by crystalline vitamin C. Journal of Experimental Medicine. 62:517-521, 1935.

50] Jungeblut, C. W. Further observations on vitamin C therapy in experimental poliomyelitis. Journal of Experimental Medicine. 65:127-146, 1937.

51] Jungeblut, C. W. A further contribution to the vitamin C therapy in experimental poliomyelitis. Journal of Experimental Medicine. 70:327, 1939.

52] Klenner, F. R. The treatment of poliomyelitis and other virus diseases with vitamin C. J Southern Med Surg. 111:210-214, 1949.

53] Levy, R., et al. Vitamin C for the treatment of recurrent furunculosis in patients with impaired neutrophil functions. J Infect Dis. 173(6):1502-1505, 1996.

54] Linder, M. C. Nutrition and metabolism of vitamins. In: Nutritional Biochemistry and Metabolism, 2nd Edition. Maria C. Linder (editor). Simon & Schuster, Connecticut, USA, 1991:146.

55] Pauling, L. Ascorbic acid and the common cold. Medical Tribune. 24:1, 1976.

56] Pauling, L. Vitamin C, the Common Cold and the Flu. W. H. Freeman & Company, San Francisco, USA. 1976.

57] Prinz, W. The effect of ascorbic acid supplementation on some parameters of human immunological defence system. International Journal of Vitamin and Nutritional Research. 47:248-256, 1977.

58] Renker, K., et al. Vitamin C-Prophylaxe in der Volkswertf Stralsund. Deutsche Gesundheitswesen. 9:702-706, 1954.

59] Rudolph, M. The immunity factor. The Energy Times. 5(6):20-25, 1995.

60] Schorah, C. J. Vitamin C intake and susceptibility to the common cold - invited commentaries. British Journal of Nutrition. 78(5):859-861, 1997.

61] Schwerdt, P. R., et al. Effect of ascorbic acid on rhinovirus in WI-38 cells. Proc Soc Biol Med. 148:1237, 1975.

62] Sirsi, M. Antimicrobial action of vitamin C on M. tuberculosis and some other pathogenic organisms. Indian J Med Sci. 6:252-255, 1952.

63] Thomas, W. R., et al. Vitamin C and immunity: an assessment of the

evidence. Clinical Experimental Immunology. 32:370-379, 1978.
64] Vallance, S. Relationships between ascorbic acid and serum proteins of the immune system. British Medical Journal. 2:437-438, 1977.
65] Washko, P., et al. Ascorbic acid and human neutrophils. American Journal of Clinical Nutrition. 54:1221S-7S, 1991
66] White, L. Cold sores be gone. Nutrition Science News. March 1999.
67] Yonemoto, R. H., et al. Enhanced lymphocyte blastogenesis by oral ascorbic acid. Proceedings of the American Association for Cancer Research. 17:288, 1976.
Vitamin C and Cancer
68] Anderson, R. Effects of ascorbate on normal and abnormal leukocyte functions. Vitamin C: New Clinical Applications in Immunology. Lipid Metabolism and Cancer. 1-178, 1982.
69] Bandera E. V., et al. Diet and alcohol consumption and lung cancer risk in the New York State Cohort. Cancer Causes Control. 8(6):828-840, 1997.
70] Bram, S., et al. Vitamin C preferential toxicity for malignant melanoma cells. Nature. 284:629-631, 1980.
71] Bruemmer, B., et al. Nutrient intake in relation to bladder cancer among middle-aged men and women. American Journal of Epidemiology. 144(5):485-495, 1996.
72] Burke, E. R. Vitamins C & E cut risk of prostate cancer cell growth. Muscular Development. 36(11):54, 1999.
73] Byers, R., et al. Epidemiologic evidence for vitamin C and vitamin E in cancer prevention. Am J Clin Nutr. 62(Supplement):1385S-1392S, 1995.
74] Graham, S., et al. Dietary factors in the epidemiology of cancer of the larynx. American Journal of Epidemiology. 113(6):675-680, 1981.
75] Greenblatt, M. Brief communication: Ascorbic acid blocking of aminopyrine nitrosation in NZO-B1 mice. Journal of the National Cancer Institute. 50(4):1055-1056, 1973.
76] Howe, G. R., et al. Dietary factors and risk of breast cancer: Combined analysis of 12-case control studies. Journal of the National Cancer Institute. 82:561-569, 1990.
77] Kurbacher, C. M., et al. Ascorbic acid (vitamin C) improves the antineoplastic activity of doxorubicin, cisplatin, and paclitaxel in human breast carcinoma cells in vitro. Cancer Letters. 103-119, 1996.
78] Maurer, K. Vitamins may prevent bladder cancer recurrence. Family Practice News. 15 December 1995:12.
79] O'Connor, H. J., et al. Effect of increased intake of vitamin C on the mutagenic activity of gastric juice and intragastric concentrations of ascorbic acid. Carcinogenesis. 6(11):1675-1676, 1985.

80] Pierson, H. F., et al. Sodium ascorbate enhancement of carbidopa-levodopa methyl ester anti-tumor activity against pigmented B16 melanoma. Cancer Research. 43:2047-2051, 1983.

81] Reed, P. I. Vitamin C, Helicobacter pylori infection and gastric carcinogenesis. Int J Vitamin Nutr Res. 69(3):220-227, 1999.

82] Shamaan, N. A., et al. Vitamin C and Aloe Vera supplementation protects from chemical hepatocarcinogenesis in the rat. Nutrition 14 (11-12):846-852, 1998

83] Schiffman, M. H. Diet and faecal genotoxicity. Cancer Surv. 6:653-672, 1987.

84] Taper, H. S., et al. Non-toxic potentiation of cancer chemotherapy by combined C and K3 vitamin pre-treatment. Int J Cancer. 40:575-579, 1987.

85] Vermeer, I. T., et al. Effect of ascorbic acid and green tea on endogenous formation of N-nitrosodimethylamine and N-nitrosopiperidine in humans. Mutation Research. 16;428(1-2):353-361, 1999.

86] Zhang, H. M., et al. Vitamin C inhibits the growth of a bacterial risk factor for gastric carcinoma: Helicobacter pylori. Cancer. 80(10):1897-1903, 1997.

87] Zheng, W., et al. Retinol, antioxidant vitamins, and cancers of the upper digestive tract in a prospective cohort study of postmenopausal women. American Journal of Epidemiology. 142(9):955-960, 1995.

COBALT AND VITAMIN B12: A MARRIAGE OF VITAMIN AND MINERAL

Vitamin B12 is a much-misunderstood vitamin. It has an unusual structure in that it contains a cobalt atom at the centre of it. This makes the mineral cobalt unusual too. When evaluating tissue mineral analysis (TMA), the cobalt level reveals much about the metabolism of Vitamin B12 within the cells. Other minerals come as salts. That is we can ingest calcium crystals, magnesium crystals, sodium crystals etc, but cobalt only enters the body buried inside the Vitamin B12 structure.

The following diagram explains the route of B12 and its activation. The process is vulnerable in several ways. Vegetarians have fewer foods with B12 in them. Those with helicobacter infection may develop low levels of "intrinsic factor" which is made in the stomach for the express purpose of B12 absorption. There are those with other forms of malabsorption due to low stomach acid such as pernicious anaemia and there are those patients who take drugs that suppress stomach acid. Some people are born with the lack of intrinsic factor (familial pernicious anaemia) and some patients (later in life) develop antibodies to the cells that make intrinsic factor.

Helicobacter infection has been linked to the later onset pernicious anaemia. Either way B12 absorption falls.

The importation of Vitamin B12 is via a tranporter protein that shuts off when the cell has adequate methylcobalamin (when it is full). It's like when you fill your car with petrol at the bowser and the flow "clicks" off. If you don't make enough methylcobalamin, the pump never stops and so inactive B12 (with it's associated cobalt) accumulates abnormally in the cell. Tissue samples show high cobalt. So, in addition to a blood level, intracellular cobalt must be performed in order to truly understand the B12-cobalt cycle.

Most B-vitamins need to be converted to their active form before they will function. Mostly, minerals such as magnesium or zinc do this. For instance Zinc and B2 are required for the activation of B6. Magnesium is required for the activation of B1. In the case of Vitamin B12, its conversion to methylcobalamin (Coenzyme B12) can be blocked by copper, lead or mercury.

The consequences of low level of methyl- cobalamin are a rise in brain homocysteine. This causes a condition called "brain fog". The symptoms include "woolly thinking". Noun substitution in sentences, transient memory loss, episodes of confusion, and even dementia. It has been shown that intramuscular Vitamin B12 can improve dementia patients even if they have normal blood levels of Vitamin b12. The reason is that by supersaturating the blood, more B12 might diffuse into the cells, which are starving for this vitamin. Of course the medical profession will always believe the blood test rather than the patient!

Contrary to what your doctor was taught, the strongest predictor of vascular disease is not cholesterol, but the level of homocysteine. This information was suppressed by the pharmaceutical industry for years because giving B6, B12 and folic acid could rectify the problem. When methionine is metabolised, the intermediate step is homocysteine, which causes collagen damage. In order to metabolise it quickly there are two paths one can take. One pathway involves folate and B12 and the other pathway needs B6 and magnesium. In the periphery, high homocysteine causes blood vessel damage and osteoporosis; in the brain it causes dementia or brain fog.

Homocysteine metabolism

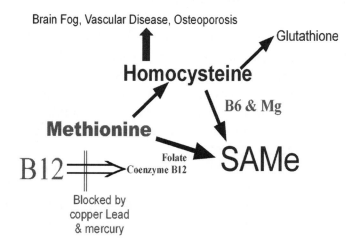

Sites for potential problems with B12- cobalt

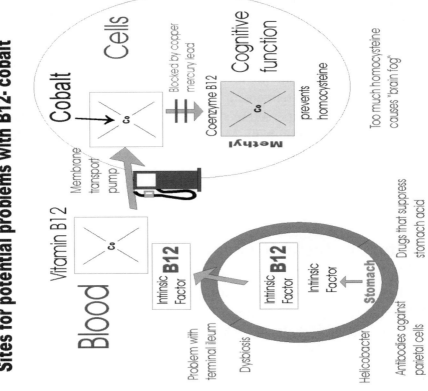

Blood

Vitamin B12

Cobalt

Cells

Membrane transport pump

Blocked by copper mercury lead

Coenzyme B12

Methyl

Cognitive function

prevents homocysteine

Too much homocysteine causes "brain fog"

Intrinsic Factor **B12**

Intrinsic Factor **B12**

Intrinsic Factor

Stomach

Problem with terminal ileum

Dysbiosis

Helicobacter

Antibodies against parietal cells

Drugs that suppress stomach acid

The most amazing personality trait of cardiologists is their double standing in looking at medical research. If drug companies carry out the studies, then the drug must have rectal solar energy. Any other studies must be rubbish.

Studies on Coenzyme Q10 date back 30 years. The range of investigation includes not only studies showing that lower levels are found in a variety of diseases, but also that therapy with Coenzyme Q10 was beneficial in a variety of diseases. An interesting story about coenzyme Q10 was about Karl Folkers the first person to synthesise it. At the time he worked for the pharmaceutical company Merck. Instead of being praised for this discovery, he was told to dump everything because Merck was about to launch a diuretic for heart failure and hypertension. The very conditions Coenzyme Q10 could have been used for! The patent was sold to a Japanese company and the rest is history.

Factors reducing Coenzyme Q10 production

1. Cholesterol Lowering agents (Pravachol, Zocor etc)
2. Betablockers (Etenolol, Metoprolol)
3. Phenothiazines (Stelazine, Chlorpromazine)
4. Tricyclic Antidepressants (Tofranil, Tryptanol etc)

Interestingly, there are many studies (never read by cardiologists) showing that certain medications lower the levels of this cofactor. What's more important however, is that this information should be present in the prescribing information of these drugs. What if patients taking prescription medication were given this supplement counteract the side effects of their drugs? Then this would mean that doctors would have to be told what Coenzyme Q10 actually was. If they knew what it was, then they would realise that this supplement could be used successfully for the very medical conditions they were being told to treat the drugs! They might be tempted to try the supplement first, which would rob the drug companies and the "specialists" of income and kudos.

Sources of Coenzyme Q10

1. Meat (only if digestion good)
2. Intestinal flora
3. Endogenous production

Mitochondrial Energy Pathway

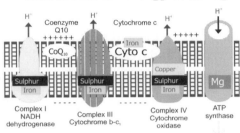

The final energy chain that drives most of the cells in the body (all except the red blood cells) needs Coenzyme Q10 as the second step. This is the energy cycle that drives the entire heart! You'd think this would be of interest to cardiologists, wouldn't you? The other steps involve iron. How many people could avoid a bypass if their iron levels were optimised? You'd think cardiologists might check a few iron levels before they suggest surgery wouldn't you? What are the sources of Coenzyme Q10? Dietary, especially red meat. Gut bacterial production (certain strains of E. Coli) and endogenous production (see diagram showing biochemical pathways.

Nutrients needed for Coenzyme Q10 production
Magnesium
Vitamin B2, B3, B5, B6, B12
Folic Acid
Vitamin C
Selenium

Coenzyme Q10 studies

Cancer prevention and treatment
Ischaemic Heart disease prevention and treatment
Heart failure prevention and treatment
Diabetes prevention and treatment
High blood pressure prevention and treatment
Stroke prevention and treatment
Glaucoma prevention and treatment
Chronic fatigue syndrome prevention and treatment
Alzheimer's disease prevention and treatment

How to make Coenzyme Q10

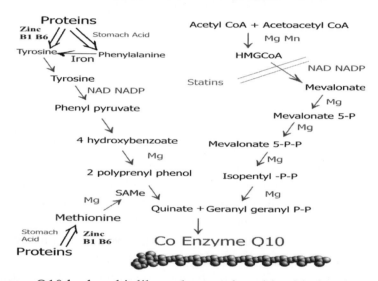

Coenzyme Q10 looks a bit like a short snake with a big head. The head is the "Q" and the tail is the "10". A Coenzyme is a cofactor, which enhances the effectiveness of an enzyme, but isn't protein based. The "Q" comes from quinate and the "10" comes from the fact that the "tail" of Coenzyme Q10 has 10 carbon atoms. So this means that Coenzyme Q10 is made in two bits. The quinate comes from Tyrosine and is bent into a ring form like a benzene molecule. (left side of the pathway). The "10" part comes from joining a 2-carbon part with a 3-carbon part to make a 5-carbon part and then joining the two 5-carbon parts to make a "10". Finally you join the head to the tail.

There are several interesting features of the biochemical pathways. Firstly, magnesium is heavily involved. This puts the pathway at risk of blockade by copper overload. Secondly a cofactor called SAMe is also required. Lastly, the cholesterol lowering agents block the pathway to make Coenzyme Q10. They block HMGCoA reductase, which is an important step in the synthesis of Coenzyme Q10. How long has medicine known this? 20 years!

The range of conditions that may respond to Coenzyme Q10 are listed. They are part of the modern "unexplained" epidemic of diseases, mostly fatal. Isn't time the medical profession woke up from their coma and started looking at the evidence in their own literature?

Negative effects of drugs on Coenzyme Q10 starting from 1975
1] Aberg F., Appelkvist E.L. & Broijersen A., et al. Gemfibrozil-induced decrease in Serum Ubiquinone and Alpha- and Gamma-Tocopherol levels in men with Combined Hyperlipidaemia. Eur J Clin Invest. 28(2):235-42, 1998
2] Appelkvist E.L., Edlund C. & Low P. et al. Effects of Inhibitors of Hydroxymethylgutaryl Coenzyme A Reductase on Coenzyme Q and Dolichol Biosynthesis. Clin Investig. 71(8 suppl):S97-102, 1993
3] Bargossi A.M. Grossi G. & Fiorella P.L., et al. Exogenous CoQ10 Supplementation Prevents Plasma Ubiquinone Reduction Induced by HMG-CoA Reductase Inhibitors. Mol Aspects Med. 15(suppl):187-93, 1994
4] Belichard P., Pruneau D. & Zhiri A. Effect of a Long-term treatment with Lovastatin or Fenofibrate on Hepatic and Cardiac Ubiquinone levels in Cardiomyopathic Hamster. Biochem Buiphys Acta. 1669(1):98-102, 1993
5] De Pinieux G., Chariot P. & Ammi-Said M., et al. Lipid-Lowering Drugs and Mitochondial Function: Effects of HMG-CoA Inhibitors on Serum Ubiquinone and Blood Lactate/Pyruvate Ration. Br J. Clin Pharmacol. 42(3):333-7, 1996
6] Folkers K., Langsjoen P. & Willis R., et al. Lovastatin decreases Coenzyme Q levels in humans. Proc Natl Acad Sci U S A. 87(22):8931-4, 1990
7] Ghirland G., Oradei A. & Manto A., et al. Evidence of plasma CoQ10-Lowering effect by HMG-CoA Reductase Inhibitors: A Double-Blind, Placebo-Controlled Study. J Clin Pharmacol. 33(3):226-9, 1993.
8] Mortensen S.A., Leth A. & Agner E., et al. Dose-related decrease

of Serum Coenzyme Q10 during treatment with HMG-CoA Reductase Inhibitors. Mol Aspects med. 18(suppl):S137-44, 1997.

9] Watts G.F., Castelluccio C. & Rice-Evans C., et al. Plasma Coenzyme Q (Ubiquinone) Concentrations n patients treated with Simvastatin. J Clin Pathol. 46(11):1055-5, 1993.

10] Willis R.A., Folkers K. & Tucker J.L., et al. Lovastatin decreases Coenzyme Q levels in rats. Proc Natl Acad Sci U S A. 87(22):8928-30, 1990

Some studies dating back to 1970

11] Brude, I.R., et al. Peroxidation of LDL from combined-hyperlipidemic male smokers supplied with omega-3 fatty acids and antioxidants. Arterioscler Thomb Vasc Biol. 17(11):2576-2588, 1997.

12] Digiesi, V., et al. mechanisms of the action of Coemzyme Q10 in essential hypertension. Curr Ther Res. 51:668-672, 1992.

13] Digiesi, V., et al. Coemzyme Q10 in essential hypertension. Mol Aspects Med. 15(supplement):257-263, 1994.

14] Folkers, K., et al. Evidence for a deficiency of coenzyme Q10 in human heart disease. Int J Vit Res. 40:380, 1970.

15] Folkers, K., et al. biochemical rationale and myocardial tissue data on the effective therapy of cardiomyopathy with coenzyme Q10. Proceedings of the National Academy of Sciences. 82:901, 1985.

16] Folkers, K., et al. Survival of cancer patients on therapy with coenzyme Q10. Biochemical and Biophysical Research Communications. 192(1):241-45, 1993.

17] Gaby, A. R. the role of coenzyme Q10 in clinical medicine. Part II. Cardiovascular disease, hypertension, diabetes mellitus and infertility. Alt Med rev. 1(2):168-175, 1996.

18] Greenberg, A., et al. Coenzyme Q10: A new drug for cardiovascular disease. Journal of Clinical Pharmacology. 30: 596-608, 1990.

19] Hanaki, Y., et al. Coenzyme Q10 and coronary artery disease. Clin Investig. 71:S112-S115, 1993.

20] Langsjoen, P.h., et al. response of patients in classes III and IV of cardiomyopathy to therapy in a blind and crossover trial with coenzyme Q10. Proceedings of the National Academy of Sciences, USA. 82(12):4240-4244, 1985.

21] Langsjoen, P.H., et al. Effective and safe therapy with coenzyme Q10 for cardiomyopathy. Klinische Wochenschrift. 66(13):583-590, 1988.

22] Langsjoen, P.H., et al. A six-year clinical study of therapy of cardiomyopathy with coenzyme Q10. Int Journal of tissue Reactions. 12(3):169-171; 1990.

23] Langsjoen, P.H., et al. Pronounced increased in survival of patients with cardiomyopathy when treated with coenzyme Q10 and conventional therapy. International Journal of Tissue Reactions. 12(3):163-168, 1990.

24] Langsjoen, P., et al Treatment of essential hypertension with coenzyme Q10. Mol Aspects Med. 15(supplement):S265-S272, 1994.

25] Langsjoen, H., et al. Usefulness of conenzyme Q10 in clinical cardiology: a long-ter study. Mol Aspects Med. 15(Supp):S165-S175, 1994.

26] Littaru, G.P., et al. Deficiency of coenzyme Q10 in human heart disease, part II. Int J Vit Nutr Res. 42:413, 1972.

27] Lockwood, K., et al. Apparent partial remission of breast cancer in 'high risk' patients supplemented with nutritional antioxidants, essential fatty acids and coenzyme Q10. Molecular Aspects of Medicine. 15(Supplement): DS231-S240, 1994.

28] Lockwood K., et al. Partial and complete regression of breast cancer in patients in relation to dosage of coenzyme Q10. Biochemical and Biophysical Research Communications. 199(3):1504-8, 1994.

29] Lockwood, K., et al. Progress on therapy of breast cancer with vitamin Q10 and the regression of metastases. Biochemical and Biophysical Research Communications. 212(1):172-177, 1995.

30] Mellstedt, H., et al. A deficiency of coenzyme Q10 (CoQ10) in cancer patients in Sweden. In: Eighth International Symposium on Biomedical and Clinical Aspects of Coenzyme Q. the Molecular Aspects of Medicine. 1994.

31] Mortensen, S. A. Perspectives on therapy of cardiovascular diseases with coenzyme Q10 (ubiquinone). Clinical Investigator. 71:S116-S123, 1993.

32] Mortensen, S.A., et al. Coenzyme Q10: Clinical benefits with biochemical correlates suggesting a scientific breakthrough in the management of chronic heart failure. Int J Tissue React. 12(3):155-162, 1990.

33] Neuzil, J., et al. Alpha-tocopherol hydroquinone is an efficient multifunctional inhibitor of radical-initiated oxidation of low density lipoprotein lipids. Proc Natl Acad Sci USA. 94:7885-7890, 1997.

34] Portakal, O., et al. Coenzyme Q10 concentrations and antioxidant status in tissues of breast cancer patients. Clin Biochem. 33:279-284, 2000.

35] Sinatra, S. Coenzyme Q10 and cancer. Sixth International Congress on Anti-Aging and Bio-Med Techn Conf Las Vegas 11-13 Dec 1998.

36] Singh, R.B., et al. Randomized, double-blind placebo-controlled trial of coenzyme Q10 in patients with acute myocardial infarction. Cardiovascular Drugs Ther. 12(40:347-353, 1998.

37] Singh, R.B., et al. Serum concentration of lipoprotein(a) decreases on treatment with hydrosoluble coenzyme Q10 in patients with coronary artery disease: discovery of a new role. Int J Cardiol. 68(1):23-29, 1999.

38] Yamagami, T., et al. Bioenergetics in clinical medicine. Studies on coenzyme Q10 and essential hypertension. Research Communications in Chemical Pathology and pharmacology. 11(2):273-278, 1975.

39] Yamagami, T., et al. Bioenergetics in clinical medicine. VIII. Administration of coenzyme Q10 to patients with essential hypertension. Research Communications in Chemical Pathology and Pharmacology. 14(4):721-727, 1976.

40] Yamagami, T., et al. Effect on Q10 on essential hypertension, a double blind controlled study. Biomed and Clin Aspects of CoQ10. 5:337-344, 1986.

41] Yu, C. A., et al. Studies on the ubiquinone-protein interaction in electron transfer complexes. Biomed and Clin Aspects of CoQ10. 4:57-68, 1984.

The Bad .....

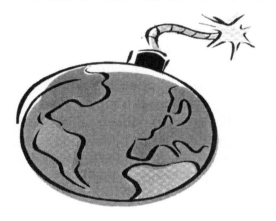

CHRONIC FATIGUE SYNDROME: COMMON THINGS OCCUR COMMONLY.

Chronic fatigue syndrome is a diagnosis made when doctors have stopped thinking. "We've done every test (? Really ?) and there's nothing we can find. It's either all in our head, or its chronic fatigue syndrome."

There are three contributors to the illness. Nutritional disturbance, digestion and infection. Two minerals that are very important in the production of symptoms in chronic fatigue syndrome are two very common minerals Iron and Magnesium.

1] A proposed mechanism of Chronic Fatigue.
The pathway on page 145 shows a common chain of events for many (50-60%) of chronic fatigue patients. (EBV is Epstein-Barr Virus, the glandular fever virus; CMV is cytomegalovirus causing a glandula fever like illness; HSV – the Herpes Simplex Virus; RRV- Ross River Virus; BFV- Barmah Forrest Virus, similar to RRV). The pivotal point is whether there are sufficient levels of immune nutrients to fight off the infection effectively. They can either be low, or be blocked by an anti-nutrient. If zinc, or the B Vitamins are involved, or if the infection involves the gut (parvovirus, Mycoplasma, Giardia, Helicobacter or Candida) or if anti-inflammatories are used, then digestion is affected. Once digestion is affected, then the slippery slope begins. Once chemical sensitivity develops, then even the foods needed to heal the person may cause adverse symptoms and at this point the vicious circle is complete.

The success of nutritional therapies depends on three factors.

a] How long ago the process started.

b] How far down the pathway have they proceeded.

c] Identifying what nutritional factors predisposed the patient to the illness. For instance, patients may have some response to Zinc, magnesium or vitamin C temporarily, but they may find that the products become ineffective or need constant dose increases to achieve the same effect, especially if digestion deteriorates, or if one is dealing with a high copper problem.

Genesis of Post infection Fatigue/ Chronic fatigue

Infection with EBV, CMV, HSV, RRV/BFV, Parvovirus B19 Influenza A/B Parainfluenza 3 candida, Giardia, Helicobacter, Mycoplasma , Rickettsia or Chlamydia.

And low levels of Zinc, Vitamin C, Selenium, Iron, Vitamin D or copper overload, presence of mercury or cadmium

Leads to unresolved , relapsing or chronic infection

May also lead to a nutritional deficiency which *prolongs* the illness

If coupled with *digestive* disturbance, the outcome takes even longer

If chemical sensitivity develops, nutritional recovery is even slower

2] Iron

You'd be amazed how many of these patients haven't even had an iron level done. To date I've found over 400 patients with iron deficiency, fifty of them with levels so low that they needed an intravenous iron infusion! So much for the thoroughness of modern medicine. Statistics are actually on my side because 12% of the world's population has iron deficiency. Common things occur commonly, but how many doctors check ferritin levels? They assume that the Haemoglobin always reflects iron levels. They are absolutely wrong, but they won't learn from their ignorance.

Let's take a look at iron deficiency and iron blockade. Iron is involved in the cytochrome system, which resides in the mitochondria (powerhouses of the cells). It is involved in 4 of the 6 steps of electron transport. Copper and mercury block iron and hence cause symptoms similar to iron deficiency. These are disrupted sleep pattern, easy fatigue, pale skin, depression, recurrent infections, and weak muscles.

Iron is needed for Carnitine production. Carnitine is the shovel that allows muscles to access their energy source of fatty acids properly. No iron, no carnitine and hence poor muscle function with pain and fatigue. Unfortunately the liver and kidney have to make carnitine for the other tissues.

Iron is needed for the white cells to kill invaders. White cells make peroxide (with Myeloperoxidase) and you need iron for this. Low Iron (and tissue iron blockade) is associated with increased infections from acne to influenza.

3] Magnesium

The second most common problem is with the mineral magnesium. The point I wish to make is that CFS is not one condition, but a multitude of conditions (some awaiting clever new names) that make up the spectrum of illness.

Many symptoms of CFS look like magnesium deficiency or tissue magnesium blockade. If a trial of magnesium is given, it should be in the form of a liquid or powder. Magnesium tablets are not the best way to give magnesium to CFS patients. The total body store is 25,000mg. The daily requirement for someone who is well, is 350 to 400mg. The strongest magnesium tablet contains 100mg of elemental magnesium (which needs good stomach acid to digest). Therefore 3-4 tablets per day for wellness and 8-10 tablets for deficiency state. The magnesium powders contain 280-300mg per teaspoon, which is easily absorbed. These are only available with a Doctor's or a naturopath's prescription. If the patient scores highly for magnesium symptoms, but does not respond to 600mg per day of the powder, then their problem is excess copper or cadmium blocking magnesium in the tissues or mercury causing blokc in the cell membrane that imports magnesium. This effect only shows up on hair analysis. Blood tests for magnesium are not very helpful in this situation, in fact they are misleading.

Let's take a detailed look at the symptoms of magnesium deficiency: We'll start with the sleep cycle. Humans have an innate clock cycle of 24 hours and 40 minutes. So, if we don't "reset" every night, we get out of synchronisation with the rest of the world. The perfect analogy is the ATM's. Every day, at 4pm (annoying as this is), all the ATM's synchronise and confirm that it is now the next working day. No arguments. Our reset chemical is melatonin. A pulse of this is made an hour before we go to sleep, like an intravenous bolus of anaesthetic. Magnesium is involved in two ways. Firstly, we need it to manufacture melatonin.

Secondly, magnesium is melatonin's private chaperone. The higher the magnesium level, the longer melatonin lasts in the body. The higher the magnesium, the better the recharge we get during our sleep. There's only one problem: magnesium falls at night. It hits rock bottom at 5am (this is why the blood pressure is highest at this time). Add the problem of low magnesium levels in CFS, and you have a recipe for insomnia (pattern 1 & 2) and poor sleep quality, unrefreshed sleep, poor concentration, daytime sleepiness and easy fatigue.

Magnesium is involved in energy cycles. To convert glucose to ATP (the energy currency), we have three main steps: Glycolysis, the Krebs cycle and oxidative phosphorylation. Magnesium is needed in 12 of the 22 steps. Hence the tendency for lactic acid to build up in muscles and cause pain. Magnesium is involved in the relaxation phase of muscles, hence tendency to cramp and stiffness. Stiff muscles use more energy, and give a feeling of heavy limbs.

Magnesium is involved in modulating the inflammatory pathways. It is needed for the production of GLA (gammalinolenic acid is the active ingredient in Evening Primrose Oil). Low GLA levels cause swelling and tenderness.

Magnesium prevents the deposits of calcium by delaying its precipitation. If this occurs in the tendons then tendonitis results.

Why do CFS patients have so much problem with magnesium? Firstly, a significant proportion of CFS patients have digestive problems, which aggravate their ability to absorb enough magnesium from the diet. This is due to hypochlorhydria (low stomach acid) and affects the absorption of calcium and iron as well. Secondly, if they have high copper, then magnesium doesn't function well in the tissues. Thirdly, many have problems storing magnesium under stress and are easily depleted by recurrent infection or the daily stresses, which get worse as the disease progresses (eg loss of income).

The deficiency or blockade of the minerals iron or magnesium cause many symptoms within the chronic fatigue spectrum. Before embarking on a journey looking for more esoteric (and untreatable) causes, a look at mineral imbalance can solve a significant number of symptoms. Because absorption of both of these minerals need good levels of stomach acid, an assessment of digestion in integral in the long-term solution. The best way to look is by hair analysis.

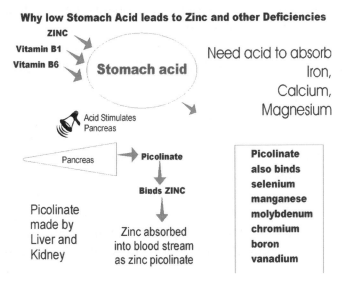

Why low Stomach Acid leads to Zinc and other Deficiencies

4] Digestion and delayed recovery
Digestive problems will aggravate the ability to absorb iron and magnesium. The diagram above shows what happens when stomach acid deteriorates. Firstly the absorption of zinc, iron, magnesium and calcium fall. This in turn further reduces stomach acid because zinc is needed to make stomach acid.

Once the dominoes fall in the game of digestion, the person cannot absorb the nutrients they need to heal their own illness. When stomach acid is consistently low, you cannot kill yeasts, hence the strong association of hypochlorhydria and candida.

Take home message;
CFS is a spectrum of disorders with similar symptomatology. Fixing it involves an analysis of why it happened. This involves looking at the period of health before the illness. Those with digestive problems have a poorer prognosis. Delay of recovery is often aggravated by the very reason the illness occurred. For instance copper excess, and the presence of mercury or cadmium are prime candidates. Those with recurrent infective symptoms have problems with the immune nutrients. (Zinc, Iron, Selenium and Vitamin C, Vitamin E and Vitamin D) either by malabsorption, tissue blockade or oxidation.

CANCER AND NUTRITION

A crash course in nutrition

The first rule of nutrition is there is no average person. The second rule is there is no average cell – each cell is a specialist cell. The third rule of nutrition is drug companies control studies and publications. They never publish negative studies in medical journals and the bulk of literature is published mostly to improve the CV's of the authors and not to improve the awareness of the collective medical consciousness. No one would fund a multi-centre trial looking at citrus rind in the treatment of cancer. Do you know why? You can't patent citrus rind. The fourth rule of nutrition is don't talk about nutrition (not in front of the specialist). When you start mentioning words like zinc and selenium, you'll bring back the trauma of the biochemistry they never understood. Have a look at the periodic table in a chemistry book for yourself. How could such little molecules make such a big difference? Try breathing in outer space, and you'll see just how important they are! Now try living without sodium. Molecules make all the difference, and this is what nutritionists (or orthomolecular medicine specialists, if you prefer) assess every day.

Why is nutrition important anyway?

Most patients I see are disappointed with the lack of information provided by their doctors. So far, all of the patients I have asked have said that their specialist never bothered to find out why they came down with the cancer. They were only interested in getting on with the prospective surgery or chemotherapy or radiotherapy. When confronted with "Should I change my diet?" the specialist usually answered "just eat what you usually eat". These patients should have immediately spoken out and said "But that's the diet on which I got cancer!"

It was most interesting to read the article about wheat and cancer in The Sunday Times recently. Fifty percent of the lymphoma patients I see have gluten sensitivity, and discovery of this fact might have changed the course of their lives if it had been detected at the start of their treatment. I'm sure I heard this "recently discovered" fact in Dr. Dominic Spagnolo's pathology lectures on lymphoma in 1980. Maybe The Sunday Times extracted the information from the medical school under the freedom of information act? Just reading any pathology textbook would have saved them time, but anyway, how do we assess nutrition?

Assessment of life history

It is important to identify all the life factors, which may have predisposed the patient to cancer. This involves taking an historical look at the life of the patient and even their parents' or children's lives. "Is it heredity that my children and I got leukaemia?" "No I said, "It may have something to do with the fact that you live next to (and downwind of) a nuclear reactor." Nutritional assessment must involve some environmental assessment. It involves looking at specific environmental exposures related to where they lived and how they lived from birth to the current time. It involves the old debate about Nature versus Nurture. Will two identical twins have exactly the same life? Will they always have exactly the same DNA from birth to death? The answers are no and no, and it's because mutations are occurring every day. They are caused by tiny subatomic particles called muons.

We are interactive organisms. We change our environment and it changes us. This interaction shapes our destiny. Back to genes. We know that there must be genes that code for cancer, but where do they come from- GM tomatoes? Just kidding. What triggers abnormal genes to start expressing themselves? Most patients with cancer will have either wheat or dairy intolerance by the time they manifest with symptoms of cancer. The best-studied association has been Coeliac disease (gluten sensitivity) and lymphoma.

Assessment of current symptoms.

What current symptoms are due to the cancer and what are due to other factors? Could their tiredness be due to iron deficiency rather than cancer? Some patients are suffering from the existing cancer, some from the toxic effects of their treatments and some from other illness. "Toxic treatments?" exclaimed the oncologist. "Our treatments aren't toxic, they're good for you!" Don't worry about the fine print at the bottom of the product information which says the side-effects of this medication may include cancer- we've got that all under control".

One very relevant example to oncologists is pre-existing zinc deficiency. You need zinc to make white cells, and low levels of this nutrient may manifest as persistent neutropenia (low white cell count) after chemotherapy. The effect of this could be threefold. It could delay the next cycle, it could make the oncologist reduce the next dose (and effectiveness) or it could predispose you to more chance of infection while your defences are down. Oh, incidentally, low Zinc is associated with an increase risk of most cancers. "Don't worry about these nutritional things Dear, they have no bearing on the outcome of your treatment". Sound familiar?

Future protection

What correctional intervention is needed to improve immunity, to address existing risk factors? What factors can affect the risk of metastasis and what can be done to reduce secondary cancers? If the patient survives this current illness what game plan can be put in place to prevent another cancer (or even other illnesses)?

These answers depend upon the information gleaned in the above assessment.

There are many protocols floating around, but the best strategy is to compile a specific program tailored to the person in front of you. Remember rule number 1. One other little problem. We need to make sure that patients are not taking too much of a nutrient. For example, too much zinc, selenium or beta-carotene can actually suppress the immune system. Food for thought?

Immunorestoration.

A good practitioner will identify the biochemical mechanisms that caused the cancer and its spread. Since early last century we have accumulated studies about the reasons cancer occurs. Even "Nutritional" doctors do not generally attempt using these studies in a clinical setting. The importance of restoring the immune system to normal involves analysing *why it failed*. Whatever the chosen mode of clearance be it surgery, radiotherapy or chemotherapy, the conditions that caused the cancer are still present in the body. This is why there are recurrences. A cancer progresses in the following steps.

1] The process be begins with a carcinogen. There are 3 groups, chemicals, metals and radiation. These compounds cause DNA mutations. The cell auditors, zinc and magnesium normally check this process.

2] The next step involves abnormal cell replication Every cell in our body has a "self-destruct button" called Apoptosis. This button should always be pushed if the cell becomes abnormal. The requirements for an intact mechanism include balance between a) Estrogen and Progesterone, b) good energy cycles, c) a balance between iron and copper and d) a balance between copper and the longevity hormone DHEA (dehydroep iandrosterone). The balance of Estrogen and Progesterone affects two important genes. P53 is an apoptosis gene. Its expression is dependent on progesterone levels. BCL-2 is a caner gene and its expression is affected by Estrogen levels (ALL estrogens, endogenous and foreign eg xenoestrogens). One of the mechanisms of apoptosis is brought about by Cytochrome C leaving the mitochondria and triggering the apoptosis "button". The availability of free cytochrome C is dependent upon iron copper balance. The more copper, or the less cytochrome C, the less apoptosis occurs. The level of free radicals to antioxidants also affects apoptosis. Since DHEA reduces copper's oxidizing power, Copper: DHEA ratio affects apoptosis. We make DHEA from Cholesterol and the rate of production is affected by Melatonin. The production of melatonin is complex and requires many steps and cofactors.

3] Any cells that attempt to migrate are controlled by a security patrol of lymphocytes. This security patrol needs zinc, iron, and selenium,

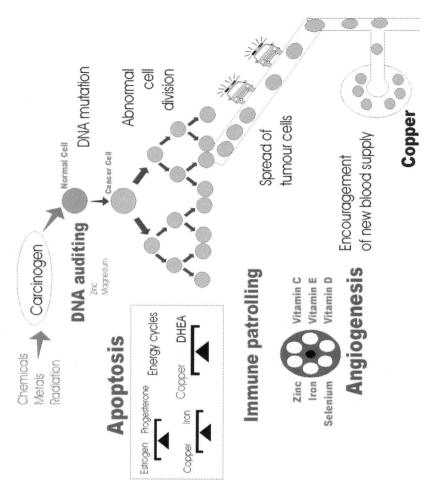

Vitamin C, Vitamin D and Vitamin E.

4] Even if the tumour cells lodge in a new environment (metastasise) they cannot survive without developing a new blood supply. This is called Angiogenesis (*angio* meaning blood vessel and *genesis* meaning new). This process is dependent upon the amount of copper in the tissues and the requirement for copper by the tumour.

So all in all, it is extremely difficult to induce a cancer in a human. Many systems have to fail. Analysing the failed systems involves blood tests, urine and hair analysis. Blood tests take a few days, but the hair analysis takes 4-5 weeks.

154

When all this information is collated, the mechanisms of the cancer become clear and the mode of repair can be planned. This involves oral supplements such as tablets, capsules and powders.

Immunostimulation

Stimulating the immune system to be more efficient can be achieved in part by correcting the defect, but also by stimulants likes cat's claw, saw palmetto, beta glucan, pectin etc.

References relating to Nutrional Medicine:

1] Abel S., et al. Changes in essential fatty acid patterns associated with normal liver regeneration and the progression of hepatocyte nodules in rat hepatocarcinogenesis. Carcinogenesis. 22(5):795-804, May, 2001

2] Abou-Issa H., et al. Basis for the anti-tumour and chemopreventive activities of glucarate and the glucarate: retinoid combination. Anticancer Res. 13(2):395-9, Mar-Apr, 1993

3] Adachi K., Nanba H. & Kuroda H. Potentiation of host-mediated antitumor activity in mice by beta-glucan obtained from Grifola frondosa (maitake). Chem Pharm Bull. 35:262-270, 1987

4] Adlercreutz H., Mazur W. Phyto-oestrogens and Western diseases. Ann Med. 29:95-120, 1997

5] Adlercreutz H., et al. Estrogen and Metabolite levels in Women at Risk for Breast Cancer. Cancer Res. 35:703, 1994

6] Ahmad N., Gupta S. & Mukhtar H. Green tea polyphenol epigallocatechin-3-gallate differentially modulates nuclear factorkappaB in cancer cells versus normal cells. Arch Biochem Biophys. 376(2):338-46, Apr 15, 2000

7] Ahmann F.R., Durie B.G. Acute myelogenous leukaemia modulated by B12 deficiency: a case with bone marrow blast cell assay corroboration. Br J Haematol. 58(1):91-4, 1984

8] Akiba S., et al. Serum ferritin and stomach cancer risk among a Japanese population. Cancer. 67:1707-12, 1991

9] Albanes D., et al. Effects of alpha-tocopherol and beta-carotene supplements on cancer incidence in the Alpha-Tocopherol Beta-Carotene Cancer Prevention Study. Am J Clin Nutr. 62(supp):1427S-30S, 1995

10] Alirezai M., et al. Clinical evaluation of topical isotretinoin in the treatment of actinic keratoses. J Am Acad Dermatol. 30(3):447-51, 1994

11] Allen J.I., et al. Association between urinary zinc excretion and lymphocyte dysfunction in patients with lung cancer. Am J Med. 79(2):209-15, 1985

12] Amer B.N. & Gold L.S. Natural chemicals, synthetic chemicals, risk assessment and caner. Princess Takamatsu Symp. 21:303-314, 1990

13] Amir H. & Karas M., et al. Lycopene and 1,25-dihydroxyvitamin D3 cooperate in the inhibition of cell cycle progression and induction of differentiation in HL-60 leukemic cells. Nutr Cancer. 33(1):105-12, 1999

14] Anderson, R. Effects of ascorbate on normal and abnormal leukocyte functions. Vitamin C: New Clinical Applications in Immunology. Lipid Metabolism and Cancer. 1-178, 1982

15] Anderson L.M., Et al. Alcohol-related cancer risk:a toxicokinetic hypothesis. Alcohol. 12(2):97-104, 1995

16] Anderson K.M. & Harris J.E. Is induction of type 2 programmed death in cancer cells from solid tumours directly related to mitochondrial mass? Med Hypotheses. 57(1):87-90. July, 2001

17] Anonymous. Alpha-tocopherol, Beta-carotene Cancer Prevention Study Group. The effect of vitamin E and beta-carotene on the incidence of lung cancer and other cancers in male smokers. N Engl J Med. 330:1029-35, 1994

18] Anonymous. Diet said to be major contributor to development of breast cancer. Primary Care and Cancer. 13, 1996

19] Anthony H.M. & Schorah C.J. Severe hypovitaminosis C in lung-cancer patients: the utilization of vitamin C in surgical repair and lymphocyte-related host resistance. Br J Cancer. 46(3):354-67, Sep, 1982

20] Anti M., et al. Effects of different doses of fish oil on rectal cell proliferation in patients with sporadic colonic adenomas. Gastroenterology. 107:1709-18, 1994

21] Anto R.J., et al. Curcumin (diferuloylmethane) induces apoptosis through activation of caspase-8, BID cleavage and cytochrome c release: its suppression by ectopic expression of Bcl-2 and Bcl-xl. Carcinogenisis. 23:143-150, 2002

22] Archimbaud E., et al. Influence of cigarette smoking on the presentation and course of chronic myelogenous leukemia. Cancer. 63:2060-2065, 1989

23] Ardier Cm. & Dees C. Xenoestrogens significantly enhance risk for breast cancer during growth and adolescence. Med Hypotheses. 50:457-464, 1998

24] Areekul S., Panatampon P. & Doungbarn J. Vitamin B12 and vitamin B12 binding proteins in liver diseases. Southeast Asian J Trop Med Public Health. 8:332-328, 1977

25] Asea A., Ara G. & Teicher B.A., et al. Effects of the flavonoid drug quercetin on the response of human prostate tumours to hyperthermia in vitro and in vivo. Int J Hyperthermia. 17(4):347-56, Jul-Aug, 2001

26] Aso Y., et al. Preventive effect of a lactobacillus casei preparation on the recurrence of superficial bladder cancer in a double-bind trial. Eur Urol. 27:104-9, 1995

27] Ausman LM. Fiber and colon cancer: does the current evidence justify a preventive policy? Nutr Rev. 51(2):57-63, 1993

28] Badary O.A. Taurine attenuates fanconi syndrome induced by ifosfamide without compromising its antitumour activity. Oncol Res. 10(7):355-60, 1998

29] Bain C., et al. Diet and melanoma. An exploratory case-control study. Ann

Epidemiol. 3(3):235-8, 1993

30] Balabhadrapathruni S. & Thomas T.J., et al. Effects of genistein and structurally related phytoestrogens on cell cycle kinetics and apoptosis in MDA-MB-468 human breast cancer cells. Oncol Rep. 7(1):3-12, Jan-Feb, 2000

31] Baldwin A.S. Control of oncogenesis and cancer therapy resistance by the transcription factor NF-kappaB. J Clin Invest. 107(3):241-6. Review. Feb, 2001

32] Barale R., et al. Vegetables inhibit, in vivo, the mutagenicity of nitrite combined with nitrosable compounds. Mutation Res. 120:145, 1983

33] Barber M.D. & Ross J.A., et al. The effect of an oral nutritional supplement enriched with fish oil weight-loss in patients with pancreatic cancer. Br J Cancer. 81(1):80-6, Sep, 1999

34] Barch D.H. Esophageal cancer and microelements. J Am Coll Nutr. 8(2):99-107, 1989

35] Barone J., et al. Dietary fat and natural-killer-cell activity. Am J Clin Nutr. 50:861-7, 1989

36] Barone J., et al. Vitamin supplement use and risk for oral and esophageal cancer. Nutr Cancer. 18:31-41, 1992

37] Baronzio G.F., et al. Tumour microcirculation and its significance in therapy: a possible role of omega-3-fatty acids as rheological modifiers. Med Hypotheses. 50(2):175-182, 1998

38] Bastide E., Almirall L. & Ordinas. A Characterisation of mechanisms involved in tumour cell induced platelet aggregation. Int J Cancer. 39:760, 1987

39] Batist G., et al. Selenium induced cytotoxicity of human leukemia cells: interaction with reduced glutathione. Cancer Research. 46(11):5482-5485, 1986

40] Batkin S., et al. Modulation of pulmonary metastasis (Lewis lung carcinoma) by bromelain, an extract of the pineapple stem (Ananas comosus). Cancer Invest. 6(2):241-2, 1988

41] Batkin S., et al. Antimetastatic effect of bromelain with or without its proteolytic and anticoagulant activity. J Cancer Res Clin Oncol. 114(5):507-8, 1988

42] Bauer G. Lactobacilli-mediated control of vaginal cancer through specific reactive oxygen species interaction. Med Hypotheses. 57(2):252-7, Aug, 2001

43] Baylin S.B. & Esteller M., et al. Aberrant patterns of DNA methylation, chromatin formation and gene expression in cancer. Hum Mol Genet. 10(7):687-92. Review. Apr, 2001

44] Beauregard D.A. & Hill S.A., et al. The susceptibility of tumours to the antivascular drug combretastatin A4 phosphate correlates with vascular permeability. Cancer Res. 61(18):6811-5, Sep 15, 2001

45] Beers E.P., Woffenden B.J. & Zhao C. Plant proteolytic enzymes: possible roles during programmed cell death. Plant Mol Biol. 44(3):399-415. Review. Oct, 2000

46] Bëgin M.E., et al. Selective killing of human cancer cells by polyunsaturated fatty acids. Prostaglandins Leukotrienes Med. 19(2):177-86, 1985

47] Bëgin M.E., et al. Differential killing of human carcinoma cells supplemented with n-3 and n-6 polyunsaturated fatty acids. J Natl Cancer Inst. 77:1053-62, 1986

48] Beier R.C. Natural pesticides and bioactive components in food. Rev Environ

Contam Toxicol. 113:47-137, 1990

49] Belanger J.T. Perillyl alcohol: application in oncology. Altern Med Rev. 3(6):448-57. Review. Dec, 1998

50] Belhoussine R., et al. Confocal-scanning microspectrofluorometry reveals specific anthracyline accumulation in cytoplasmic organelles of multidrug-resistant cancer cells. J Histochem Cytochem. 46(12):1369-76. Dec, 1998

51] Belhoussine R., et al. Characterization of intracellular pH gradients in human multidrug-resistant tumor cells by means of scanning microspectrofluorometry and dual-emission-ratio probes. Int J Cancer. 81(1):81-9, 1999

52] Bell M. C., et al. Placebo-controlled trial of indole-3-carbinol in the treatment of CIN. Gynecol Oncol. 78(2):123-129, 2000

53] Ben-Eliyahu S., et al. Stress increases metastatic spread of a mammary tumour in rats: evidence for mediation by the immune system. Brain Behav Immun. 5(2):193-205, Jun, 1991

54] Beniston R.G., et al. Quercetin, E7 and p53 in papillomavirus oncogenic cell transformation. Carcinogenesis. 22(7):1069-76, Jul, 2001

55] Benner S.E., et al. Regression of oral leukoplakia with alpha-tocopherol: a community clinical oncology program chemoprevention study. J Natl Cancer Inst. 85:44-7, 1993

56] Bernardi P. & Pace V. Correlations between folic acid, human papilloma virus (HPV) and cervix neoplasms. Minerva Ginecol. 46(5):249-55, May, 1994

57] Beuth J., et al. Impact of complementary oral enzyme application on the postoperative treatment results of breast cancer patients-results of an epidemiological multicentre retrolective cohort study. Cancer Chemother Pharmacol. 47 Suppl:S45-54, Jul, 2001

58] Beutler E., Gelbart T. Plasma glutathione in health and in patients with nakignant disease. J Lab Clin Med. 105:581-4, 1985

59] Bingham S.A., et al. Does increased endogenous formation of N-nitroso compounds in the human colon explain the association between red meat and colon cancer? Carcinogenesis. 17:515-23, 1996

60] Block G., et al. Fruit, vegetables, and cancer prevention: a review of the epidemiological evidence. Nutr Cancer. 18:1-20, 1992

61] Blondell J.M. The anticarcinogenic effect of magnesium. Med Hypotheses. 6:863-71, 1980

62] Blutt .E. & Weigel N.L. Vitamin D and prostate cancer. Proc Soc Exp Biol Med. 221(2):89-98, Jun, 1999

63] Böing H., et al. Regional nutritional pattern and cancer mortality in the Federal Republic of Germany. Nutr Cancer. 7(3):121-30, 1985

64] Böing H., et al. Dietary carcinogens and the risk for glioma and meningioma in Germany. Int J Cancer 53:561-5, 1993

65] Bond G.G., et al. Dietary vitamin A and lung cancer: Results of a case-control study among chemical workers. Nutr Cancer. (:109-21, 1987

66] Booyens J., Katzeff IE. Cancer: A simple metabolic disease? Med Hypotheses 12(3):195-201, 1983

67] Booyens J., et al. Dietary fats and cancer. Med Hypotheses 17:351-62, 1985

68] Boros L.G., et al. Thiamine supplementation to cancer patients: a double edged sword. Anticancer Res. 18(1B):595-602, 1998

69] Boros L.G. & Bassilian S., et al. Genistein inhibits nonoxidative ribose synthesis in MIA pancreatic adenocarcinoma cells: a new mechanism of controlling tumour growth. Pancreas. 22(1):1-7, Jan, 2001

70] Bostick R., et al. Relation of calcium, vitamin D, and dairy food intake to incidence of colon cancer among older women. Am J Epidemiol. 137:1302-17, 1993

71] Bostick R.M., et al. Sugar, meat, and fat intake, and non-dietary risk factors for colon cancer incidence in Iowa women (United States). Cancer Causes Control. 5:38-52, 1994

72] Bounous D.G., et al. Whey proteins in cancer prevention. Cancer Lett. 57:91-4, 1991

73] Bourantas K.L., Tsiara S. & Christou L. Treatment of 34 patients with myelodysplastic syndromes with 13-cis retinoic acid. Eur J Haematol. 55:235-239, 1995

74] Boyd N.F., McGuire V. The possible role of lipid peroxidation in breast cancer risk. Free Rad Biol Med. 10(3-4):185-90, 1991

75] Bradlow H. L., et al. Indole-3-carbinol. A novel approach to breast cancer prevention. Annals of the New York Academy of Sciences USA. 768:180-200, 1995

76] Bradlow et al. Effects of pesticides on rates of 16 alpha/2 hydroxyestrone: A Biological marker for breast cancer risk. Environ Health Persp. 103:147-50, 1995

77] Bram, S., et al. Vitamin C preferential toxicity for malignant melanoma cells. Nature. 284:629-631, 1980.

78] Brand R.F. & McCormack J.J., et al. Effects of folate deficiency on the metastatic potential of murine melanoma cells. Cancer Res. 48(16):4529-34, Aug 15, 1988

79] Branda R.F. & Nigels E., et al. Nutritional folate status influences the efficacy and toxicity of chemotherapy in rats. Blood. 92(7):2471-6, Oct 1, 1998

80] Braverman E.R. Reversal of pre-leukemia with antioxidants: a case report. J Nutr Med 2:313-15, 1991

81] Brewer et al Treatment of metastatic cancer with tetrathiomolybdate, an anticopper , antiangiogenic agent. Phase I study. Clin Cancer res 6(1): 1-10 2000

82] Brewer G.J. Copper control as an antiangiogenic anticancer therapy: lessons from treating Wilson's disease. Exp Biol Med (Maywood). 226(7):665-73, Jul, 2001

83] Britteden J., et al. L-arginine stimulates host defenses in patients with breast cancer. Surgery. 115(2):205-12, 1994

84] Brizel D.M. & Schroeder T., et al. Elevated tumour lactate concentrations predict for an increased risk of metastases in head-and-neck cancer. Int J Radiat Oncol Biol Phys. 51(2):349-53, Oct 1, 2001

85] Broghamer W.L., et al. Relationship between serum selenium levels and patients with carcinoma. Cancer. 37:1384, 1976

86] Brohult A., et al. Reduced mortality in cancer patients after administration of alkoxylglycerols. Acta Obstet Gynecol Scand. 65(7):779-85, 1986

87] Brohult A., et al. Effect of alkoxylglycerols on the frequency of fistulas following radiation therapy for carcinoma of carcinoma of the uterine cervix. Acta Obstet Gynercol Scand. 58(2):203-07, 1979

88] Brown R.R., et al. Correlation of serum retinol levels with response to chemotherapy in breast cancer. Meeting abstract. Proc Am Assoc Cancer Res. 22:184, 1981

89] Bruce W.R., Dion PW. Studies relation to a fecal mutagen. Am J Clin Nutr. 33:2511-12, 1980

90] Bruemmer B., et al. Nutrition intake in relation to bladder cancer among middle-aged men and women. Am J Epidemiol 144(5):485-95, 1996

91] Bryan B.T. The influence of niacin and niacinamide on in vivo carcinogenesis. Adv Exp Med Biol. 206:331-8, 1986

92] Budas R.R. Vitamin D receptors in breast cancer cells. Breast Cancer Res Treat. 31(2-3):191-202, 1994

93] Bueno-de-Mesquita HB., Gonzalez CA. Main hypotheses on diet and cancer investigated in the EPIC study. Eur J Canc Prev. 6:1-7-17, 1997

94] Buolamwini J.K. Cell cycle molecular targets in novel anticancer drug discovery. Curr Pharm Des. 6:379-392, 2000

95] Burnley P.G.J., et al. Serologic precursors of cancer: Serum micronutrients and the subsequent risk of pancreatic cancer. American Journal of Clinical Nutrition. 49:895-900, 1989

96] Burns C.P. & Halabi S., et al. Phase I clinical study of fish oil fatty acid capsules for patients with cancer cachexia: cancer and leukemia group B study 9473. Clin Cancer Res. 5(12):3942-7, Dec, 1999

97] Butterworth C.E. Jr., et al. Improvement in cervical dysplasia associated with folic acid therapy in users of oral contraceptives. Am J Clin Nutr. 35:73-82, 1982

98] Butterworth C.E. Jr. Effect of folate on cervical cancer. Synergism among risk factors. Ann N Y Acad Sci. 669:293-9, 1992

99] Butterworth C.E., et al. Folate status, women's health, pregnancy outcome and cancer. J Am Coll Nutr. 12(4):438-41. Review. Aug, 1993

100] Byers, R., et al. Epidemiologic evidence for vitamin C and vitamin E in cancer prevention. Am J Clin Nutr. 62(Supplement):1385S-1392S, 1995.

101] Camagna A., et al. The synergistic effect of simultaneous addition of retinoic acid and vitamin D3 on the in-vitro differentiation of human promyelocytic leukemia cell? Could be efficiently transposed in vivo. Med Hypotheses. 50:253-257, 1998

102] Cambier N., et al. All-trans retinoic acid in adult chronic myelomonocytic leukemia: results of a pilot study. Leukemia. 10:1164-1167, 1996

103] Cameron E., et al. The orthomolecular treatment of cancer.III. Reticulum cell sarcoma: double complete regression induced by high-dose ascorbic acid therapy. Chem Biol Interact. 11(5):387-93, 1975

104] Cameron E., Pauling L. Supplemental ascorbate in the supportive treatment of cancer: Reevaluation of prolongation of survival times in terminal human cancer. Proc Nat Acad Sci USA. 75:4538-42, 1978

105] Cameron E. Protocol for the use of vitamin C in the treatment of cancer. Med hypotheses. 36(3):190-4, 1991

106] Campbell A., et al. Reticulum cell sarcoma: two complete 'spontaneous' regressions, in response to high-dose ascorbic acid: a report on subsequent progress. Oncology. 48(6):495-7, 1991

107] Cao G.H., et al. A study of the relationship between trace element Mo and gastric cancer. World J Gastroenterol Feb. 4(1): 55-56, 1998

108] Carroll K.K. Dietary factors in hormone-dependent cancers, in M Winick, Ed. Current Concepts in Nutrition, Volume 6: Nutrition and Cancer. New York, John Wiley & Sons, 25-40, 1977

109] Carroll K.K. Lipid oxidation and carcinogenesis. Prog Clin Biol Res. 206:237-44, 1986

110] Carroll K.K. Dietary fats and cancer. Am J Clin Nutr. 53:1064S-7S, 1991

111] Carroll P.E. & Okuda M., et al. Centrosome hyperamplification in human cancer: chromosome instability induced by p53 mutation and/or Mdm2 overexpression. Oncogene. 18(11):1935-44, Mar 18, 1999

112] Casciari J.J & Riordan N.H., et al. Cytotoxicity of ascorbate, lipoic acid and other antioxidants in hollow fibre in vitro tumours. Br J Cancer. 84(11):1544-50, June 1,2001

113] Casinus S., et al. Neuroprotective effect of reduced glutathione on cisplatin-based chemotherapy in advanced gastric cancer: a randomized double-bind placebo-controlled trial. J Clin Oncol. 13:26-32, 1995

114] Cats A., et al. Randomized, double-binded, placebo-controlled intervention study with supplemental calcium in families with hereditary nonpolyposis colorectal cancer. J Natl Cancer Inst. 87(8):598-603, 1995

115] Chan F.L. & Choi H.L., et al. Induction of apoptosis in prostate cancer cell lines by a flavonoid, baicalin. Cancer Lett. 160(2):219-28, Nov 28, 2000

116] Cavelier G. Theory of malignant cell transformation by superoxide fate coupled with cytoskeletal electron-transport and electron-transfer. Med Hypotheses. 54(1):95-8, Jan, 2000

117] Check W.A. Folate for oral contraceptive users may reduce cervical cancer risk. JAMA. 244(7):633-4, Aug 15, 1980

118] Chen C-J., et al. Arsenic and cancer. Letter. Lancet i:414-15, 1988

119] Chen C., et al. Activation of antioxidant-response element (ARE), mitogen-activated protein kinases (MAPKs) and caspases by major green tea polyphenol components during cell survival and death. Arch Pharm Res. 23(6):605-12, 2000

120] Chen H. & Zhang Z.S., et al. Curcumin inhibits cell proliferation by interfering with the cell cycle and inducing apoptosis in colon carcinoma cells. Anticancer Res. 19(5A):3675-80, Sep-Oct, 1999

121] Chen Y., et al. A mechanism for tamoxifen-mediated inhibition of acidification. J Biol Chem. 274(26):18364-73, 1999

122] Chen Y., et al. Tamoxifen can inhibit the acidification of cytoplasmic organelles in mammalian cells. It inhibits ATP dependent acidification or organelles by increasing proton leakage. J Biol Chem. 274(26):1864-73, 1999

123] Cheng K.K., et al. Stopping drinking and risk of oesophageal cancer. Br Med J.

310:1094-7, 1995

124] Cheng K.K., et al. Nutrition and oesophageal cancer. Cancer Causes and Control. 7:33-40, 1996

125] Chigbrow M. & Nelson M. Inhibition of mitotic cyclin B and cdc2 kinase activity by selenomethionine in synchronized colon cancer cells. Anticancer Drugs. 12(1):43-50, Jan, 2001

126] Chinery R., et al. Antioxidants enhance the cytotoxicity of chemotherapeutic agents in colorectal cancer: A p53-independent induction of p21 WAF1/CIP1 via C/EBPb. Nature Med. 3(11):1233-41, 1997

127] Chinje E.C., Stratford IJ. Role of nitric oxide in growth of solid tumours: a balancing act. Essays Biochem 32:61-72, 1997

128] Chinni S.R. & Li Y., et al. Indole-3-carbinol (13C) induced cell growth inhibition, GI cell cycle arrest and apoptosis in prostate cancer cells. Oncogene. 20(23):2927-36, May 24, 2001

129] Chiu B C-H., et al. Diet and risk of non-Hodgkin lymphoma in older women. JAMA 275(17):1315-31, 1996

130] Chlebowski R.T., et al. New directions in the nutritional management of the cancer patient. Nutr Res. 13:3-21, 1993

131] Choi J.A. & Kim J.Y., et al. Induction of cell cycle arrest and apoptosis in human breast cancer cells by quercetin. Int J Oncol. 19(4):837-44, Oct, 2001

132] Christley B.M., et al. Vitamin B6 status of a group of cancer patients. Nutr Res. 6(9):1023-30, 1986

133] Clark L. The epidemiology of selenium and cancer. Federation Proceedings. 44:2584-2589, 1985

134] Clark L.C., et al. Plasma selenium and skin neoplasms: A case control study. Nutr Cancer. 6:13, 1985

135] Clark L.C., et al. Effects of selenium supplementation for cancer prevention in patients with carcinoma of the skin. JAMA. 276(24):1957-63, 1996

136] Clark L.C., et al. Decreased incidence of prostate cancer with selenium supplementation: results of double-blind cancer prevention trial. Br J Urol. 81:730-734, 1998

137] Clement M.V. & Hirpara J.L., et al. Chemopreventive agent resveratrol, a natural product derived from grapes, triggers CD95 signaling-dependent apoptosis in human tumour cells. Blood. 92(3):996-1002, Aug 1, 1998

138] Clinton S.K. Lycopene:chemistry, biology and implications for human health and disease. Nutr Rev. 56(2 part I):35-51, 1998

139] Colditz G.A., et al. Increased green and yellow vegetable intake and lowered cancer deaths in an elderly population. Am J Clin Nutr 41(1):32-6, 1985

140] Coldsitz G.A. Selenium and cancer prevention: promising results indicate further trials required. The Journal of the American Medical Association. 276(24):1984, 1996

141] Collins K. & Jacks T., et al. The cell cycle and cancer. Proc Natl Acad Sci USA. 94(7):2776-8, Apr 1, 1997

142] Colquhoun-Flannery W. Diet modified sex hormone metabolism: Is it the way forward in recurrent respiratory papillomatosis and squamous carcinoma prophylaxis. J Laryngology and Otology. 109:873-75, 1995

143] Colston K.W., et al. Possible role for vitamin D in controlling breast cancer proliferation. Lancet i:188-91, 1989

144] Colucci M. & Delaini F., et al. Warfarin inhibits both procoagulant activity and metastatic capacity of Lewis lung carcinoma cells. Role of vitamin K deficiency. Biochem Pharmacol. 32(11):1689-91, Jun 1, 1983

145] Combs G.F., et al. Can dietary selenium modify cancer risk? Nutr. Rev. 43:325-331, 1985

146] Combs G.F. Jr., et al. Reduction of cancer mortality and incidence by selenium supplementation. Med Klin. 92(Supplement 3):42-45, 1997

147] Comee J., et al. A Case-control study of gastric cancer and nutrutuinal factors in Marseille, France. Eur J Epidemiol. 11:55-65, 1995

148] Conklin K.A. Dietary antioxidants during cancer chemotherapy: impact on chemotherapeutic effectiveness and development of side effects. Nutr Cancer. 37(1):1-18. Review. 2000

149] Conner E.M & Grisham M.B. Inflammation, free radicals and antioxidants. Nutrition. 12(4):274-7. Review. April, 1996

150] Cooley M.E. & Kaiser L.R., et al. The silent epidemic: tobacco and the evolution of lung cancer and its treatment. Cancer Invest. 19(7):739-51, 2001

151] Contreras V. National cancer institute spotlights nutrients: prestigious panel focuses on substances found in plants. Journal of Longevity. #48, 1999

152] Copeland E.M. 3rd et al. Nutrition and cancer. Int Adv Surg Oncol. 4:1-13, 1981

153] Cordova C., Musca A. & Violi F., et al. Influence of ascorbic acid on platelet aggregation in vitro and in vivo. Atherosclerosis. 41:15, 1982

154] Couch D.B. Carcinogenesis: basic principles. Drug Chem Toxicol. 19(3):133-48, August, 1996

155] Cover C. M., et al. Indole-3-carbinol and tamoxifen cooperate to arrest the cell cycle of MCF-7 human breast cancer cells. Cancer Research. 59:1244-1251, 1999

156] Cowan L.D., Gordis L., Tonascia J.A. and Jones G.S. Breast Cancer Incidence in Women with a History of Progesterone Deficiency. Am J Epidemiol. 114:209-217, 1981

157] Cox C et al The role of copper suppression as an antiangiogenic strategy in head and neck squamous cell carcinoma Laryngoscope apr 111 (4 pt 1) : 696-701 2001

158] Cravo M., et al. DNA methylation as an intermediate biomarker in colorectal cancer: modulation by folic acid supplementation. Eur J Cancer Prev. 3(6):473-9, 1994

159] Cross J.H., et al. Effect of quercetin on the genotoxic potential of cisplatin. Int J Cancer. 66:404-9, 1996

160] Cucuianu A. Cell darwinism, apoptosis, free radicals and haematological malignancies. Med Hypotheses. 56(1):52-7, Jan, 2001

161] Cuendet M. & Pezzuto J.M. The role of cyclooxygenase and lipoxygenase in cancer chemoprevention. Drug Metabol Drug Interact. 17(1-4):109-57, 2000

162] Curier C., Jang A. & Hill R.P. Exposure to hypoxia, glucose starvation and acidosis: effect on invasive capacity of murine tumour cells and correlation with cathepsin (L+B) secretion. Clin Exp Metastasis. 15(1):19-25, Jan, 1997

163] Damiens E., et al. Anti-mitotic properties of indirubin-3'-monoxime, a CDK/GSK-3 inhibitor: induction of ensoreplication following prophase arrest. Oncogene. 20:3786-3797, 2001

164] Damiens E. & Meijer L. Chemical inhibitors of cyclic-dependent kinases: preclinical and clinical study. Pathol Biol (Paris).(Article in French) 48:340-351, 2000

165] De Jaeger K. & Kavanagh M.C., et al. Relationship of hypoxia to metastatic ability in rodent tumours. Br J Cancer. 84(9):1280-5. May 4, 2001

166] Dale P.S., et al. Co-medication with hydrolytic enzymes in radiation therapy of uterine cervix: evidence of the reduction of acute side effects. Cancer Chemother Pharmacol. 47 Suppl:S29-34, Jul, 2001

167] Dalhoff K., et al. Glutathione treatment of hepatocellular carcinoma. Liver. 12:341-3, 1992

168] Daou D.L. Natural anticarcinogens, carcinogens and changing patterns in cancer: some speculations. Enviro Res. 50(2):322-40, 1989

169] D'Avanzo B., et al. Alcohol consumption and the risk of gastric cancer. Nutr Cancer. 22:57-64, 1994

170] Davies P. Bailey J. & Goldenburg M.M. The role of arachidonic acid oxygenation products in pain and inflammation. Ann Rev Immunol. 2:325-57, 1984

171] Davis C.D., et al. The chemical form of selenium influences 3,2'-dimethyl-4-aminobiphenyl-DNA adduct formation in rat colon. Journal of Nutrition. 129(1):63-69, 1999

172] Davis C.D., et al. Dietary selenium and arsenic affect DNA methylation in vitro in Caco-2 cells and in vivo in rat liver and colon. Journal of Nutrition. 130:2903-2909, 2000

173] Davis D.L., Bradlow H.L., Wolff M., Woodruff T., Hoel D.G. and Anton-Culver H. Medical Hypothesis: Xenohormones as Preventable Causes of Breast Cancer. Env Health Persoectuves. 101:372-377, 1993

174] Davis S.R. & Dalais F., et al. Phytoestrogens in health and disease. Recent Prog Horm Res. 54:185-210; discussion 210-1. Review. 1999

175]DeCosse J.J., et al. Effect of wheat fiber and vitamins C and E on rectal polyps in patients with familial adenomatous polyposis. J Natl Cancer Inst. 81(17):1290-7, 1989

176] De Flora S., et al. In vivo effects of N-acetylcysteine on glutathione metabolism and on the biotransformation of carcinogenic and/or mutagenic compounds. Carcinogenesis 6:1735-45, 1985

177] De Flora S. & Izzotti A., et al. Multiple points of intervention in the prevention of cancer and other mutation-related diseases. Mutat Res. 480-481:9-22. Review. Sep 1, 2001

178] De Jaeger K. & Kavanagh M.C., et al. Relational of hypoxia to metastatic

164

ability in rodent tumours. Br J Cancer. 84(9):1280-5, May 4, 2001

179] Del Giudice M.E., et al. Insulin and Related Factors in Premenopausal Breast Cancer Risk. Breast Cancer Res Treat. 47(2):111-120, 1998

180] Delmore G. Assessment of nutritional status in cancer patients: widely neglected? Support Care Cancer. 5(5):376-80, 1997

181] DeLuca H.F., et al. Mechanisms and functions of vitamin D. Nutr Rev. 56(2): S1-S10, 1998

182] De Maria D., et al. Adjuvant radiotherapy of the pelvis with or without reduced glutathione: a randomized trial in patients operated on for endometrial cancer. Tumori. 78:374-6, 1992

183] Demark-Wahnefried W., et al. Pilot study of dietary fat restriction and flaxseed supplementation in men with prostate cancer before surgery: exploring the effects on hormonal levels, prostate-specific antigen, and histopathologic features. Urology. 58(1):47-52, Jul, 2001

184] Denekamp J., et al. Low ATP levels are a characteristic of solid tumours. Acta Oncol. 38(7):903-18, 1999

185] Desser L., Rehberger A. Induction of tumor necrosis factor in human peripheral-blood mononuclear cells by proteolytic enzymes. Oncology. 47(6):475-7, 1990

186] Desser L., et al. Oral therapy with proteolytic enzymes decreases excressive TGF-beta levels inhuman blood. Cancer Chemother Pharmacol. 47 Suppl:S10-5, Jul, 2001

187] Dewys W.D., et al. Prognostic effect of weight loss prior to chemotherapy in cancer patients. Am J Med. 69:491-7, 1980

188] Dich J., et al. Pesticides and cancer. Cancer cayses control. 8(3):420-443, 1997

189] Dinarello C.A. & Endres S., et al. Interleukin-1, anorexia and dietary fatty acids. Ann N Y Acad Sci. 587:332-8. Review. 1990

190] Ding G.S. Important Chinese herbal remedies. Clin Ther. 9:345-357, 1987

191] Dippenaar N., et al. The reversibility of cancer: Evidence that malignancy in melanoma cells is gamma-linolenic acid deficiency-dependent. S Afr Med J. 62:505-9, 1982

192] Dische S., et al. Tumour regression as a guide to prognosis: a clinical study. Br J Radiol. 53(629):454-61, May, 1980

193] Dokal I.S., et al. Vitamin B-12 and folate deficiency presenting as leukeamia. Br Med J. 300:1263-4, 1990

194] Doll R., et al. Cancers of the lung and nasal sinuses in nickel workers. Br J Cancer. 24:623-32, 1970

195] Domellof L. Gastric carcinoma promoted by alkaline reflux gastritis – with special reference to bile and other surfactants as promoters of postoperative gastric cancer. Med Hypotheses. 5(4):463-76, 1979

196] Dupont J., et al. Food uses and health effects of com oil. Am J Clin Nutr. 9(5):438-70, 1990

197] Durie B.G., et al. Antitumor activity of bovine cartilage (Catrix-S) in the human tumor stem cell assay. J Biol Response Mid. 4(6):590-95, 1985

198] Durlach J., Bara M. Magnesium and its relationship to oncology, in H. Sigel, A. Sigel, Eds. Metal Ions in Biological Systems. Vol. 26: Compendium on magnesium and its role in biology. New York-Basel, Marcek Dekker, 1990

199] Dyke G.W., et al. Effect of vitamin C supplementation on gastric mucosal damage. Carcinogenesis. 15(2):291-5, 1994

200] Eckert K., et al. Effects of oral bromelain administration on the impaired immunocytotoxicity of mononuclear cells from mammary tumour patients. Oncol Eep. 6(6):1191-9, Nov-Dec, 1999

201] Eichhlozer M., et al. Prediction of male cancer mortality by plasma levels of interacting vitamins: 17 year follow-up of the prospective Basal study. Int J Cancer. 66:145-50, 1996

2021] Elattar T.M. & Virgi A.S. Biphasic action of vitamin E on the growth of human oral squamous carcinoma cells. Anticancer Res. Jan-Feb. 19(1A):365-8, 1999

203] Elinder C.G., et al. Cancer mortality of cadmium workers. Br J Ind Med. 42(10):651-5, 1985

204] Ellis L.M. & Liu W., et al. Role of angiogenesis inhibitors in cancer treatment. Oncology (Huntingt). 15(7 Suppl 8):39-46, Jul, 2001

205] Engin K., et al. Extracellular pH distribution in human tumors. Int J Hyperthermia. 11(2):211-6, 1995

206] Enig M.G., et al. Dietary fat and cancer trends – A critique. Fed Proc. 37:2215-20, 1978

207] Enwonwu C.O. & Meeks V.I. Bionutrition and oral cancer in humans. Crit Rev Oral Biol Med. 6:5-17, 1995

208] Eskin B.A. Iodine and breast cancer. A 1982 update. Biol Trace Elem Res. 5:399-412, 1983

209] Esteve J., et al. Diet and cancers of the larynx and hypopharynx: the IARC multi-center study in southwestern Europe. Cancer causes Control. 7:240-52, 1996

210] Faber M., et al. Lipid peroxidation products, and vitamin and trace element status in patients with cancer before and after chemotherapy, including adriamycin: a preliminary study. Biol Trace Elem Res. 47:117;24, 1995

211] Fearson K.C. Nutritional pharmacology in the treatment of neoplastic disease. Bailieres Clin Gastroenterol. 2(4):941-9, Oct, 1988

212] Fearson K.C. & Borland W., et al. Cancer cachexia: influence of systemic ketosis on substance levels and nitrogen metabolism. Am J Clin Nutr. 47(1):42-8, Jan, 1988

213] Fearon K.C., et al. An open-label phase I/II does escalation study of the treatment of pancreatic cancer using lithium gammalinolenate. Anticancer Res. 16(2):867-74, 1996

214] Fenaux P., Chomienne C. & Degos L. All-trans retinoic acid and chemotherapy in the treatment of acute promyelocytic leukemia. Semin Hematol. 38:13-25, 2001

215] Fenech M. & Ferguson L.R. Vitamins/minerals and genomic stability in humans. Mutat Res. 475(1-2):1-6, Apr 18, 2001

216] Ferguson L.R. Role of plant polyphenols in genomic stability. Mutat Res. 475(1-2):89-111, 2001

217] Fernandes G. Dietary lipids and risk of autoimmune disease. Clin Immunol Immunopathol. 72(2):193-7, Aug, 1994

218] Ferraroni M., et al. Selected micronutrient intake and the risk of colorectal cancer. Br J cancer. 70(6):1150-5, 1994

219] Ferrigno D., Buccheri G., Camilla T. Serum copper and zinc content in non-small cell lung cancer: abnormalities and clinical correlates. Monaldi Arch Chest Dis (Italy), Jun. 54(3) p204-8, 1999

220] Feustel A. & Wennrich R. Zinc and cadmium in cell fractions of prostatic cancer tissues of different histological grading in comparison to BPH and normal prostate. Urol Res. 12(2):147-50, 1984

221] Fico M.E., et al. Differential Effects of Selenium on normal and neoplastic canine mammary cells. Cancer Research. 46:3384-3388, 1986

222] Fife R.S., et al. Effects of vitamin D3 on proliferation of cancer cells in vitro. Cancer Lett. 120(1):65-9, 1997

223] Finley J.W., et al. Selenium from high selenium broccoli protects rats from colon cancer. Journal of Nutrition. 130(9):2384-2389, 2000

224] Fisher S. & Weber P.C. Prostaglandin I3 is formed in vivo in men after dietary eicosapentaenoic acid. Nature. 307:165, 1984

225] Flagg E.W., et al. Dietary glutathione intake and the risk of oral and pharyngeal cancer. Am J Epidemiol. 139:453-65, 1994

226] Flaten T.P. Chlorination of drinking water and cancer incidence in Norway. Int J Epidemiol. 21(1):6-15. 1992

227] Folkers K., et al. Survival of cancer patients on therapy with coenzyme Q10. Biochem Biophys Res Commun. 192(1):241-5, 1993

228] Folkers K., et al. Activities of vitamin Q10 in animal models and a serious deficiency in patients with cancer. Biochem Biophys Res Commun. 234(2):296-9, 1997

229] Formby B. and Wiley T.S. Progesterone Inhibits Growth and Induces Apoptosis in Breast Cancer Cells: Inverse Effect on Expression of p53 and Bcl-2. Ann Clin Lab Sc. 28(6):360-9, 1998

230] Formenti S. & Felix J., et al. Expression of metastases-associated genes in cervical cancers resected in the proliferative and secretory phases of the menstrual cycle. Clin Cancer Res. 6(12):4653-7, Dec, 2000

231] Fraker P.J., et al. Interrelationships between zinc and immune function. Fed Proc. 45:1474-1479, 1986

232] Franca D.S. & Souza A.L., et al. B vitamins induce an antinociceptive effect in the acetic acid and formaldehyde models of nociception in mice. Eur J Pharmacol. 421(3):157-64, Jun 15, 2001

233] Franceschi S., et al. Dietary factors and non-Hodgkin's lymphoma: a case-control study in the north-eastern part of Italy. Nurt Cancer. 12:333-41, 1989

234] Franceschi S. I., et al. Food groups and risk of colorectal cancer in Italy. Int J Cancer. 72:56-61, 1997

235] Frentzel-Beyme R. & Chang-Claude J. Vegetarian diets and colon cancer: the

German Experience. Am J Clin Nutr. 59(suppl):1143S-52S,1994

236] Freudenheim J.L., et al. Diet, smoking and alcohol in cancer of the larynx: a case-control study. Nutr Cancer. 17:33-45, 1992

237] Fuch C.S., et al. Dietary fiber and the risk of colorectal cancer and adenoma in women. N Engl J Med. 230(3):169-76, 1999

238] Fujiki H., et al. Inhibition of tumor promotion by flavonoids, in Plant Flavonoids in Biology and Medicine, vol. 1. New York, Alan R. Liss. 429-40, 1986

239] Fullerton S.A. & Samadi A.A. Induction of apoptosis in human prostatic cancer cells with beta-glucan (Maitake mushroom polysaccharide). Mol Urol. 4(1):7-13, Spring, 2000

240] Funahashi H., et al. Seaweed prevents breast cancer? Jpn J Cancer Res. 92(5):483-7, May, 2001

241] Funaki N.O., et al. Membrane fluidity correlates with liver cancer cell proliferation and infiltration potential. Oncol Rep. 8(3):527-32, May-Jun, 2001

242] Fyles A.W. & Milosevic M., et al. Anemia, hypoxia and transfusion in patients with cervix cancer: a review. Radiother Oncol. 57(1):13-9. Review. Oct, 2000

243] Gale A.J. & Gordon S. G. Update on tumour cell procoagulant factors. Acta Haematol. 106(1-2):25-32. Review. 2001

244] Galli C. & Butrum R. Dietary omega-3 fatty acids and cancer: an overview, in AP Simopoulos et al, Eds. Health Effects of omega-3 polyunsaturated Fatty Acids in Seafoods. World Rev Nutr Diet. 66:3446-61, 1991

245] Gao W.C. & Qiao J.T. Nitric oxide contributes to both spinal nociceptive transmission and its descending inhibition in rats: An immunocytochemical study.

246] Gao Y.T., et al. Risk factors for esophageal cancer in Shanghai, China. II. Role of diet and nutrients. Int J Cancer. 58(2):197-202, 1994

247] Garewal H.S. Potential role of -carotene in prevention of oral cancer . Am J Clin Nutr. 53:294S-7S, 1991

248] Garland C., et al. Dietary vitamin D and calcium and risk of colorectal cancer: A 19-year prospective study in men. Lancet i:307-9, 1985

249] Garland C.F., et al. Serum 25-hydroxyvitamin D and colon cancer. Eight-year prospective study. Lancet i:176-8, 1989

250] Garland F.C., et al. Geographic variation in breast cancer mortality in the United States: A hypothesis involving exposure to solar radiation. Prev Med. 19:614-22, 1990

251] Garland M., et al. Prospective study of toenail selenium levels and cancer among women. J Natl Cancer Inst. 87(7):497-505, 1995

252] Gasic G.J. Role of plasma, platelets and endothelial cells in tumor metastasis. Cancer Metast Rev. 3:99, 1984

253] Gastpar H. Platelet aggregation inhibitors and cancer metastasis. Ann Chir Gynaecol. 71:142, 1982

254] Gerald G. Anticancer treatment and bromelains. Agressologie. 13(4):261-74, 1972

255] Gerber G.B. & Leonard A. Mutagenicity, carcinogenicity and teratogenicity of germanium compounds. Mutat Res. 387(3):141-6. Review. Dec, 1997

256] Gerhardsson de Verdier M. Epidemiologic studies on fried foods and cancer in Sweden. Princess Takamatsu Symp. 23:292-8, 1995

257] Gerweck L.E. Tumor pH: implications for treatment and novel drug design. Semin Radiat Oncol. 1998

258] Gey K.F., et al. Plasma levels of antioxidant vitamins in relation to ischemic heart disease and cancer. Am J Clin Nutr. 45(5 Suppl):1368-77, 1987

259] Ghadirian P., et al. International comparisons of nutrition and mortality from pancreatic cancer. Cancer Detect Prev. 15(5):357-62, 1991

260] Ghadirian P., et al. Nutritional factors and colon carcinoma: a case-control study involving French canadians in Montreal, Quebec, Canada. Cancer. 80:858-64, 1997

261] Ghalaut P.S., Singh V. & Gupta S. Serum vitamin E levels in patients of chronic myeloid leukaemia. J Assoc Physician India. 47:703-704, 1999

262] Ghent W.R., et al. Iodine replacement in fibrocystic disease of the breast. Can J Surg. 36(5):453-60, Oct, 1993

263] Giannoulaki E.E. & Kalpaxis D.L., et al. Lactate dehydrogenase isoenzyme pattern in sera of patients with malignant diseases. Clin Chem. 35(3):396-9, Mar, 1989

264] Gilmore M.A. Phases in Wound Healing. Dimens Oncol Nurs. 5(3):32-4, Fall, 1991

265] Giovannucci E., et al. A prospective study of dietary fat and risk of prostate cancer. J Natl Cancer Inst. 85(19):1571-9, 1993

266] Giovannucci E., et al. Alcohol, low-methionine-low-folate diets, and risk of colon cancer in men. J Natl Cancer Inst. 87(4):265-73, 1995

267] Gogos C.A., et al. Dietary omega-3 polyunsaturated fatty acids plus vitamin E restore immunodeficiency and prolong survival for severely ill patients with generalized malignancy: a randomized control trial. Cancer. 82(2):395-402, 1998

268] Goldberg D.M. Structural, functional and clinical aspects of gamma-glutamyltransferase. CRC Crit Rev Clin Lab Sci. 12(1):1-58, 1980

269] Goldhirsch A. & Gelber R.D., et al. Menstrual cycle and timing of breast surgery in premenopausal node-positive breast cancer: results of the International Breast Cancer Study Group (IBCSG) Trial VI. Ann Oncol. 8(8):751-6, Aug, 1997

270] Goldin B.R., et al. Effect of diet and Lactobacillus acidophilus supplements on human fecal bacterial enzymes. J Natl Cancer Inst. 64(2):255-61, 1980

271] Goldin B.R., et al. Estrogen excretion patterns and plasma levels in vegetarian and omnivorous women. N Engl J Med. 307:1542-7, 1982

272] Goldin B.R. & Gorbach S.L. The effect of milk and lactobacillus feeding on human intestinal bacterial enzyme activity. Am J Clin Nutr. 39(5):756-61, 1984

273] Gompel A., Malet C., Spritzer P., La Lardrie J.-P., et al. Progestin Effect on Cell Proliferation and 17 -hydroxysteroid Dehydrogenase Activity in Normal Human Breast Cells in Culture. J Clin Endocrinol Metab 63:1174, 1986

274] González C.A., et al. Nutritional factors and gastric cancer in Spain. Am J Epidemiol. 139:466-73, 1994

275] Goodman M.T., et al. Diet, body size, physical activity and the risk of endometrial cancer. Cancer Res. 57:077-85, 1997a

276] Goodman M.T., et al. Association of soy and fiber consumption with the risk of endometrial cancer. Am J Epidemiol. 146(4):294-306, 1997b

277] Gorbach S.L. The intestinal microflora and its colon cancer connection. Infection. 10(6):379-84, 1982

278] Gould M.N. Cancer chemoprevention and therapy by monoterpenes. Enviro Health Perspect. 105 Suppl 4:977-9. Review. June, 1997

279] Graf E & Eaton J. Suppression of colon cancer by dietary phytic acid. Nutr Cancer. 19(1):11-19, 1993

280] Graham S., et al. Dietary factors in the epidemiology of cancer of the larynx. Am J Epidemiol. 113(6):675-80, 1981

281] Greenberg E.R., et al. A clinical trial of antioxidant vitamins to prevent colorectal adenoma. N Engl J Med. 331:141-7, 1994

282] Gridley G., et al. Vitamin supplement use and reduced risk of oral and pharyngeal cancer. Am J Epidemiol. 135(10):1083-92, 1992

283] Grimble R.F. & Tappia P.S. Modulation of pro-inflammatory cytokine biology by unsaturated fatty acids. Z Ernahrungswiss. 37 Suppl 1:57-65. Review. 1998

284] Grimble R.F. Nutritional modulation of cytokine biology. Nutrition. 14(7-8):634-40. Review. Jul-Aug, 1998

285] Griffin B.E. Epstein-Barr virus (EBV) and human disease: facts, opinions and problems. Mutat Res. 462(2-3):395-405, Apr, 2000

286] Grimble R.F. Nutritional antioxidants and the modulation of inflammation: theory and practice. New Horiz. 2(2):175-85. Review. May, 1994

287] Groopman J. & Ellman L. Acute promyelocytic leukemia. Am J Hematol. 7(4):395-408, 1979

288] Gubareva A.A. The use of enzymes in treating patients with malignant lymphoma with a large tumour mass. Lik Sprava. 6:141-3, Aug, 1998

289] Gujral M.S., et al. Efficacy of hydrolytic enzymes in preventing radiation therapy-induced side effects in patients with head and neck cancers. Cancer Chemother Pharmacol. 47 Suppl:S23-8, Jul, 2001

290] Guo How-Ran et al. Arsenic in drinking water and incidence of urinary cancers. Epidemiology. 8(5):545-50, 1997

291] Gupta S. Effect of radiotherapy on plasma ascorbic acid concentration in cancer patients. Unpublished thesis-summarized in Hanck AB. Vitamin C and cancer. Prog Clin Biol Res. 259:307-20, 1988

292] Ha C., et al. The effect of B-6 on host susceptibility to Moloney Sarcoma Virus-induced tumor growth in mice. J Nutr. 114:938-45, 1984

293] Haag J.D., et al. Limonene-induced regression of mammary carcinoma. Cancer Res. 52(4):4021-4026, 1992

294] Habib F.K., et al. Metal-androgen interrelationships in carcinoma and hyperplasia of the human prostate. J Endocrinol. 71(1):133-41, 1976

295] Hageman G.J. & Stierum R.H. Niacin, poly (ADP-ribose) polymerase-1 and genomic stability. Mutat Res. 475(1-2):45-56. Review. Apr 18, 2001

296] Hague A., et al. The role of butyrate in human colonic epithelial cells: an energy source or inducer of differentiation and apoptosis? Proc Nutr Soc. 55:937-43, 1996

297] Hakim I.A. & Harris R.B., et al. Citrus peel use is associated with reduced risk of squamous cell carcinoma of the skin. Nutr Cancer. 37(2):161-8, 2000

298] Hallivell B. & Gutteridge J.M. Oxygen free radicals and iron in relation to biology and medicine: Some problems and concepts. Arch Biochem Biophys. 246:501-14, 1986

299] Hamburger A.W. & White C.P. Growth factors for human tumour clonogenic cells elaborated by macrophages isolated from human malignant effusions. Cancer Immunol. Immunother. 22:186-90, 1986

300] Han R. Highlight on the studies of anticancer drugs derived from plants in China. Stem Cells. 12:53-63, 1994

301] Han J. Traditional Chinese medicine and the search for new antineoplastic drugs. J Ethnopharmacol. 24:1-17, 1988

302] Han Y.P. & Tuan T.L., et al. TNF-alpha stimulates activation of pro-MMP2 in human skin through NF(kappa)B mediated induction of MT1-MMP. J Cell Sci. 114(Pt 1):131-139. Jan, 2001

303] Hankinson S.E. Circulating Concentrations of Insulin-like Growth Factor-I and Risk of Breast Cancer. The Lancet. 351(9113):1393-1396, 1998

304] Hansen-Algenstaedt N. & Stoll B.R., et al. Tumour oxygenation in hormone-dependent tumours during vascular endothelial growth factor receptor-2 blockade, hormone ablation and chemotherapy. Cancer Res. 60:4556-60, Aug, 2000

305] Hanul V.L., et al. Application of systemic enzyme therapy in combined treatment of patients with pulmonary cancer and malignant thymoma. Klin Khir. 6:17-9, Jun, 2000

306] Harimaya K. & Tanaka K., et al. Antioxidants inhibit TNFalpha-induced motility and invasion of human osteosarcoma cells: possible involvementof NFkappaB activation. Clin Exp Metastasis. 18(2):121-9, 2000

307] Harrison L.E., et al. The role of dietary factors in the intestinal and diffuse histologic subtypes of gastric adenocarcinoma: a case-control study in the U.S. Cancer. 80(6):1021-8, 1997

308] Hartman T.J., et al. Association of the B-vitamins pyridoxal 5'-phosphate (B(6)), B(12), and folate with lung cancer risk in older men. Am J Epidemiol. 153(7):688-94, Apr 1, 2001

309] Hartwig A. Role of magnesium in genomic stability. Mutat Res. 475(1-2):113-21. Review. Apr 18, 2001

310] Hayashi A., Gillen A.C. & Lott J.R. Effects of daily oral administration of quercetin chalcone and modified citrus pectin. Altern Med Rev. 5(6):546-52, Dec, 2000

311] Head K. Ascorbic acid in the prevention and treatment of cancer. Altern Med Rev. 3(3):174-186, 1998

312] Hebert J. & Rosen A. Nutritional, Socioeconomic and reproductive factors in relation to female breast cancer mortality: findings from a cross-national study. Cancer Detect Preven. 20(3):234-44, 1996

313] Hedberg K., et al. Alcoholism and cancer of the larynx: a case-control study in western Washington (United States). Cancer Causes and Control. 5:3-8, 1994

314] Heerdt A.S., et al. Calcium glucarate as a chemopreventive agent in breast cancer. Isr J Med Sci. 31(2-3):101-5, Feb-Mar, 1995

315] Heerdt B.G. Mitochondrial Membrane Potential in the coordination of p53 independent proliferation and apoptosis pathways in human colonic carcinoma cells. Cancer Research. 58:2869-2875, 1998

316] Heimburger D.C., et al. Improvement in bronchial squamous metaplasia in smokers treated with folate and vitamin B12: Report of a preliminary randomized, double-bind intervention trial. JAMA. 259(10):1525-30, 1988

317] Heimburger D.C. Localized deficiencies of folic acid in aerodigestive tissues. Ann NY Acad Sci. 669:87-96, 1992

318] Heinonen O.P., et al. Prostate cancer and supplementation with alpha-tocopherol and beta-carotene: incidence and mortality in a controlled trial. J Natl Cancer Inst. 90(6):440-6, 1998

319] Hellstrand K. & Brune M., et al. Alleviating oxidative stress in cancer immunotherapy: a role for histamine? Med Oncol. 17:258-69, Nov, 2000

320] Hellstrom & Hellstrom, in Salinas and Hanna, Eds. Immune Complexes and Cancer. Vol. 15, 1985

321] Hennekens C.H., et al. Lack of effect of ling-term supplementation with beta carotene on the incidence of malignant neoplasms and cardiovascular disease. N Engl J Med. 334(18):1145-9, 1996

322] Hennig B. & Diana J.N., et al. Influence of nutrients and cytokines on endothelial cell metabolism. J Am Coll Nutr. 13(3):224-31. Review. Jun, 1994

323] Herak-Kramberger C.M., et al. Cadmium inhibits vacuolar H(+)-AT Pase and endocytosis in rat kidney cortex. Kidney Int. 53(6):1713-26, 1998

324] Herak-Kramberger C.M., et al. Cadmium impairs acidification in cell organelles by (a) causing a loss of V-ATPase protein (V= vacuole) in their limiting membrane, (b) inhibiting the intrusive V-ATPase activity, (c) dissipating the transmembrane pH gradient. Kidney Int. 53(6):1783-26, 1998

325] Heron D.S., et al. Alleviation of drug withdrawal symptoms by treatment with a potent mixture of natural lipids. Eur J Pharmacol. 83(3-4):253-61, Sep 24, 1982

326] Herr R., et al. Cigarette smoking, blast crisis and survival in chronic myeloid leukemia. Am J Hematol. 34:1-4, 1990

327] Hertog M.G.L., et al. Dietary flavonoids and cancer risk in the Zutphen Elderly Study. Nutr Cancer. 22:175-84, 1994

328] Hibbs J.B., et al. L-arginine is required for the expression of the activated macrophage effector mechanism causing selective metabolic inhibition in target cells. J Immunol. 138:550-65, 1987

329] Hidalgo M., et al. Development of matrix metalloproteinase inhibitors in cancer therapy. J Natl Cancer Inst. 93(3):178-93, Feb 7, 2001

330] Hill M. Epidemiology of meat and colorectal cancer – historical aspects. Eur Cancer Prevent News. 31:8-10, 1997

331] Hinds M.W., et al. Dietary cholesterol and lung cancer among men in Hawaii.

Am J Clin Nutr. 37:192-3, 1983

332] Hishida I., Nanba H. & Kuroda H. Antitumor activity exhibited by orally administered extract from fruit body of Grifola frondosa (maitake). Chem Pharm Bull. 36:1819-1827, 1988

333] Hocman G. Chemoprevention of cancer: Selenium. Int J Biochem. 20(2):123-132, 1988

334] Hockel M. & Schlenger K., et al. Association between tumour hypoxia and malignant progression in advanced cancer of the uterine cervix. Cancer Res. 56:4509-15, Oct, 1996

335] Hoehn S.K. & Carroll K.K. Effects of dietary carbohydrate on the incidence of mammary tumors induced in rats by 7,12-dimethylbenz(a)-anthracene. Nutr Cancer. 1(3):27-30, Spring, 1979

336] Hoessel R., et al. Indirubin, the active constituent of a Chinese antileukaemia medicine, inhibits cyclin-dependent kinases. Nat Cell Biol. 1:60-67, 1999

337] Hoffer A. & Pauling L. Hardin Jones biostatistical analysis of mortality data for a second set of cohorts of cancer patients with a large fraction surviving at the termination of the study and a comparison of survival times of cancer patients receiving large regular doses of vitamin C and other nutrients with similar patients not receiving these doses. J Orthomol Med . 8(3);157-67, 1993

338] Hoffman R., et al. Enhanced anti-proliferative action of busulphan by quercetin on the human leukaemia cell line K562. Br J Cancer. 59:347-8, 1989

339] Hoirsemann M.R., et al. Reducing acute and chronic hypoxia in tumours by combining nicotinamide with carbogen breathing. Acta Oncol. 33:(4)371-6, 1994

340] Holtzman E.J., et al. Serum cholesterol and the risk of clorectal cancer. N Engl J Med. 9:114, July, 1987

341] Honn K.V., Cicone B. & Skoff A. Prostacyclin: a potent anti metastatic agent. Science. 212:1270, 1981

342] Honn K.V. & Dunn J.R. Nafazatron (BAYg6575) inhibition of tumour cell lipoxygenase activity and cellular proliferation. FEBSLett. 139:65, 1982

343] Horsman M.R., et al. Combretastatins novel vascular targeting drugs for improving anti-cancer therapy. Combretastatins and conventional therapy. Adv Exp Med Biol. 476:311-23, 2000

344] Howe G., et al. Dietary factors and risk of pancreatic cancer: Results of a Canadian population-based case-control study. Int J Cancer. 45:604-8, 1990

345] Hrelia S., et al. The role of delta-6- and delta-9-desaturase in the fatty acid metabolism of hepatomas with different growth rate. Biochem Mol Biol Int. 34(3):449-55, 1994

346] Hrelia S., et al. Gamma-Linolenic acid supplementation can affect cancer cell proliferation via modification of fatty acid composition. Biochem Biophys Res Commun. 225(2):441-7, 1996

347] Hrushesky W.J.M. Breast Cancer, Timing of Surgery, and the Menstrual Cycle: Call for Prospective Trial. J Women's Health. 5:555-566, 1996

348] Hrushesky W.J. Menstrual Cycle Timing of Breast Cancer Resection: Prospective Study is Overdue. J Natl Cancer Inst. 87(2):143-4, 1995

349] Hsu B. The use of herbs as anticancer agents. Am J Chin Med. 8:301-306, 1980

350] Hu Y-J., et al. The protective role of selenium on the toxicity of cisplatin-contained chemotherapy regimen in cancer patients. Biol Trace Elem Res. 56:331-41, 1997

351] Huang Y-C., et al. N-3 fatty acids decrease colonic epithelial cell proliferation in the high-risk bowel mucosa. Lipids. 31(suppl):S313-S317, 1996

352] Huang Z. Bcl-2 family proteins as targets for anticancer drug design. Oncogene. 19(56):6627-31. Review. Dec 27, 2000

353] Huang S. & Pettaway C.A., et al. Blockade of NF-kappaB activity in human prostate cancer cells is associated with suppression of angiogenesis, invasion and metastasis. Oncogene. 20(31):4188-97, Jul 12, 2001

354] Hunter J.E. & Applewhite T.H. Isomeric fatty acids in the US diet: Levels and health perspectives. Am J Clin Nutr. 44(6):707-17, 1986

355] Hursting S., et al. Types of dietary fat and the incidence of cancer at five sites. Prev Med. 19:242-53, 1990

356] Hyder S.M. & Chiappetta C., et al. Pharmacological and endogenous progestins induce vascular endothelial growth factor expression in human breast cancer cells. Int J Cancer. 92(4):469-73, May 15, 2001

357] Iitaka M. et al. Induction of apoptosis and necrosis by zinc in human thyroid cancer cell lines. J Endocrinol. 169(2):417-24, 2001

358] Ingram D., et al. Case-control study of phyto-oestrogens and breast cancer. Lancet. 350:990-4, 1997

359] Inoh A., Kamiya K., Fujii Y. and Yokoro K. Protective Effect of Progesterone and Tamoxifen in Estrogen-induced Mammary Carcinogenesis in Ovariectomized W/Fu Rats. Jpn J Cancer Res. 76:699-704, 1985

360] Inoue A. & Kunitoh H., et al. Radiation pneumonitis in lung cancer patients: a retrospective study of risk factors and the long-term prognosis. Int J Radiat Oncol Biol Phys. 49:649-55, Mar, 2001

361] Ip C. Selenium inhibition of chemical carcinogenesis. Federation Proceedings. 44:2573-2578, 1985

362] Ip C. Interaction of vitamin C and selenium supplementation in the modification of mammary carcinogenesis in rats. J N C I. 77:299, 1986

363] Ip C. & Scimeca J.A. Conjugated linoleic acid and linoleic acid are distinctive modulators of mammary carcinogenesis. Nutr Cancer. 27(2):131-5, 1997

364] Iseki T. Vitamin B12 and transcobalamin in chronic myeloproliferative disorders. Rinsho Byori. (Article in Japanese) 41:1310-1321, 1993

365] Israels L.G. & Israels E.D. Apoptosis. Stem Cells. 17(5):306-13. Review, 1999

366] Israel K. & Yu W., et al. Vitamin E succinate induces apoptosis in human prostate cancer cells: role for Fas in vitamin E succinate-triggered apoptosis. Nutr Cancer. 36(1):90-100, 2000

367] Jaakkola K., et al. Treatment with antioxidant and other nutrients in combination with chemotherapy and irradiation in patients with small-cell lung cancer. Anticancer Res. 12:599-606, 1992

368] Jacobs D.R. Jr., et al. Whole grain intake and cancer: a review of the literature.

Nutr Cancer. 24(3):221-9, 1995

369] Jacobson E.L. & Jacobson M.K. A biomarker for the assessment of niacin nutriture as a potential preventive factor in carcinogenesis. J Intern Med. 233:59-62, 1993a

370] Jacobson E.L. Niacin deficiency and cancer in women. J Am Coll Nutr. 12(4):412-16, 1993b

371] Jacobson E.L., et al. Evaluating the role of niacin in human carcinogenesis. Biochemic. 77(5):394-398, 1995

372] Jaga K. & Duvvi H. Risk reduction for DDT toxicity and carcinogenesis through dietary modification. J R Soc Health. 121(2):107-13. Review. Jun, 2001

373] Jajoo A., et al. Mg(2+)-induced lipid phase transition in thylakoid membranes is reversed by anions. Biochem Biophys Res Commun. 202(3):1724-30, Aug 15, 1994

374] Janssen G., et al. Boswellic acids in the palliative therapy of children with progressive or relapsed brain tumours. Klin Padiatr. 212(4):189-95, Jul-Aug, 2000

375] Jayasunder R., et al. Hyperthermia decreases pH. Magan Reson. Med. 43(1):1-8, 2000

376] Jha M.N. & Bedford J.S., et al. Vitamin E (d-alpha-tocopheryl succinate) decreases mitotic accumulation in gamma-irradiated human tumour, but not in normal cells. Nutr Cancer. 35(2):189-94, 1999

377] Ji X., et al. Pharmacological studies of meisoindigo: absorption and mechanism of action. Biomed Environ Sci. 4:332-337, 1991

378] Jiang C. & Wang Z., et al. Caspases as key executors of methyl selenium-induced apoptosis (anoikis) of DU-145 prostate cancer cells. Cancer Res. 61(7):3062-70, Apr 1, 2001

379] Jiang Y. & Cui L., et al. Inhibition of anchorage-independent growth and lung metastasis of A549 lung carcinoma cells by IkappaBbeta. Oncogene. 20(18):2254-63, Apr 26, 2001

380] John A.P. Dysfunctional mitochondria, not oxygen insufficiency, cause cancer to produce inordinate amounts of lactic acid: the impact of this on the treatment of cancer. Med Hypotheses. 57(4):429-431, 2001

381] Joossens J.V., et al. Dietary salt, nitrate and stomach cancer mortality in 24 countries. Int J Epidemiol. 25(3);494-502, 1996

382] Juhl J.H. Fibromyalgia and the serotonin pathway. Altern Med Rev. 3(5):367-75. Review. Oct, 1998

383] Kamei T., et al. Experimental study of the therapeutic effects of folate, vitamin A and vitamin B12 on squamous metaplasia of the bronchial epithelium. Cancer. 71(8):2477-83, 1993

384] Kandaswami, C., et al. Differential inhibition of proliferation of human squamous cell carcinoma, gliosarcoma and embryonic fibroblast-lung cells in culture by plant flavonoids. Anticancer Drugs. 3(5):525-530, 1992

385] Kandouz M., Siromachkova M., Jacob D., Marquet B.C., et al. Antagonism between Estradiol and Progestin on Bcl-2 Expression in Breast Cancer Cells. Int J Cancer. 68:120-125, 1996

386] Kapadia G.J. & Tokuda H., et al. Chemoprevention of lung and skin cancer by Beta vulgaris (beet) root extract. Cancer Lett. 100(1-2):211-4, Feb 27, 1996

387] Kaplan S., et al. Nutritional factors in the etiology of brain tumors. Am J Epidemiol. 146(10):832-41, 1997

388] Karas M. & Amir H., et al. Lycopene interferes with cell cycle progression and insulin-like growth factor I signaling in mammary cancer cells. Nutr Cancer. 36(1):101-11. 2000

389] Karmali R.A. Historical perspective and potential use of omega-3 fatty acids in therapy of cancer cachexia. Nutrition. 12(1) suppl:S2-S4, 1996

390] Katdare M., et al. Prevention of mammary preneoplastic transformation by naturally-occurring tumor inhibitors. Cancer Letters. 111(1-2):141-147, 1997

391] Kaul L., et al. The role of diet in prostate cancer. Nutr Cancer. 9:123-8, 1987

392] Kearney R. Acceleration and Prevention of Tumour Growth: Effects of inflammation, obesity, age, essential fatty acids, caloric restriction and frequency of eating on cancer risk. Proc. 1st Oceania Symposium On Complementary Medicine Brisbane Australia. 1:1-35, 1990

393] Kelly G.S. Conjugated linoleic acid: a review. Altern Med Rev. 6(4):367-82. Review. Aug, 2001

394] Kemen M. & Senkal M., et al. Early postoperative enteral nutrition with arginine, omega-3-fatty acids and ribonucleic acid-supplemented diet verses placebo in cancer patients: an immunologic evaluation of impact.

395] Kerr P.E. & DiGiovanna J.J. From vitamin to Vesanoid: systemic retinoids for the new millennium. Med Health R.I. 84(7):228-31, Jul, 2001

396] Kim J.A., et al. Topical use of N-acetylcysteine for reduction of skin reaction to radiation therapy. Semin Oncol. 10(1 Suppl 1):86-88, 1983

397] Kim J-P. et al. Effects on rosette forming T-lymphocyte level in immunochemotherapy using Picibanil and Wobe-Mugos in gastric cancer patients. J Korean Surg Soc. 23, 1981

398] Kim Y-I., et al. Folate, epithelial dysplasia and colon cancer. Proc Assco Am Physicians. 107:218-27, 1995

399] Kim Y.I. Methylenetetrahydrofolate reductase polymorphisms, folate and cancer risk: a paradigm of gene nutrient interaction in carcinogenesis. Nutr Rev. 58(1):205-17, 2000

400] Kinscherf R. & Hack V., et al. Low plasma glutamine in combination with high glutamate levels indicate risk for loss of body cell mass in healthy individuals: the effect of N-acetyl-cysteine. J Mol Med. 74(7):393-400, Jul, 1996

401] Kinsella J.E., et al. Metabolism of trans fatty acids with emphasis on the effects of trans, trans-octadecadienoate on lipid composition, essential fatty acid, and prostaglandins: an overview. AM J Clin Nutr. 34:2307, 1981

402] Kirchholf D. & Kirchhof E. The successful Use of Bovine Tracheal Cartilage in the Treatment of Cancer. Belgrade, Montana, Kriegel & Assoc., 1995

403] Kirkpatrick C.S., et al. Case-control study of malignant melanoma in Washington States. II. Diet, alcohol and obesity. Am J Epidemiol. 139:869-80, 1994

404] Kirsch M. & Schackert G., et al. Anti-angiogenic treatment strategies for

176

malignant brain tumours. J Neurooncol. 50(1-2):149-63, Oct-Nov, 2000

405] Kirschner M.A. The Role of Hormones in the Etiology of Human Breast Cancer. Cancer. 39(6):2716-2726, 1977

406] Kitai R., et al. Sensitization to hyperthermia by intracellular acidification of C6 glioma cells. J Neuro Oncol. 39(3):197-203, 1998

407] Kitomura K., et al. Toxic effects of arsenic (As 3+) and other metal ions on acute promyelocytic leukemia cells. Int J Haematology. 65(2):179-185, 1997

408] Klein G. & Kullich W. Reducing pain by oral enzyme therapy in rheumatic diseases. Wien Med Wochenschr. 149(21-22):577-80. Review. 1999

409] Klimberg V.S. Prevention of radiogenic side effects using glutamine-enriched elemental diets. Recent Results Cancer Res. 121:283-5, 1991

410] Klimberg V.S., et al. Glutamine suppresses PGE2 synthesis and breast cancer growth. J Surg Res. 63(1):293-7, 1996a

411] Klimberg V.S., McClellan J.L. Glutamine, cancer and its therapy. Am J Surg. 172(5):418-24, 1996b

412] Klurfeld D.M. & Kritchevsky D. Wistar Institute, Philadelphia-quoted in Med World News. April 25, 1988

413] Knekt P., et al. Serum selenium and subsequent risk of cancer among Finnish men and women. J National Cancer Institute. 82:864-868, 1990

414] Knekt P., et al. Body iron stores and risk of cancer. Int J Cancer. 56(3):379-82, 1994

415] Knekt P., et al. Dietary flavonoids and the risk of lung cancer and other malignant neoplasms. Am J Epidemiol. 146(3):223-30, 1997

416] Kobayashi M., et al. Inhibitory effect of dietary selenium on carcinogenesis in rat glandular stomach induced by N-Methyl-N'-nitro-N-nitro. Cancer Research. 46:2266-2270, 1986

417] Kobryn C.E. & Fishum G. Differential sensitivity of AS-30 D rat hepatoma cells and normal hepatocytes to anoxic cell damage. Am J Physiol. 262(6 Pt 1): C1384-7, Jun, 1992

418] Kohshi K. & Kinoshita Y., et al. Effects of radiotherapy after hyperbaric oxygenation on malignant gliomas. Br J Cancer. 80:236-41, Apr, 1999

419] Kokron O. Österr Zschr Onkol. 4:82-5, 1977 (in German)

420] Kolonel L.N., et al. Nutrient intakes in relation to cancer incidence in Hawaii. Br J Cancer. 44(3);332-9, 1981

421] Komada K., et al. Effects of dietary molybdenum on esophageal carcinogenesis in rats induced by N-methyl-N-benzylnitrosamine. Cancer Res. 50:2418-2422, 1990

422] Konety B.R. & Lavelle J.P., et al. Effects of vitamin D (calcitriol) on transitional cell carcinoma of the bladder in vitro and in vivo. J Urol. 165(1):253-8, Jan, 2001

423] Kong A.N., et al. Pharmacodynamics and toxicodynamics of drug action: signaling in cell survival and cell death. Pharm Res. 16(6):790-8, 1999

424] Kong A.N., et al. Signal transduction events elicited by natural products: role of MAPK and caspase pathways in homeostatic response and induction of apoptosis.

Arch Pharm Res. 23(1):1-16, Feb, 2000
425] Kong A.N., et al. Signal transduction events elicited by cancer prevention compounds. Mutat Res. 480-481:231-41, 1, 2001
426] Korsmeyer S.J. & Yin X.M., et al. Reactive oxygen species and the regulation of cell death by the Bcl-2 gene family. Biochim Biophys Acta. 1271(1):63-6, May 24, 1995
427] Knowles L.M., et al. Allyl sulfides modify cell growth. Drug Metabol Drug Interact. 17(1-4):81-107, 2000
428] Krimsky S. Hormonal Chaos: The Scientific and Social Origins of the Environmental Endocrine Hypothesis. Baltimore, Md.: Johns Hopkins University Press, 2000
429] Kirsh M. & Schackert G., et al. Anti-angiogenic treatment strategies for malignant brain tumours. J Neurooncol. 50(1-2):149-63, Oct-Nov, 2000
430] Krishnaswamy K. & Raghuramulu N. Bioactive phytochemicals with emphasis on dietary practices. Indian J Med Res. 108:167-81. Review. Nov, 1998
431] Kritchevsky D. Antimutagenic and some other effects of conjugated linoleic acid. Br J Nutr. 83(5):459-65. Review. May, 2000
432] Kritz H., et al. Low cholesterol and cancer. J Clin Oncol. 14(11):3043-8, 1996
433] Kubo K., Aoki H. & Nanba H. Anti-diabetic activity present in the fruit body of Grifola frondosa (maitake). I. Biol Pharm Bull. 17:1106-1110, 1994
434] Kubo K. & Nanba H. Anti-hyperliposis effect of maitake fruit body (Grifola frondosa). I. Biol Pharm Bull. 20:781-785, 1997
435] Kubo K. & Nanba H. Modification of cellular immune responses in experimental autoimmune hepatitis in mice by mistake (Grifola frondosa). Mycoscience. 39:351-360, 1998
436] Kuhnau J. The flavonoids A class of semi-essential food components: their role in human nutrition. World Rev Nutr Diet. 24:117-91, 1976
437] Kumakura S., Yamashita M. & Tsurufuji S. Effect of bromelain on kaolin-induced inflammation in rats. Eur J Pharmacol. 150(3):295-301, Jun 10, 1988
438] Kumar P. Tumour hypoxia and anemia: impact on the efficacy of radiation therapy. Semin Hematol. 37(4 Suppl 6):4-8, Oct, 2000
439] Kumerova A., et al. Anaemia and antioxidant defence of the red blood cells. Mater Med Pol. 30:12-15, 1998
440] Kune G., et al. Dietary sodium and potassium intake and colorectal cancer risk. Nutr Cancer. 12:351-9, 1989
441] Kune G.A., Vitetta L. Alcohol consumption and the aetiology of colorectal cancer; a review of the scientific evidence from 1957 to 1991. Nutr Cancer. 18:97-111, 1992
442] Kunikata T., et al. Indirubin inhibits inflammatory reactions in delayed-type hypersensitivity. Eur J Pharmacol. 410:93-100, 2000
443] Kuo M.L., Huang T.S. & Lin J.K. Curcumin, an antioxidant and anti-tumor promoter, induces apoptosis in human leukemia cells. Biochim Biophys Acta. 1317:95-100, 1996
444] Kurbacher C.M., et al. Ascorbic acid (vitamin C) improves the antineoplastic

178

activity of doxorubicin, cisplatin and paclitaxel in human breast carcinoma cells in vitro. Cancer Lett. 103:183-9, 1996

445] Kurzer M.S., et al. Dietary phytoestrogens. Annu Rev Nutr. 17:353-81, 1997

446] Labadarios D., Walker A.R.P. Dietary avoidance of coronary heart disease-How practicable is the Mediterranean Diet? Cardiovasc J So Afr Cardiovascular Suppl. 1: C30-C36, 1996

447] Lackey B.R., Gray S.L. & Henricks D.M. Synergistic approach to cancer therapy: exploiting interactions between anti-estrogens, retinoids, monoterpenes and tyrosine kinase inhibitors. Med Hypotheses. 54(5):832-6. Review. May, 2000

448] Laganiere S., Femandes G. High peroxidizability of subcellular membrane induced by high fish oil diet is reversed by vitamin E. Clin Res. 35:A565, 1987

449] Lajer H. & Daugaard G. Cisplatin and hypomagnesemia. Cancer Treat Rev. 25(1):47-58. Review. Feb, 1999

450] Lamm D.L., et al. Megadose vitamins in bladder cancer: a double-blind clinical trial. J Urol. 151(1):21-6, 1994

451] Lamson D.W. & Brignall M.S. Antioxidants and cancer therapy II: quick reference guide. Altern Med Rev. 5(2):152-63, Apr, 2000

452] Lane I. W. & Contreras E. Jr. High rate of bioactivity (reduction in gross tumor size) observed in advanced cancer patients treated with shark cartilage material. J Naturopath Med. 3(1):86-8, 1992

453] Langer R. & Murray J. Angiogenesis inhibitors and their delivery systems. Appl Biochem Biotechnol. 8(1):9-24, 1983

454] Larocca L.M., et al. Quercetin and the growth of leukemic progenitors. Leuk Lymphoma. 23(1-2):49-53, 1996

455] Lashner B.A., et al. The effect of folic acid supplementation on the risk for cancer or dysplasia in ulcerative colitis. Gastroenterology. 112(1):29-32, 1997

456] Lasky S.R., et al. Effects of 1 alpha, 25-dihydroxyvitamin D3 on the human chronic myelogenous leukemia cell line RWLeu-4. Cancer Res. 50:3087-3094, 1990

457] Lathia D. & Blum A. Role of vitamin E as nitrite scavenger and N-nitrosamine inhibitor: a review. Int J Vitam Nutr Res. 59(4):430-8, 1989

458] La Vecchia C., et al. Intake of selected micronutrients and risk of colorectal cancer. Int J Cancer. 73:525-30, 1997

459] Leake A., et al. Subcellular distribution of zinc in the benign and malignant human prostate: evidence for a direct zinc androgen interaction. Acta Endocrinol (Copenhagen). 105:281-288, 1984

460] Le Bon A.M. & Siess M.H. Organosulfur compounds from Allium and the chemoprevention of cancer. Drug Metabol Drug Interact. 17(1-4):51-79, 2000

461] Leclerc S, et al. Indirubins inhibit glycogen synthase kinase-3 beta and CDK5/ p25, two protein kinases involved in abnormal tau phosphorylation in Alzheimer's dissease. A property common to most cyclin-dependent kinase inhibitors? J Biol Chem. 276:251-260, 2001

462] Lee A. & Langer R. Shark cartilage contains inhibitors of tumor angiogenesis. Science. 221:1185-7, 1983

463] Lee J.R. Fluoridation and bone cancer. Editorial. Fluoride. 26(2):79-82, 1993

464] Lee-Feldstein A. A comparison of several measures of exposure to arsenic. Matched case-control study of copper smelter employees. Am J Epidemiol. 129(1):112-24, 1989

465] Lefkowitz E.S. & Garland C.F. Sunlight, vitamin D and ovarian cancer mortality rates in US women. Epidemiol. 23(6):1133-6, 1994

466] Leipner J. & Saller R. Systemic enzyme therapy in oncology: effect and mode of action. Drugs. 59(4):769-80, Apr, 2000

467] Leis H.P. Endocrine Prophylaxis of Breast Cancer with Cyclic Estrogen and Progesterone. Intern Surg. 45:496-503, 1966

468] Lemon H.M. & Rodriguez-Sierra J.F. Timing of breast cancer surgery during the luteal menstrual phase may improve prognosis. Nebr Med J. 81(4):110-5, Apr, 1996

469] Levi F., et al. Dietary factors and the risk of endometrial cancer. Cancer. 71:3575-81, 1993

470] Leviton A. & Allred E.N. Correlates of decaffeinated coffee choice. Epidemiology. 5:537-40, 1994

471] Levonen A.L., et al. Mechanisms of cell signaling by nitric oxide and peroxynitrite: from mitochondria to MAP kinases. Antioxid Redox Signal. 3(2):215-29, Apr, 2001

472] Levy L. & Vredevoe D.L. The effect of N-acetyl cysteine on cyclophosphamide immunoregulation and antitumor activity. Semin Oncol. 10(1 Suppl 1):7-16, 1983

473] Liang J.Y., et al. Inhibitory effect of zinc on human prostatic carcinoma cell growth. Prostate. 40(3):200-207, 1999

474] Liehr J.G. Catechol Estrogens as Mediators of Estrogen-induced Carcinogenesis. Cancer Res. 35:704, 1994

475] Liehr J.G. Genotoxic Effects of Estrogens. Mutat Res. 238(3):269-276, 1990

476] Liehr J.G. Mechanisms of Metabolic Activation and Inactivation of Catecholestrogens: A Basis of Genotoxicity. Polycyclic Aromatic Compounds. 6:229-239, 1994

477] Liehr J.G., et al. 4-Hydroxylation of Estradiol by Human Uterine Myomerium and Myoma Microsomes: Implications for the Mechanism of Uterine Turmorigenesis. Proc Nat Acad Sci. 92:1229-1233, 1995

478] Ling-Wei X., et al. Trace element content of drinking water of nasopharyngeal carcinoma patients. Trace Elements in Medicine. %(3):93-6, 1988

479] Lipkin M. & Newmark H. Effect of added dietary calcium on colonic epithelial-cell proliferation in subjects at high risk for familial colonic cancer. N Engl J Med. 313:1381-4, 1985

480] Lipman T., et al. Esophageal zinc content in human squamous esophageal cancer. J am Coll Nutr. 6:41-6, 1987

481] Lipworth L., et al. Olive oil and human cancer: an assessment of the evidence. Prev Med. 26:181-90, 1997

482] Litaka M., et al. Induction of apoptosis and necrosis by zinc in human thyroid cancer cell lines. J Endocrinol. 169(2):417-24, May, 2001

483] Liu N. & Lapcevich R.K., et al. Metastatin: a hyaluronan-binding complex from cartilage that inhibits tumour growth. Cancer Res. 61(3):1022-8, Feb, 2001

484] Liu X.M., et al. Induction of differentiation and down-regulation of c-myb gene expression in ML-1 human myeloblastic leukemia cells by the clinically effective anti-leukemia agent meisoindigo. Biochem Pharmacol. 51:1545-1551, 1996

485] Llang J., et al. Indole-3-carbinol prevents cervical cancer in human papilloma virus type 16 (HPV16) transgenic mice. Cancer Research. 59:3991-3997, 1999

486] Locigno R. & Castronovo V. Reduced glutathione system: role in cancer development, prevention and treatment (review). Int J Oncol. 19(2):221-36. Review. Aug, 2001

487] Lockwood K., et al. Partial and complete regression of breast cancer in patients in relation to dosage of coenzyme Q10. Biochem Biophys Res Commun. 199(3):1504-8, 1994a

488] Lockwood K., et al. Apparent partial remission of breast cancer in 'high risk' patients supplemented with nutritional antioxidants, essential fatty acids and coenzyme Q10. Molec Aspects Med. 15(suppl):S231-S240, 1994b

489] Lockwood K., et al. Progress in therapy of breast cancer with vitamin Q10 and the regression of metastases. Biochem Biophys Res Commun. 212(1):172-7, 1995

490] Longnecker M.P. Alcoholic beverage consumption in relation to risk of breast cancer: meta-analysis and review. Cancer Causes Control. %(1):73-82, 1994

491] Losonczy K.G., et al. Vitamin E and vitamin C supplement use and risk of all-cause and coronary heart disease mortality in older persons: the Established Populations for Epidemiologic Studies of the Elderly. Am J Clin Nutr. 64:190-6, 1996

492] Lotz-Winter H. On the pharmacology of bromelain: an update with special regard to animal studies on dose-dependent effects. Planta Med. 56(3):249-53. Review. Jun, 1990

493] Lund E.L. & Spang-Thomsen M., et al. Tumour angioenesis-a new therapeutic target in gliomas. Acta Neurol Scand. 97(1):52-62. Review. Jan, 1998

494] Luo X.M., et al. Molybdenum and oesophageal cancer in China. Federation Proceedings. Federation of the American Society for Experimental Biology. 46:928, 1981

495] Luo X.M., et al. Inhibitory effects of molybdenum on esophageal and forestomach carcinogenesis in rats. J Natl. Cancer Inst. 71:75-80, 1983

496] MacDonald H.B. Conjugated linoleic acid and disease prevention: a review of current knowledge. J Am Coll Nutr. 19(2 suppl):111S-118S. Review. Apr, 2000

497] MacGregor J.T., et al. Cytogenetic damage induced by folate deficiency in mice is enhanced by caffeine. Proc Natl Acad Sci USA. 87(24):9962-5, 1990

498] Mahon F.X., et al. All-trans retinoic acid potentiates the inhibitory effects of interferon alpha on chronic myeloid leukemia progenitors in vitro. Leukemia. 11:667-673, 1997

499] Malafa M.P. & Neitzel L.T. Vitamin E succinate promotes breast cancer tumour dormancy. J Surg Res. 93(1):163-70, Sep, 2000

500] Malloy V. L., et al. Interaction between a semisynthetic diet and indole-3-carbinol on mammary tumor incidence in Balb/cfC3H mice. Anticancer Research.

17(6D):4333-4337, 1997

501] Malter M., et al. Natural killer cells, vitamins and other blood components of vegetarian and omnivorous men. Nutr Cancer. 12(3):271-8, 1989

502] Malvy D.J.M., et al. Assessment of serum antioxidant micronutrients and biochemical indicators of nutritional status in children with cancer in search of prognostic factors. Int J Vitam Nutr Res. 67:267-71, 1997

503] Mann J. Position statement: nutrition options when reducing saturated fat intake. J Am Coll Nutr. 11(S):82S-83S, 1992

504] Mantovani G., et al. Restoration of functional defects in peripherial blood mononuclear cells isolated from cancer patients by thiol antioxidants alpha-ipoic acid and N-acetyl cysteine. Int J Cancer. 86(6):842-7, Jun 15, 2000

505] Marino A.A. & Iliev I.G., et al. Association between cell membrane potential and breast cancer. Tumour Biol. 15(2):82-9, 1994

506] Marko D., et al. Inhibition of cyclin-dependent kinase 1 (CDK1) by indirubin derivatives in human tumour cells. Br J Cancer. 84:283-289, 2001

507] Martinez M.E. & Willett W.C. Calcium, vitamin D and colorectal cancer: a review of the epidemioligic evidence. Cancer Epidemiol Biomarkers Prev. 7(2):163-8, 1998

508] Martin-Himenez M., et al. Failure of high-dose tocopherol to prevent alopecia induced by doxorubicin. Letter. N Engl J Med. 315(14):894-5, 1986

509] Matikainen S. & Hurme M. Comparison of retinoic acid and phorbol myristate acetate as inducers of monocytic differentiation. Int J Cancer. 57:98-103, 1994

510] Matthews J. Sharks still intrigue cancer researchers. J Natl Cancer Inst. 84(13):1000-2, 1992

511] Matzkin H., et al. Immunohistochemical evidence of the existence and localization of aromatase in human prostatic tissues. Prostate. 21:309-314, 1992

512] Maurer H.R. Bromelain: biochemistry, pharmacology and medical use. Cell Mol Life Sci. 58(9):1234-45. Review. Aug, 2001

513] Mayne S.T. Nutrition intake and risk of subtypes of esophageal and gastric cancer. Cancer Epidemiol Biomarkers Prev. 10(10):1055-62, Oct, 2001

514] McCarty M.F. An anti thrombotic role for nutritional antioxidants: Implications for tumour metastasis and other pathologies. Med Hypotheses. 19:345-57, 1986

515] McCarty M.F. Fish oil may impede tumour angiogenesis and invasiveness by down-regulating protein kinase C and modulating eicosanoid production. Med Hypotheses. 46(2):107-15. Review. Feb, 1996

516] McCarty M.F. Polyphenol-mediated inhibition of AP-1 transactivating activity may slow cancer growth by impeding angiogenesis and tumour in invasiveness? Med Hypotheses. 50:511-514, 1998

517] McCarty M.F. Current prospects for controlling cancer growth with non-cytotoxic agents-nutrients, phytochemicals, herbal extracts and available drugs. Med Hypotheses. 56(2):137-54, Feb, 2001

518] McCarthy M. Selenium linked to lower prostate cancer risk [letter]. Lancet. 352:713, 1998

519] McConnell K.P., et al. The relationship between dietary selenium and breast cancer. Journal of Surgical Oncology. 15(1):67-70, 1980

520] McKeown-Eyssen G., et al. A randomized trial of vitamins C and E in the prevention of recurrence of colorectal polyps. Cancer Res. 48(16):4701-5, 1988

521] McIllmurray M.B. & Turkie W. Controlled trial of gamma linolenic acid in Dukes's C colorectal cancer. Br Med J. 294:1260, 1987

522] Medina V., et al. Sodium butyrate inhibits carcinoma development in a 1,2-dimethylhydrazine-induced rat colon cancer. JPEN J Parenter Enteral Nutr. 22(1):14-17, 1998

523] Meguid M., et al. Plasma carotenoid profiles in normals and patients with cancer. J Parenter Enteral Nutr. 12(2):147-51, 1988

524] Mellibovsky L., et al. Long-standing remission after 25-OH D3 treatment in a case of chronic myelonomocytic leukaemia. Br J Haematol. 85:811-812, 1993

524] Meng Q., et al. Indole-3-carbinol is a negative regulator of estrogen receptor-signaling in human tumor cells. Journal of Nutrition. 130:2927-2931, 2000

525] Meng Q., Qi M. & Chen D.Z., et al. Suppression of breast cancer invasion and migration by indole-3-carbinol: associated with up-regulation of BRCA1 and E-cadherin/catenin complexes. J Mol Med. 78(3):155-65, 2000

526] Menkes M.S., et al. Serum beta-carotene, vitamins A and E, selenium and the risk of lung cancer. NEJM. 315:1250, 1986

527] Menter D.G., Sabichi A.L. & Lippman S.M. Selenium effects on prostate cell growth. Cancer Epidemiol Biomarkers Prev. 9(11):1171-82, Nov, 2000

528] Messina M.J., et al. Soy intake and cancer risks: a review of the in vitro and in vivo data. Nutr Cancer. 21:113:31, 1994

529] Mettlin C.J., et al. Patterns of milk consumption and risk of cancer. Nutr Cancer. 12:89-99, 1990

530] Meydani S.N. & Dinarello C.A. Influence of dietary fatty acids on cytokine production and its clinical implications. Nutr Clin Pract. 8(2):65-72. Review. 1993

531] Meysken F.L. Jr., et al. Effects of vitamin A on survival in patients with chronic myelogenous leukemia: a SWOG randomixed trial. Leuk Res. 19:605-612, 1995

532] Mikhail M.S, Palan P.R. & Romney S.L. Coenzyme Q10 and alpha-tocopherol concentrations in cervical intraepithelial neoplasia and cervic cancer. Obstet Gynecol. 97(4 Suppl 1):S3, Apr, 2001

533] Milde et al. Serum levels of selenium, manganese, copper and iron in colorectal patients. Biol Trace Elem Res (USA) .79 (2) 107-14, 2001

534] Milenic D.E., et al. Comparison of methods for the generation of immunoreactive fragments of a monoclonal antibody (B72.3) reactive with human carcinomas. JimmunolMethods. 120(1):71-83, 2, 1989

535] Miller A.L. Therapeutic considerations of L-glutamine: a review of the literature. Altern Med Rev. 4(4):239-48, Aug, 1999

536] Milner J.A. A historical perspective on garlic and cancer. J Nutr. 131(3s):1027S-31S, Mar, 2001

537] Ming X., Yin H. & Zhu Z. Effect of dietary selenium and germanium on the precancerous lesion in rat glandular stomach induced by N-methyl-N'-nitro-N-nitrosoguanidine. Zhonghua Wai Ke Za Zhi. 34(4):221-3, Apr, 1996

538] Miyazawa K. & Yaguchi M., et al. Apoptosis/differentiation-inducing effects of vitamin K2 on HL-60 cells: dichotomous nature of vitamin K2 in leukemia cells. Leukemia. 15(7):1111-7, Jul, 2001

539] Mizegewski G.J. Role of integrins in cancer: survey of expression patterns. Pros Soc Exp Biol Med. 222(2):124-38, Nov, 1999

540] Moerman C.J., et al. Consumption of foods and micronutrients and the risk of cancer of the biliary-tract. Prev Med. 24(6):591-602, 1995

541] Moertel C.G., et al. High-dose vitamin C versus placebo in the treatment of patients with advanced cancer who have had no prior chemotherapy: A randomized double-blind comparison. N Engl J Med. 312:137-41, 1985

542] Mohr P.E., Wang D.Y., Gregory W.M., Richards M.A. and Fentiman I.S. Serum Progesterone and Prognosis in Operable Breast cancer. Brit J Cancer. 73:1552-1555, 1996

543] Molinari M. Cell cycle checkpoints and their inactivation in human cancer. Cell Prolif. 33(5):261-74. Review. Oct, 2000

544] Momparler R.L. & Bovenzi V. DNA methylation and cancer. J Cell Physiol. 183(2):145-54. Review. May, 2000

545] Moon T.E., et al. Retinoids in prevention of skin cancer. Cancer Lett. 114:203-5, 1997

546] Moore W.E. & Moore L.H. Intestinal floras of populations that have a high risk of colon cancer. Appl Environ Microbiol. 61(9):3202-7, 1995

547] Mori K., et al. Anti-tumor action of fruit body of edible mushrooms orally administered to mice. Mushroom Sci. XII:653-660, 1987

548] Morrow D.M & Fitzsimmons P.E., et al. Dietary supplementation with the anti-tumour promoter quercetin: its effects on matrix metalloproteinase gene regulation. Mutat Res. 480-481:269-76, Sep 1, 2001

549] Morton M.S., et al. Lignans and isoflavonoids in plasma and prostatic fluid in men: samples from Portugal, Hong Kong and the United Kingdom. Prostate. 32:122-8, 1997

550] Motoo Y. & Sawabu N. Antitumour effects of saikosaponins, baicalin and baicalein on human hepatoma cell lines. Cancer Lett. 86(1):91-5, Oct 28, 1994

551] Moulder J.E. & Rockwell S. Tumour hypoxia: its impact on cancer therapy. Cancer Metastasis Rev. 5(4):313-41. Review. 1987

552] Mufti S.I. Alcohol acts to promote incidence of tumors. Cancer Detect Prev. 16(3):157-62, 1992

553] Muindi J.R. Retinoids in clinical cancer therapy. Cancer Treat Res. 87:305-42, 1996

554] Muñoz N., et al. No effect of riboflavine, retinol and zinc on prevalence of precancerous lesions of lesions of oestophagus. Randomised double-blind intervention study in high-risk population of China. Lancet. ii:111-14, 1985

555] Murono S. & Yoshizaki T., et al. Aspirin inhibits tumour cell invasiveness induced by Epstein-Barr virus latent membrane protein 1 through suppression of matrix metalloproteinase-9 expression. Cancer Res. 60(9):2555-61. May 1, 2000

556] Muscaritoli M., et al. Oral glutamine in the prevention of chemotherapy-induced gastrointestinal toxicity. Eur J Cancer. 33:319-20, 1997

557] Muto Y., et al. Prevention of second primary tumors by an acyclic retinoid, polyprenoic acid, in patients with hepatocellular carcinoma. N Engl J Med. 334:1561-7, 1996

558] Myers C., et al. A randomized controlled trial assessing the prevention of doxorubicin cardiomyopathy by N-acetylcysteine. Semin Oncol 10(1 Suppl 1):53-5, 1983

559] Nagabhushan M. & Bhide S.V. Curcumin as an inhibitor of cancer. J Am Coll Nutr. 11:192-198, 1992

560] Nagata C., et al. Relations of Insulin Resistance and Serum Concentrations of Estradiol and Sex Hormone-binding Globulin to Potential Breast Cancer Risk Factors. Jpn J Cancer Res. 91(9):948-953, 2000

561] Nair P.P., et al. Diet, nutrient intake and metabolism in populations at high and low risk for colon cancer: Dietary cholesterol, beta-sitosterol and stigmasterol. Am J Clin Nutr. 40(4 suppl):927-30, 1984

562] Nakadaira H., et al. Distribution of selenium and molybdenum and cancer mortality in Niigata, Japan. Arch Envir Health Sep. 50:5 374-80, 1995

563] Nakakoshi T. Copper and hepatocellular carcinoma. Radiology (United States), Jan. 214(1) p304-6, 2000

564] Nanba H., Hamaguchi A. & Kuroda H. The chemical structure of an antitumor polysaccharide in fruit bodies of Grifola frondosa (maitake). Chem Pharm Bull. 35:1162-1168, 1987

565] Nanba H. Antitumor activity of orally administered "D-Fraction" from maitake mushroom (Grifola frondosa). J Naturopathic Med. 1:10-15, 1993

566] Nebeling L.C. & Lerner E. Implementing a ketogenic diet based on medium-chain triglyceride oil in pediatric patients with cancer. J Am Diet Assoc. 95(6):693-7. Review. Jun, 1995

567] Nebeling L.C. & Miraldi F., et al. Effects of a ketogenic diet on tumour metabolism and nutritional status in pediatric oncology patients: two case reports. J Am Coll Nutr. 14(2):202-8, Apr, 1995

568] Negri I., et al. Intake of selected micronutrients and the risk of breast cancer. Int J Cancer. 65:140-4, 1996

569] Nehlig A. & Debry G. Coffee and cancer: a review of human and animal data. World Rev Nutr Diet. 79:185- 221, 1997

570] Nelson R.L. Is the changing pattern of colorectal cancer caused by selenium deficiency? Dis Colon Rectum. 459-461, 1984

571] Nelson R.L., et al. Serum selenium and colonic neoplastic risk. Diseases of the Colon and Rectum. 38:1306-1310, 1995

572] Neuzil J. & Weber T., et al. Selective cancer cell killing by alpha-tocopheryl succinate. Br J Cancer. 84(1):87-9, Jan 5, 2001

573] Newmark H.L., et al. Colon cancer and dietary fat, phosphate and calcium: A hypothesis. J Natl Cancer Inst. 72(6):1323-5, 1984

574] Newmark H.K. Vitamin D adequacy. A possible relationship to breast cancer. Adv Exp Med Biol. 364:109-114, 1994

575] Niakan B. Repression of the enzyme lactate dehydrogenase and the spontaneous remission or regression of cancer. Med Hypotheses. 56(5):693-4, May, 2001

576] Nicolodi M. & Sicuteri F. Fibromyalgia and migraine, two faces of the same mechanism. Serotonin as the common clue for pathogenesis and therapy. Adv Exp Med Biol. 398:373-9, 1996

577] Nicolodi M. & Sicuteri F. L-5-hydroxytrypotophan can prevent nociceptive disorders in man. Adv Exp Med Biol. 467:177-82, 1999

578] Nieswandt B., et al. Lysis of tumour cells by natural killer cells in mice is impeded by platelets. Cancer Res. 59(6):1295-300, Mar 15, 1999

579] {No authors listed}. American Institute for Cancer Research 10th annual research conference: The role of nutrition in preventing and treating breast and prostate cancer. Washington, DC, USA. August 31-September 1, 2000. Abstracts J Nutr. 131⊗1):151S-203S, Jan, 2001

580] {No auther listed}. Beetroot: substitution of oxidative enzymes. Schweiz Rundsch Med Prax. 76(42):1162-4, Oct 13, 1987

581] Nomura A.M., et al. Serum micronutrients and upper aerodigestive tract cancer. Cancer Epidemiol Biomark Prevent. 6:407-12, 1997

582] Nordsmark M. & Overgaard M., et al. Pretreatment oxygenation predicts radiation response in advanced squamous cell carcinoma of the head and neck. Radiother Oncol. 41:31-9, Oct, 1996

583] Nordsmark M., et al. Hypoxia in human soft tissue sarcomas: adverse impact on survival and no association with p53 mutations. Br J Cancer. 84(8):1070-5, 20, 2001

584] Norie I.H. & Foster H.D. Water quality and cancer of the digestive tract: The Canadian experience. J Orthomol Med. 4(2):59-69, 1989

585] Normnan A., et al. Antitumor activity of sodium linoleate. Nutr Cancer. 11(2):107-15, 1988

586] Novi A.M. Regression of aflatoxin B1-induced hepatocellular carcinoma by reduced glutathione. Science. 212:541-2, 1981

587] Nwankwo J.O. Mechanism of chemical carcinogenesis: an alternative hypothesis. Med Hypotheses. 35(4):330-6, August, 1991

588] Nydegger U.E. & Davis J.S. Soluble immune complexes in human disease. Crit Rev Clin Lab Sci. 12;123, 1980

589] Oberringer M. & Lothschutz D., et al. Centrosome multiplication accompanies a transient clustering of polyploid cells during tissue repair. Mol Cell Biol Res Commun. 2(3):190-6, Sep-Dec, 1999

590] Obrador E. & Carretero J., et al. Possible mechanisms for tumour cell sensitivity to TNF-alpha and potential therapeutic applications. Curr Pharm Biotechnol. 2:119-30, Jun, 2001

591] O'Conner H.J., et al. Effect of increased intake of vitamin C on the mutagenic activity of gastric juice and intragastric concentrations of ascorbic acid. Carcinogenesis. 6(11):1675-6, 1985

592] Odeleye O.E. & Watson R.R. Health implications of the n-3 fatty acids. Letter.

Am J Clin Nutr. 53:177-81, 1991

593] O'Flaherty T.J. Biology of Disease-lipid mediators of inflammation and allergy. Lab Invest. 47:314-29, 1982

594] Ogawa K. & Hirai M., et al. Suppression of cellular immunity by surgical stress. Surgery. 127(3):329-36, Mar, 2000

595] Omenn G.S., et al. Effects of a combination of beta carotene and vitamin A on lung cancer and cardiovascular disease. N Engl J Med. 334:1150-5, 1996

596] Ono K. & Han J. The p38 signal transduction pathway: activation and function. Cell Signal. 12(1):1-13. Review. Jan, 2000

597] Opal S.M. & DePalo V.A. Anti-inflammatory cytokines. Chest. 117)4):1162-72. Review. Apr, 2000

598] Orr J.W. Jr., et al. Nutritional status of patients with untreated cervical cancer. II. Vitamin assessment. Am J Obstet Gynecol. 151(5):632-5, 1985

599] Osborne M.P., et al. Upregulation of Estradiol C16-alpha-hydroxylation in HumanBreast Tissue: A Potential Biomarker of Breast Cancer Risk. J Nat Cancer Inst. 85(23):1917-1993, 1993

600] O'Toole P. & Lombard M. Vitamin C and gastric cancer: Supplements for some or fruit for all? Gut. 39:345-7, 1996

601] Overgaard J. & Horsman M.R. Modification of Hypoxia-Induced Radioresistance in Tumours by the Use of Oxygen and Sensitizers. Semin Radiat Oncol. 6(1):10-21, Jan, 1996

602] Owen R.W., et al. Analysis of calcium-lipid complexes in faeces. Eur J Cancer Prev. 43(3):247-55, 1995

603] Owen R.W. Faecal steroids and colorectal carcinogenesis. Scand J Gastroenterol Suppl. 222:76-82, 1997

604] Ozeki Y. & Mitsui Y., et al. Ribose 1,5-bisphosphate regulates rat kidney cortex phosphofructokinase. Comp Biochem Physiol B Biochem Mol Biol. 124(3):327-32, Nov, 1999

605] Page G.G. & Ben-Eliyahu S., et al. Morphine attenuates surgery-induced enhancement of metastatic colonization in rats. Pain. 54(1):21-8, Jul, 1993

606] Pagnanelli G.M., et al. Effect of vitamin A, C and E supplementation on rectal cell proliferation in patients with colorectal adenomas. J Natl Cancer Inst. 84:47-51, 1992

607] Pais R.C., et al. Abnormal vitamin B6 status in childhood leukemia. Cancer. 66(11):2421-8, 1990

608] Palan P., et al. Decreased b-carotene tissue levels in uterine leiomyomas and cancers of reproductive and nonreproductive organs. Am J Obstet Gynecol. 161:1649-52, 1989

609] Palmierei-Sevier A., et al. Case report: long-term remission of parathyroid cancer: possible relation to vitamin D and calcitriol therapy. Am J Med Sci. 306(5):309-12, 1993

610] Pan W.H., et al. Vitamin A, vitamin E, or beta-carotene status and hepatitis B-related hepatocellular carcinoma. Ann Epidemiol. 3:217-24, 1993

611] Parazzini F., et al. Alcohol and endometrial cancer risk: findings from an Italian case-controlled study. Nutr Cancer. 23(1):55-61, 1995

612] Park C.J., et al. Sweet's syndrome during the treatment of acute promyelocytic leukemia with all-trans retinoic acid. Korean J Intern Med. 16:218-221, 2001

613] Park H.J., et al. Nodular hidradenocarcinoma with prominent squamous differentiation: case report and immunohistochemical study. Eur J Cancer. 32A(3):540-6, 1996

614] Park J.S., et al. Zinc finger of replication protein A, a non-DNA binding element, regulates its DNA binding activity through redox. J Biol Chem. 274(41):29075-29080, 1999

615] Park K., et al. Stimulation of human breast cancers by dietary L-arginine. Clin Sci. 82:413-17, 1992

616] Pascoe G.A. & Reed D.J. Vitamin E protection against chemical-induced cell injury. II. Evidence for a threshold effect of cellular alpha-tocopherol in prevention of adriamycin toxicity. Arch Biochem Biophys. 256:159-66, 1987

617] Pearson C.A. & Prozialeck W.C. E-Cadherin, beta-Catenin and cadmium carcinogenesis. Med Hypotheses. 56(5):573-81. Review. May, 2001

618] Peng Q., Wei Z. & Lau B.H. Pycnogenol inhibits tumour necrosis factor-alpha-induced nuclear factor kappa B activation and adhesion molecule expression in human vascular endothelial cells. Cell Mol Life Sci. 57(5):834-41, May, 2000

619] Perdikis D.A., et al. Differential effects of mucosal pH on human (Caco-2) intestinal epithelial cell motility, proliferation and differentiation. Dig Dis Sci. 43(7):1537-46, 1998

620] Pervaiz S. Resveratrol-from the bottle to the bedside? Leuk Lymphoma. 40(5-6):491-8. Review.Feb, 2001

621] Petrek J.A., et al. Fatty acid composition of adipose tissue, an indication of dietary fatty acids, and breast cancer prognosis. J Clin Oncol. 15(4):1377-84, 1997

622] Peters J.M., Preston-Martin S. & London S.J., et al. Processed meats and risk of childhood leukemia. Cancer Causes Control. 5(2):195-202, 1994

623] Petzinger E. & Ziegler K. Ochratoxin A from a toxicological perspective. J Vet Pharmacol Ther. 23(2):91-8, Apr, 2000

624] Picurelli L., et al. Determination of serum Fe in prostatic pathology. Actas Urol Esp. 14(4):262-3, 1990 (in Spanish)

625] Pearce M.L. & Dayton S. Incidence of cancer in men on a diet high in polyunsaturated fats. Lancet I:464-7, 1971

626] Pinsolle V. & Ravaud A., et al. Does surgery promote the development of metastasis in melanoma? Ann Chir Plast Esthet. 45(4):485-93. Review. Aug, 2000

627] Planelle-Cases R. & Aracil A., et al. Arginine-rich peptides are blockers of VR-1 channels with analgesic activity. FEBS Lett. 481(2):131-6, Sep 15, 2000

628] Plate K.H. & Breier G., et al. Molecular mechanisms of developmental and tumour angiogenesis. Brain Pathol. 4(3):207-18. Review. Jul, 1994

629] Pokotny J. Natural toxic substances in food. Cas Lek Cesk. 136(9):267-270, 1997

630] Popiela T., et al. Double-blind pilot-study on the efficacy of enzyme therapy in advanced colorectal cancer. Przegl Lek. 57 Suppl 5:142, 2000

631] Popiela T., et al. Influence of a complementary treatment with oral enzymes on patients with colorectal cancers-an epidemiological retrolective cohort study. Cancer Chemother Pharmacol. 47 Suppl:S55-63, Jul, 2001

632] Popov A.I. Effect of the nonspecific prevention of thrombogenic complications on late results in the combined treatment of bladder cancer. Med Radiol (Mosk). 32(2):42-45, 1987

633] Porcelli B., et al. Levels of folic acid in plasma and red blood cells of colorectal cancer patients. Biomed Pharmacother. 50(6-7):303-5, 1996

634] Portenoy R.K. & Lesage P. md. Management of cancer pain. The Lancet. April 21, 2001

635] Potter J.D. & McMichael A.J. Alcohol, beer and lung cancer: A meaningful relationship? Int J Epidemiol. 13(2):240-2, 1984

636] Potischman N., et al. A case-control study of serum folate levels and invasive cervical cancer. Cancer Res. 51(18):4785-9, 1991

637] Pozniak P.C. The carcinogenicity of caffeine and cancer: A review. J Am Diet Assoc. 85(9):1127-33, 1985

638] Prasad K.N., et al. Sodium ascorbate potentiates the growth inhibitory effect of certain agents on neuroblastoma cells in culture. Proc Natl Acad Sci USA. 76(2):829-32, 1979

639] Prasad K.N. Modulation of the effects of tumor therapeutic agents by vitamin C. Life Sci. 27(4):275-80, 1980a

640] Prasad K.N., et al. Vitamin E increases the growth inhibitory and differentiating effects of tumor therapeutic agents on neuroblastoma and glioma cells in culture. Proc Soc Exp Biol Med. 164(2):158-63, 1980b

641] Prasad K.N. & Edwards-Prasad J. Vitamin E and cancer prevention: recent advances and future potentials. J Am Coll Nutr. 11(5):487-500, 1992

642] Preston T. & Slater C., et al. Fibrinogen synthesis is elevated in fasting cancer patients with an acute phase response. J Nutr. 128(8):1355-60, Aug, 1998

643] Pribluda V.S. & Gubish E.R. Jr., et al. 2-Methoxyestradiol: an endogenousantiangiogenic and antiproliferative drug candidate. Cancer Metastasis Rev. 19(1-2):173-9. Review. 2000

644] Prinz-Lingenohl R., Fohr I. & Pictrzik K. Beneficial role for folate in the prevention of colorectal and breast cancer. Nutr 40(3):98-105, Jun, 2001

645] Prior F. Theoretical involvement of vitamin B6 in tumor initiation. Med Hypotheses. 16:421-8, 1985

646] Pritchard G.A., et al. Lipids in breast carcinogenesis. Br J Surg. 76(10):1069-73, 1989

647] Prudden J.F. The treatment of human cancer with agents prepared from bovine cartilage. J Biol Response Mod. 4(6):551-84, 1985

648] Pujol P., Hilsenbeck S.G., Chamness G.C. and Elledge R.M. Rising Levels of Estrogen Receptor in Breast Cancer over 2 Decades. Cancer. 74:1601-1606, 1994

649] Rabsberger K. & Maehder K. The significance of proteolytic enzyme therapy as a component of cancer treatment. Osterr Z Erforsch Bekampf Krebskr. 28(5-6):187-93, 1973(in German)

650] Rao A.V., et al. Effect of fiber-rich foods on the composition of intestinal flora. Nutr Res. 14(4):523-35, 1994

651] Rasmussen L.B., et al. Effect of diet and plasma fatty acid composition on immune status in elderly men. Am J Clin Nutr. 59:572-7, 1994

652] Rato A.G. & Pedrero J.G., et al. Melatonin blocks the activation of estrogen receptor for DNA binding. FAS EB J. 13(8):857-68, May, 1999

653] Redman C., et al. Involvement of polyamines in selenomethionine induced apoptosis and mitotic alterations in human tumour cells. Carcinogenesis. 18(6):1195-1202, 1997

654] Redman C., et al. Inhibitory effect of selenomethionine on the growth of three selected human tumour cell lines. Cancer Letters. 125(1-2):103-110, 1998

655] Reddy V.G. & Khanna N., et al. Vitamin C augments chemotherapeutic response of cervical carcinoma HeLa cells by stabilizing P53. Biochem Biophys Res Commun. 282(2):409-15, Mar 30, 2001

656] Reed M.J. and Purohit A. Breast Cancer and the Role of Cytokines in Regulating Estrogen Synthesis: An Emerging Hypothesis. Endocrine Rev. 18:701-715, 1997

657] Reich R., et al. Eicosapentaenoic acid reduces the invasive and metastatic activities of malignant tumor cells. Biochem Biophys Res Commun. 160:559-64, 1989

658] Reichel H., et al. The role of the vitamin D endocrine system in health and disease. N Engl J Med. 320(15):980-91, 1989

659] Reinacher-Schick A. & Petrasch S., et al. Helicobacter pylori induces apoptosis in mucosal lymphocytes in patients with gastritis. Z Gastroenterol. 36(12):1021-6, Dec, 1998

660] Reynolds J., et al. Arginine as an immunomodulator. Abstract. Surg Forum. 38:415-18, 1987

661] Rhodes E.L., Misch K.J. & Edwards J.M., et al. Dipyridamole for treatment of melanoma. Lancet. 1(8430):693, 1985

662] Rickles F.R. & Falanga A. Molecular basis for the relationship between thrombosis and cancer. Thromb Res. 102(6):V215-V224, Jun 15, 2001

663] Riordan N.H., et al. Intravenous ascorbate as a tumor cytotoxic chemotherapeutic agent. Med Hypotheses. 44:207-13, 1995

664] Riordan H.D., et al. High dose intravenous vitamin C in the treatment of a patient with renal cell carcinoma of the kidney. J Orthomo Med. 13(2):72-73, 1998

665] Risch H.A., et al. Dietary fat intake and risk of epithelial ovarian cancer. J Natl Cancer Inst. 86(18):1409-15, 1994

666] Rivadeneira D.E., et al. Nutritional support of the cancer patient. CA Cancer J Clin. 48(2):69-80, 1998

667] Rock C.L. Carotenoids: biology and treatment. Pharmacol Ther. 75(3):185-97, 1997

668] Rodriquez C., Calle E.E., Coates R.J., Miracle-McMahill H.L., Thun M.J. and Heath C.W. Estrogen Replacement Therapy and Fatal Ovarian Cancer. Am J Epidemiol. 141:828-834, 1995

669] Rodrigue C.M., et al. Resveratrol, a natural dietary phytoalexin, possesses similar properties to hydroxyurea towards erythroid differentiation. Br J Haematol. 113(2):500-7, May, 2001

670] Rofstad E.K. & Sundfor K., et al. Hypoxia-induced treatment failure in advanced squamous cell carcinoma of the uterine cervix is primarily due to hypoxia-induced radiation resistance rather than hypoxia-induced metastasis. Br J Cancer. 83:354-9, Aug, 2000

671] Rokitansky O. Präoperative tumortherapie zur Verbessrung der Heilungsergebnisse beim Mammakarzinom. Krevegescgehan. 12:127-30, 1980(in German)

672] Roncucci L., et al. Antioxidant vitamins or lactulose for the prevention of the recurrence of colorectal adenomas. Dis Colon Rectum. 36:227-34, 1993

673] Rood J.C., et al. Helicobacter pylori-associated gastritis and the ascorbic acid concentration in gastric juice. Nutr Cancer. 22:65-72, 1994

674] Rose D.P. & Hatala M.A. Dietary fatty acids and breast cancer invasion and metastasis. Nutr Cancer. 21:103-11, 1994

675] Rose D.P. & Connolly J.M. Omega-3 fatty acids as cancer chemopreventive agents. Pharmacol Ther. 83(3):217-44. Review. Sep, 1999

676] Rose D.P. & Connolly J.M. Regulation of tumour angiogenesis by dietary fatty acids and eicosanoids. Nutr Cancer. 37(2):119-27. Review. 2000

677] Ross J., et al. Dietary and hormonal evaluation of men at different risks for prostate cancer: Fiber intake, excretion and composition, with in vitro evidence for an association between steroid hormones and specific fiber components. Am J Clin Nutr. 51:365-70, 1990

678] Roubenoff R. & Roubenoff R.A., et al. Abnormal vitamin B6 status in rheumatoid cachexia. Association with spontaneous tumour necrosis factor alpha production and markers of inflammation. Arthritis Rheum. 38(1):105-9, Jan, 1995

679] Rouse K., et al. Glutamine enhances selectivity of chemotherapy through changes in glutathione metabolism. Ann Surg. 221(4):420-6, 1995

680] Sacchi S., et al. All-trans retinoic acid in hematological malignancies, and update. GER (Gruppo Ematologico Retinoidi). Haematologica. 82:106-121, 1997

681] Sagayadan G.E., et al. Effect of retinoic acid and interferon alpha on granulocyte-macrophage colony forming cells in chronic myeloid leukemia: increased inhibition by all-trans- and 13-cis-retinoic acids in advanced stage disease. Leuk Res. 18:741-748, 1994

682] Saito M.,Kato H. & Tsuchida T., et al. Chemoprevention effects on bronchial squamous metaplasia by folate and vitamin B12 in heavy smokers. Chest. 102(2):496-9, 1994

683] Sakagami H. & Sato K. Effect of ascorbate oxidase on radical intensity and cytotoxic activity of ascorbate. Anticancer Res. 17(2A):1163-6, 1997

684] Sakalova A., et al. Retrolective cohort study of an additive therapy with an oral enzyme preparation in patients with multiple myeloma. Cancer Chemother Pharmacol. 47 Suppl:S38-44, Jul, 2001

685] Salminen E., et al. Preservation of intestinal integrity during radiotherapy using live Lactobacillus acidophilus cultures. Clin Radiol. 39:435-7, 1988

686] Salminen E., et al. Adverse effect of pelvic radiotherapy. Fifth Int. Mtg. Progress in Radio-Oncology. May. 10-14:501-4, 1995

687] Sandler R.S., et al. Diet and risk of colorectal adenomas: macronutrients, cholesterol and fiber. J Natl Cancer Inst. 85(11):846-8, 1993

688] Sankaranarayanan R. & Mathew B. Retinoids as cancer-preventive agents. IARC Sci Publ. 139:47-5, 1996

689] Santamaria L. & Bianchi-Santamaria A. Carotenoids in cancer chemoprevention and therapeutic interventions. J Nutr Sci Vitaminol (Tokyo)Spec No:321-6, 1992

690] Santisteban G.A., et al. Glycemic modulation of tumor tolerance in a mouse model of breast cancer. Biochem Biophys Res Commun. 132(3):1174-9, 1985

691] Salonen J.T., et al. Association between serum selenium and the risk of cancer. American Journal of Epidemiology. 120:342, 1984

692] Salonen J.T., et al. Risk of cancer in relation to serum concentrations of selenium and vitamins A and E: matched case control analysis of prospective data. British Medical Journal. 290:417-420, 1985

693] Sarasua S. & Savitz D.A. Cured and broiled meat consumption in relation to childhood cancer: Denver, Colorado (United States). Cancer Causes Control. 5(2):141-8, 1994

694] Sasai K. & Ono K., et al. The effect of arterial oxygen content on the results of radiation therapy for epidermoid bronchogenic carcinoma. Int J Radiat Oncol Bio Phys. 1477-81, Jun 16, 1989

695] Satoh K., et al. Enhancement of radical intensity and cytotoxic activity of ascorbate by hyperthermia. Anticancer Res. 16(5A):2987-91, 1996

696] Sauer L.A. & Dauchy R.T., et al. Mechanism for the antitumour and anticachectic effects of n-3 fatty acids. Cancer Res. 60(18):5289-95, Sep 15, 2000

697] Scambia G. & Ranelletti F.O., et al. Quercetin potentiates the effects of adriamycin in a multidrug-resistant MCF-7 human breast-cancer cell line: P-glycoprotein as a possible target. Cancer Chemother Pharmacol. 34(6):459-64, 1994

698] Schairer C., et al. Menopausal Estrogen and Estrogen-Progestin Replacement Therapy and Breast Cancer Risk. JAMA 283:485-491, 2000

699] Schlegel J.U., et al. The role of ascorbic acid in the prevention of bladder tumor formation. J Urol. 103(2):155-9, 1970

700] Schmitt-Gräff A. & Scheulen M.E. Prevention of adriamucin cardiotoxicity by niacin, isocitrate or N-acetyl-cysteine in mice. A morphological study. Pathol Res Pract. 181(2):168-74, 1986

701] Schner H.W., et al. Oestrogen and endothelial cell angiogenic activity. Clin Exp Pharmacol Physiol. 23(3):247-250, 1996

702] Schrauzer G.N. Selenium and cancer: A review. Bioinorganic Chemistry. 5:275-281, 1976

703] Schrauzer G.N., et al. Cancer mortality correlation studies III: Statistical associations with dietary selenium intakes. Bioinorganic Chemistry. 7:23-34, 1977

704] Schrauzer G.N. Anticarcinogenic effects of selenium. Cell Mol Life Sci. 57(13-

14):1864-73, Dec, 2000

705] Schwartz G.G. & Hulka B.S. Is vitamin D deficiency a risk factor for prostate cancer? Anticancer Res. 10(5A):1307-11, 1990

706] Schwartz D. & Rotter V. p53-dependent cell cycle control: response to genotoxic stress. Semin Cancer Biol. 8(5):325-36. Review. 1998

707] Sciaudone M.P., et al. Chelation of zinc amplifies induction of growth hormone mRNA levels in cultured rat pituitary tumour cells. J Nutr. 130(2):158-63, Feb, 2000

708] Seely S. & Horrobin D.F. Diet and breast cancer: The possible connection with sugar consumption. Med Hypotheses. 11(3):319-27, 1983

709] Seelig M.S. Magnesium and other nutritional clinical deficiencies in immunologic abnormalities including allergies and neoplasms. Abstract. J Am Coll Nutr. 12:579, 1993

710] Sengupta A. & Das S. The anti-carcinogenic role of lycopene, abundantly present in tomato. Eur J Cancer Prev. 8(4):325-30. Review. August, 1999

711] Senie R.T. & Tenser S.M. The timing of breast cancer surgery during the menstrual cycle. Oncology (Huntingt). 11(10):1509-17, Oct, 1997

712] Shamsuddin A.M., et al. IP6: a novel anti-cancer agent. Life Sci. 61(4):343-54, 1997

713] Shao W., et al. Arsenic trioxide as an inducer of apoptosis and loss of PML/RAR alpha protein in acute promelocytic leukemia cells. J Natl Cancer Inst. 90(2):124-133, 1998

714] She Q.B., et al. Resveratrol-induced activation of p53 and apoptosis is mediated by extracellular-signal-regulated protein kinases and p38 kinase. Cancer Res. 61(4):1604-10, 15, 2001

715] Shering S.G., et al. Thyroid Disorders and Breast Cancer. Eur J Cancer Prev. 5(6):504-506, 1996

716] Shertzer H.G. & Senft A.P. The micronutrient indole-3-carbinol: implications for disease and chemoprevention. Drug Metabol Drug Interact. 17(1-4):159-88, 2000

717] Sherwin R.W., et al. Serum cholesterol levels and cancer mortality in 361,662 men screened for the mulitple risk factor intervention trial. JAMA. 257(7):943-8, 1987

718] Shi-Zhong Bu, De-Ling Yin, Xiu-Hai Ren, Li-Zhen Jiang, et al. Progesterone Induces Apoptosis and Up-regulation of p53 Expression in Human Ovarian Carcinoma Cell Lines. Am Cancer Soc. 1944-1950, 1997

719] Shklar G. Mechanisms of cancer inhibition by anti-oxidant nutrients. Oral Oncol. 34:24-9, Jan, 1998

720] Shultz T.D. & Howie B.J. In vitro binding of steroid hormones by natural and purified fibers. Nutr Cancer. 8(2):141-7, 1986

721] Siguel E.N. Cancerostatic effect of vegetarian diets. Nutr Cancer. 4(4):285-91, 1983

722] Silbergeld E.K., Waalkes M. & Rice J.M. Lead as a carcinogen: experimental evidence and mechanisms of action. Am J Ind Med. 38(3):316-23. Review. Sep, 2000

723] Silver J., et al. Regulation of parathyroid cell proliferation. Curr Opin Nephrol

Hypertens. 6(4):321-6, 1997

724] Sim A.K. & McCraw A.P. The activity of linolenate and dihomo- - linolenate methyl esters in vitro and in vivo on plateler function in non-human primates and in man. Thromb Res. 10:385, 1977

725] Singh R.B., et al. Dietary intake and plasma levels of antioxidant vitamins in health and disease: a hospital-based case-control study. J Nutr Environ Med. 5:235-42, 1995

726] Singh V.N. & Gaby S.K. Premalignant lesion: role of antioxidant vitamins and beta-carotene in risk reduction and prevention of malignant transformation. Am J Clin nutr. 53:386S-90S, 1991

727] Singh V., et al. Serum vitamin E in chronic myeloid leukaemia. J Assoc Physicians India. 48:201-203, 2000

728] Skubitz K.M., et al. Oral glutamine to prevent chemotherapy-induced stomatitis: a pilot study. J Lab Clin Med. 127:223-8, 1996

729] Smith J.R. & Herrera J.L. Chronic hepatitis C: implications for the primary care clinician. JAAPA. 14(2):41-4,63. Review. Feb, 2001

730] Smolanka II. Systemic enzyme therapy with the preparation Wobe-Mugos E in the combined treatment of lung cancer patients. Lik Sprave. 5:121, Jul-Aug, 2000

731] Smyth J.F., et al. Glutathione reduces the toxicity and improves quality of life of women diagnosed with ovarian cancer treated with cisplatin: results of a double-blind, randomised trial. Ann Oncol. 8(6):569-73, 1997

732] Smyth P.P. The Thyroid and Breast Cancer: A Significant Association? Ann Med. 29(3):189-191, 1997

733] Snowdon D.A. Diet and ovarian cancer. Letter to the Editor. JAMA. 254(3):356-57, 1985

734] Sobala G.M., et al. Levels of nitrite, nitrate, N-nitroso compounds, ascorbic and total bile acids in gastric juice of patients with and without precancerous conditions of the stomach. Carcinogenesis. 12(2);193-8, 1991

735] Soignet S.L., et al. Complete remission after treatment of acute promyelocytic leukemia with arsenic trioxide. N Eng J Med. 339(19):1341-1348, 1998

736] Sokoloski J.A. & Hodnick W.F., et al. Induction of the differentiation of HL-60 promyelocytic leukemia cells by vitamin E and other antioxidants in combination with low levels of vitamin D3: possible relationship to NF-Kappa B. Leukemia. 11(9):1546-53, Sep, 1997

737] Sokoloski J.A. & Sartorelli A.C. Induction of the differentiation of HL-60 promyelocytic leukemia cells by nonsteroidal anti-inflammatory agents in combination with low levels of vitamin D3. Leuk Res. 22:153-161, 1998

738] Sola M.M. & Oliver F.J., et al. Citrate inhibition of rat-kidney cortex phosphofructokinase. Mol Cell Biochem. 135(2):123-8, Jun 29, 1994

739] Soldatenkov V.A., et al. Poly (ADP-ribose) polymerase in DNA damage-response pathway: implications for radiation oncology. Int J Cancer. 90(2):59-67, Apr 20, 2000

740] Song C.W., et al. Association of pseudoachalasia with advancing cancer of the gastric cardia. Int J Radiat Oncol Biol Phys. 30(5):1161-9, 1994

741] Song M.K., et al. Effect of different levels of dietary zinc on longevity of Balb/ c mice inoculated with plasmacytoma MOPC 104E. J Natl Cancer Inst. 72:647-52, 1984

742] Song M.K., et al. Zinc, calcium and magnesium metabolism: effects on plasmacytomas in Balb/c mice. Am J Clin Nutr. 49:701-7, 1989

743] Spigelman A.D., et al. Vitamin C levels in patients with familial adenomatous polyposis. Br J Surg. 77(5):508-9, 1990

744] Sprietsma J.E. Modern diets and diseases: NO-zinc balance. Under Th1, zinc and nitrogen monoxide (NO) collectively protect against viruses, AIDS, autoimmunity, diabetes, allergies, asthma, infectious diseases, atherosclerosis and cancer. Med Hypotheses. 53(1):6-16. Review. Jul, 1999

745] Srivastava M., et al. Nutritional risk factors in carcinoma of the esophagus. Nutr Res. 15(2):177-85, 1995

746] Stadel V.V. Dietary iodine and the risk of breast, endometrial and ovarian cancer. Lancet i:890-1, 1976

747] Stavric B. Quercetin in our diet: from potent mutagen to probable anticarcinogen. Clin Biochem. 27(4):245-8, 1994

748] Steele V.E. & Holmes C.A., et al. Potential use of lipoxygenase inhibitors for cancer chemoprevention. Expert Opin Investig Drugs. 9(9):2121-38, Review. Sep, 2000

749] Steinhausen D., et al. Evaluation of systemic tolerence of 42.0 degree C infrared-A whole-body hyperthermia in combination with hyperglycemia and hyperoxemia. A Phase-1 study. Strahlenther Onkol. 170(6):322-34, June, 1994

750] Steinmetz K.A. & Potter J.D. Vegetables, fruit and cancer prevention: a review. J Am Diet Assoc. 96:1027-9, 1996

751] Stern R.G. Carcinogenesis and the plasma membrane. Med Hypotheses. 52(5):367-72, May, 1999

752] Stevens R.G., et al. Iron-binding proteins and risk of cancer in Taiwan. J Natl Cancer Inst. 76:605-10, 1986

753] Stich H.F., et al. Remission of precancerous lesions in the oral cavity of tobacco chewers and maintenance of the protective effect of -carotene or vitamin A. Am J Clin Nutr. 53:298S-304S, 1991

754] Stoll B.A. Can supplementary dietary fiber suppress breast cancer growth? Br J Cancer. 73:557-9, 1996

755] Stoll B.A. Eating to beat breast cancer: potential role for soy supplements. Ann Oncol. 8:223-5, 1997

756] Stoll B.A. Dietary Supplements of Dehydroepiandrosterone in Relation to Breast Cancer Risk. Eur J Clin Nutr. 53(10):771-775, 1999

757] Stoll B.A. Alcohol intake and late-stage promotion of breast cancer. Eur J Cancer. 35(12):1653-8. Review. Nov, 1999

758] Stoll B.A. Adiposity as a Risk Determinant for Postmenopausal Breast Cancer. Int J Obes Relat Metab Disord. 24(5): 527-533, 2000

759] Stubbs M., et al. Increased intracellular pH gives advantages to tumour cells for growth, decreased extracellular pH promotes invasiveness. Mol Med Today. 6(1):15-

9, 2000

760] Sugihava T. & Hattori Y., et al. Preferential impairment of nitric oxide-mediated endothelium-dependent relaxation in human cervical arteritis after irradiation. Circulation. 100(6):635, Aug 10, 1999

761] Sun A.S. & Yeh H.C., et al. Pilot study of a specific dietary supplement in tumour-bearing mice and in stage IIIB and IV non-small cell lung cancer patients. Nutr Cancer. 39(1):85-95, 2001

762] Sun L.K. & Yoshii Y., et al. Cytotoxic effect through fas/APO-1 expression due to vitamin K in human glioma cells. J Neurooncol 47(1):31-8, March, 2000

763] Sundaram N. & Pahwa A.K., et al. Selenium causes growth inhibition and apoptosis in human brain tumour cell lines. J Neurooncol. 46(2):125-33, 2000

764] Sundstrom H., et al. Serum selenium in patients with ovarian cancer during and after therapy. Carcinogenesis. 5(6):731-734, 1984

765] Sundstrom H., et al. Supplementation with selenium, vitamin E and their combination in gynaecological cancer during cytotoxic chemotherapy. Carcinogenesis. 10:273-8, 1989

766] Surh Y.J., et al. Inhibitory effects of curcumin and capsaicin on phorbol ester-induced activation of eukaryotic transcription factors, NF-kappaB and AP-1. Biofactors. 12:107-112, 2000

767] Sutherland R.M. Tumour hypoxia and gene expression- implications for malignant progression and therapy. Acta Oncol. 37(6):567-74, 1998

768] Sutton P.R. Sodium fluoride as an oral carcinogen. Letter. N Z Med J. 98(775):207, 1985

769] Takashima T. & Fujiwara Y., et al. PPAR-gamma ligands inhibit growth of human esophageal adenocarcinoma cells through induction of apoptosis, cell cycle arrest and reduction of ornithine decarboxylase activity. Int J Oncol. 19(3):465-71, Sep, 2001

770] Takigawa M. & Shirai E., et al. Cartilage-derived anti-tumour factor (CATF) inhibits the proliferation of endothelial cells in culture. Cell Biol Int Rep. 9(7):619-25, Jul, 1985

771] Talamini R. Selected Medical Conditions and Risk of Breast Cancer. Brit J Cancer. 75(11):1699-1703, 1997

772] Tallman M.S., et al. Acute promyelocytic leukemia: evolving therapeutic strategies. Blood. 99:759-767, 2002

773] Tashiro T. & Yamamori H., et al. N-3 polyunsaturated fatty acids in surgical nutrition. Nippon Geka Gakkai Zasshi. 99(4):256-63, Apr, 1998

774] Taussig S.J., et al. Bromelain, the enzyme complex of pineapple (Ananas comosus) and its clinical application. An update. J Ethnopharmacol. 22(2):191-203, Feb-Mar, 1988

775] Taylor J.A., et al. Association of prostate cancer with vitamin D receptor gene polymorphism. Cancer Res. 56(18):4108-10, 1996

776] Taylor P.R., et al. Effect of nutrition intervention on intermediate endpoints in esophageal and gastric carcinogenesis. Am J Clin Nutr. 62(suppl):1420S-3S, 1995

777] Taylor T.V., Rimmer S. & Day B., et al. Ascorbic acid supplementation in the treatment of pressure sores. The Lancet. 2(7881):544-6, Sep 7, 1974

778] Teicher B., et al. Antiangiogenic agents potentiate cytotoxic cancer cell therapies against primary and metastatic disease. Can Res. 52:6702-4, 1992

779] The Leukemia and Lymphoma Society. http://13.leukemia-lymphoma.org./all

780] The American Cancer Society. www.cancer.org

781] The International Lymphoma Study Group. http://13.leukemia-lymphoma.org./all

782] Thomas M.G., et al. Vitamin D and its metabolites inhibit cell proliferation in human rectal mucosa and colon cancer cell line. Gut. 33(12):1660-3, 1992

783] Thompson H., et al. Morphological and biochemical status of the mammary gland as influenced by conjugated linoleic acid: implication for a reduction in mammary cancer risk. Cancer Res. 57(22):5067-72, Nov 15, 1997

784] Thorgeursson V.P., et al. Tumour incidence in a chemical carcinogenesis study of non-human primate. Regul Toxicol Pharmacol.19(2):130-151, 1994

785] Thornes R.D. Oral anticoagulant therapy of human cancer. J Med. 5:83, 1974

786] Tisch M. & Lohmeier A., et al. Genotoxic effect of the insecticides pentachlorophenol and lindane on human nasal mucosal epithelium. Dtsch Med Wochenschr. 126(30):840-4, Jul 27, 2001

787] Tisdale M.J. & Brennan R.A. Metabolic substrate utilization by a tumour cellline which induces cachexia in vivo. Br J Cancer. 54(4):601-6, Oct, 1986

788] Tisdale M.J. & Brennan R.A. A comparison of long-chain triglycerides and medium-chain triglycerides on weight loss and tumour size in a cachexia model. Br J Cancer. 58(5):580-3, Nov, 1988

789] Tisdale M.J. & Dhesi J.K. Inhibition of weight loss by omega-3 fatty acids in an experimental cachexia model. Cancer Res. 50(16):5022-6, Aug 15, 1990

790] Tisdale M.J. Role of prostaglandins in metastatic dissemination of cancer. Exp Cell Biol. 51:250, 1983

791] Tisdale M.J. Wasting in cancer. J Nutr. 129(1 S Suppl):243S-246S. Review. Jan, 1999

792] Toke G.B.& Dhamne B.K. A study of serum copper, serum zinc and Cu/Zn ratio as diagnostic and prognostic index in cases of head, neck and face tumors. Indian J Pathol Microbiol Apr. 33(2):171-4, 1990

793] Tokunaga A. & Senba E. Molecular mechanisms of chronic pain. Masui. 45(5):547-57. Review. May, 1996

794] Tomono Y., et al. Pharmacokinetic study of deuterium-labelled coenzyme Q10 in man. Int J Clin Pharmacol Ther Toxicol. 24(10):536-41, 1986

795] Trebukhina R.V., et al. Metabolism of vitamins B1 and PP and their use in oncological practice. Vopr Med Khim. 38(5):33-6, 1992 (in Russian)

796] Trickler D., et al. Inhibition of oral carcinogenesis by glutathione. Nutr Cancer. 20:139-44, 1993

797] Trouillas P. & Honnorat J., et al. Redifferentiation therapy in brain tumours: long-lasting complete regression of glioblastomas and an anaplastic astrocytoma under long term 1-alpha-hydroxycholecalciferol. J Neurooncol. 51(1):57-66, Jan, 2001

798] Tully D.B. & Allgood V.E., et al. Modulation of steroid receptor-mediated gene expression by vitamin B6. FASEB J. 8(3):343-9. Review. Mar 1, 1994

799] Tvedt K.E., et al, Intracellular distribution of calcium and zinc in normal, hyperplastic, and neoplastic human prostate: x-ray microanalysis of freeze-dried cryosections. Prostate. 15:41-51, 1989

800] Ujiie S., et al. Serum selenium contents in cancer patients. Gan To Kagaku Ryoho. 24(4):401-5, 1997

801] Umansky V. & Ushmorov A., et al. Nitric oxide-mediated apoptosis in human breast cancer cells requires changes in mitochondrial functions and is independent of CD95 (APO-1/Fas). Int J Oncol. 16(1):109-17, Jan, 2000

802] Umegaki K., et al. Beta-carotene prevents x-ray induction of micronuclei in human lymphocytes. Am J Clin Nutr. 53:238S-46S, 1991

803] Vahdat L. & Papadopoulos K., et al. Reduction of paclitaxel-induced peripheral neuropathy with glutamine. Clin Cancer Res. 7(5):1192-7, May, 2001

804] Vanchieri C. Cutting copper curbs angiogenesis, studies show. J Natl Cancer Inst. 92(15):1202-3, Aug 2, 2000

805] Van Der Merwe C.F., et al. Oral gamma-linoleic acid in 21 patients with untreatable malignancy. An ongoing pilot open clinical trial. Br J Clin Pract. 41(9):907-15, 1987

806] Van Der Merwe C.F. The reversibility of cancer. S Afr Med J. 65:712, 1984

807] Van Der Merve L.F. Evening primrose oil in cancer treatment. Following up of an ongoing pilot open clinical trial. Proc. 7th Int. Conf. Prostaglandins related compound Florence. 279, May 28th 1990

808] Van Helden P.D., et al. Esophageal cancer: vitamin and lipotrope deficiencies in an at-risk South African population. Nutr Cancer. 10(4):247-55, 1987

809] Van Loon A.J., et al. Nitrate intake and gastric cancer risk: results from the Netherlands cohort study. Cancer Lett. 114:259-61, 1997

810] Van Zandwijk N. N-acetylcysteine for lung cancer prevention. Chest. 107(5):1437-41, 1995

811] Vand Der Merve L.F. Evening primrose oil in cancer treatment. Following up of an ongoing pilot open clinical trial. Proc. 7th Int. Conf. Prostaglandins related compound Florence. 279, May 28th 1990

812] Vanderwalle B., et al. Vitamin D3 derivatives and breast tumour cell growth. Effect on intracellular calcium and apoptosis. Int J Cancer. 61(6):806-11, 1995

813] Vartak S. & McCaw R., et al. Gamma-linolenic acid (GLA) is cytotoxic to 36B10 malignant rat astrocytoma cells but not to 'normal' rat astrocyes. Br J Cancer. 77(10):1612-20, May, 1998

814] Vaupel P. & Hockel M. Blood supply, oxygenation status and metabolic micromilieu of breast cancers: characterization and therapeutic relevance. Int J Oncol. 17(5):869-79. Review. Nov, 2000

815] Vaupel P. & Kelleher D.K., et al. Oxygen status of malignant tumours: pathogenesis of hypoxia and significance for tumour therapy. Semin Oncol. 28(2 Suppl 8):29-35. Review. Apr, 2001

816] Velazquez M.C., et al. Butyrate and the colonocyte: implications for neoplasia.

Dig Dis Sci. 41(4):727-39, 1996

817] Verma S.P. & Salamone E., et al. Curcumin and genistein, plant natural products, show synergistic inhibitory effects on the growth of human breast cancer MCF-7 cells induced by estrogenic pesticides. Biochem Biophys Res Commun. 233(3):692-6, Apr 28, 1997

818] Verreault R., et al. A case-control study of diet and invasive cervical cancer. Int J Cancer. 43:1050-4, 1989

819] Vlajinac H.D., et al. Diet and prostate cancer: a case-control study. Eur J Cancer. 33(1):101-7, 1997

820] Von Ardenne M. Adaptation of anticancer strategies to progress in tumour immunology. Med Hypothesis. 25(3):163-173, Mar, 1988

821] Vucenik I., et al. Comparison of pure inositol hexaphosphate and high-bran diet in the prevention of DMBA-induced rat mammary carcinogenesis. Nutr Cancer. 28(1):7-13, 1997

822] Wadleigh R.G., et al. Vitamin E in the treatment of chemotherapy- induced mucositis. Am J Med. 92(5):481-4, 1992

823] Wainwright M. Highly pleomorphic staphylococci as a cause of cancer. Med Hypotheses. 54(1):91-4, Jan, 2000

824] Walaszek Z., et al. Metabolism, uptake and excretion of a D-glucaric acid salt and its potential use in cancer prevention. Cancer Detect Prev. 21(2):178-90, 1997

825] Wald M., et al. Mixture of trypsin, chymotrypsin and papain reduces formation of metastases and extends survival time of C57B16 mice with syngeneic melanoma B16. Cancer Chemother Pharmacol. 47 Suppl:S16-22, Jul, 2001

826] Wang G.Q., et al. Effects of vitamin/mineral supplementation on the prevalence of histological dysplasia and early cancer of the esophagus and stomach: results from the General Population Trial in Linxian, China. Cancer Epidemiol Biomarkers Prev. 3(2):161-6, 1994

827] Wargovich M.J. Calcium and colon cancer. J Am Coll Nutr. 7(4):295-300, 1988

828] Wasan H.S. & Goodlad R.A. Fibre-supplemented foods may damage your health. Viewpoint. Lancet. 348:319-20, 1996

829] Watrach A.M., et al. Inhibition of human breast cancer cells by selenium. Cancer Lett. 25:41-7, 1984

830] Watson R.A. Ifosfamide: Chemotherapy with new promise and new problems for the urologist. Urology. 24(5):465-8, 1984

831] Watson W.H. & Cai J., et al. Diet and apoptosis. Annu Rev Nutr. 20:485-505. Review. 2000

832] Wattenburg L.W., et al. Inhibition of polycyclic aromatic hydrocarbon-induced neoplasia by naturally occurring indoles. Cancer Research. 38(5):1410-1413, 1978

833] WCRF Panel. Diet, Nutrition and the Prevention of Cancer. A Global Perspective. Washington, DC, World Cancer Research Fund/American Institute for Cancer Research, 1997

834] Webb S.D., et al. Alterations in proteolytic activity at low pH and its association with invasion: a theoretical model. J Theor Biol. 196(2):237-50, 1999

835] Webber M.M. Effects of zinc and cadmium on the growth of human prostatic epithelium in vito. Nutr Res. 6:35-40, 1986

836] Wei H. J., et al. Effect of molybdenum and tungsten on mammary carcinogenesis in Sprague-Dawley (SD) rats Chung Hua Liu Tsa Chih. 9:204-207, 1987

837] Weide M., et al. Study of immune function of cancer patients influenced by supplemental zinc or selenium-zinc combination. Biol Trace Elem Res. 28:11-20, 1991

838] Weinberg E.D. The role of iron in cancer. Eur J Cancer Prev. 5(1):19-36, 1996

839] Weinburger J.H., et al. Protective mechanisms of dietary fibers in nutritional carcinogenesis. Basic Life Sci. 61:45-63, 1993

840] Weisburger J.H. Dietary fat and risk of chronic disease: mechanistic insights from experimental studies. J Am Diet Assn. 97(Suppl):S16-S23, 1997

841] Weisel C.P. & Chen W.J. Exposure to chlorination by-products from hot water uses. Risk Anal. 14(1):101-6, 1994

842] Wheeler M.D., et al. Glycine: a new anti-inflammatory immunonutrient. Cell Mol Life Sci. 56(9-10):843-56, Nov 30, 1999

843] Whelen P., et al. Zinc, vitamin A and prostatic cancer. Br J Urol. 55(5):525-8, 1983

844] Whigham L.D., Cook M.E. & Atkinson R.L. Conjugated linoleic acid: implications for human health. Pharmacol Res. 42(6):503-10. Review. Dec, 2000

845] White W.S., et al. Pharmacokinetics of beta-carotene and canthaxanthin after individual and combined doses by human subjects. J Am Coll Nutr. 12:665-71, 1994

846] Wigmore S.J. & Fearon K.C, et al. Down-regulation of the acute-phase response in patients with pancreatic cancer cachexia receiving oral eicosapentaenoic acid is mediated via suppression of interleukin-6. Clin Sci (Lond). 92(2):215-21, Feb, 1997

847] Wigmore S.J. & Barber M.D., et al. Effect of oral eicosapentaenoic acid on weight loss in patients with pancreatic cancer. Nutr Cancer. 36(2):177-84, 2000

848] Wilkens L.R., et al. Risk factors for lower urinary tract cancer: the role of total fluid consumption, nitrites and nitrosamines, and selected foods. Cancer Epidemiol Biomark Prevent. 5:161-6, 1996

849] Wilkinson J. 4th et al. Detoxication enzymes and chemoprevention. Proc Soc Exp Biol Med. 216(2):192-200, Nov, 1997

850] Willett W.C. & MacMahon B. Diet and cancer: An overview. N Engl J Med. 310(11):697-703, 1984

851] Winking M. & Sarikaya S., et al. Boswellic acids inhibit glioma growth: a new treatment option? J Neurooncol. 46(2):97-103, 2000

852] Wisdom R. AP-1: one switch for many signals. Exp Cell Res. 253(1):180-5. Review. Nov 25, 1999

853] Witte J.S., et al. Diet and premenopausal bilateral breast cancer: a case-control study. Breast Cancer Res Treat. 42:243-51, 1997

854] Wood L. Possible prevention of adriamycin-induced alopecia by tocopherol. N Engl J Med. 312:1060, 1985

855] Yaguchi M., et al. Vitamin K2 and its derivatives induce apoptosis in leukemia cells and enhance the effect of all-trans retinoic acid. Leukemia. 11:779-787, 1997

856] Yamamoto H. Interrelation of differentiation, proliferation and apoptosis in cancer cells. J Osaka Dent Univ. 29:51-60, 1995

857] Yang C. S. Research on esophageal cancer in China: a review. Cancer Research. 40:2633-2644, 1980

858] Yang C.Y., et al. Calcium and magnesium in drinking water and risk of death from colon cancer. Jpn J Cancer Res. 88(10):928-33, 1997

859] Yang C.Y., et al. Calcium, magnesium and nitrate in drinking water and gastric cancer mortality. Jpn J Cancer Res. 89(2):124-130, 1998

860] Yang G.Y. & Shamsuddin A.M. IP6-induced growth inhibition and differentiation of HT-29 human colon cancer cells: involvement of intracellular inositol phosphates. Anticancer Res. 15(6B):2479-87, 1995

861] Yeum K-J et al. -carotene intervention trial in premalignant gastric lesions. Abstract. J Am Coll Nutr. 14(5):536, 1995

862] Yiomouyiannis J.A. Fluoridation and cancer – the biology and epidemiology of bone and oral cancer related to fluoridation. Fluoride. 26(2):83-96, 1993

863] Yoon S.O. & Kim M.M., et al. Inhibitory effect of selenite on invasion of HT1080 tumour cells. J Biol Chem. 276(23):20086-92, Jun 8, 2001

864] Yoshizawa K., et.al. Study of prediagnostic selenium level in toenails and the risk of advanced prostate cancer. J Natl Can Inst. 90:1219-24, 1998

865] Yu M.W., et al. Plasma selenium levels and the risk of hepatocellular carcinoma among men with chronic hepatitis virus infection. Am J Epidemiol. 150:367-374, 1999

866] Yu R., et al. Role of a mitogen-activated protein kinase pathway in the induction of phase II detoxifying enzymes by chemicals. J Biol Chem. 274(39):27545-52, 24, 1999

867] Yu S.Y., et al. A preliminary report on the intervention trials of primary liver cancer in high-risk populations with nutritional supplementation of selenium in China. Biol Trace Element Research. 29:289-294, 1991

868] Yu S. Y., et al. Protective role of selenium against hepatitis B virus and primary liver cancer in Qidong. Biol Tr Elem Res. 56(1):117-124, 1997

869] Yu S-Y, et al. Intervention trial in selenium for the prevention of lung cancer among tin miners in Yunnan, China. Bio Tr El Res24:105-108, 1990

870] Yuan F., et al. Anti-estrogenic activities of indole-3-carbinol in cervical cells: implications for prevention of cervical cancer. Anticancer Research. 19:1673-1680, 1999

871] Zaffaroni N. & Fiorentini G., et al. Hyperthermia and hypoxia: new developments in anticancer chemotherapy. Eur J Surg Oncol. 27(4):340-2. Review. Jun, 2001

872] Zaichick Vye et al. Zinc in the human prostate gland: normal, hyperplastic and cancerous. Int Urol Nephrol. 29(5):565-74, 1997

873] Zhang D. & Holmes W.F., et al. Retinoids and ovarian cancer. J Cell Physiol. 185(1):1-20. Review. Oct, 2000

874] Zhang L., et al. Serum micronutrients in relation to pre-cancerous gastric lesions. Int J Cancer. 56(5):650-4, 1994

875] Zhang X., Xu Q. & Saiki I. Quercetin inhibits the invasion and mobility of murine melanoma B16-BL6 cells through inducing apoptosis via decreasing Bcl-2 expression. Clin Exp Metastasis. 18(5):415-21, 2000

876] Zheng W., et al. Retinol, antioxidant vitamins and cancer of the upper digestive tract in a prospective cohort study of postmenopausal women. Am J Epidemiol. 142:955-60, 1995

877] Zhou S., et al. Effect of dietary fatty acids on tumourigenesis of colon cancer induced by methyl nitrosourea in rats. J Environ Pathol Toxicol Oncol. 19(1-2):81-6, 2000

878] Zhu Z. & Kimura M., et al. Apoptosis induced by selenium in human glioma cell lines. Biol Trace Elem Res. 54(2):123-34, August, 1996

879] Zhu K. & Williams S.M. Methyl-deficient diets, methylated ER genes and breast cancer: an hypothesized association. Cancer Causes Control. 9(6):615-20, Dec, 1998

STRANGERS IN THE NIGHT: XENOESTROGENS AND HEALTH.

What is Estrogen dominance? This refers to the balance of Estrogen and Progesterone. In a normal menstrual cycle (see Fig 1), Estrogen is the dominant hormone up until ovulation day (usually day 14). Then progesterone is the dominant hormone until the period. Progesterone rises to increase the store of Magnesium, Zinc and Vitamin B6. It also brings down the copper, which has gradually risen to a mid-cycle peak. Overall there is no net gain of copper, if progesterone kicks in properly. If there is a lack of progesterone (see fig2), then Magnesium, Zinc and B6 tend to be low and copper tends to rise.

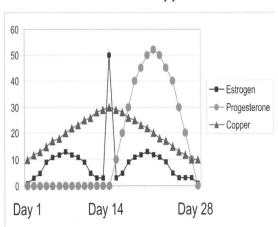

Figure 1. Normal Cycle

Another example is the oral contraceptive pill. The Estrogens in these pills have Estrogenic effects, but the progesterone (being synthetic) tends not to have true progesterone effect (see Fig 4).

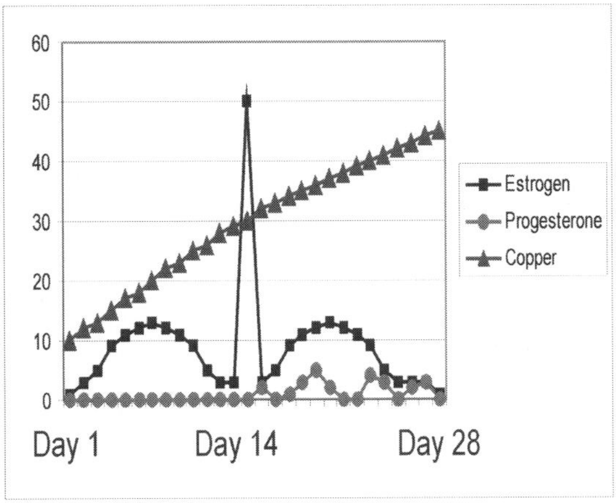

Figure 2. Low Progesterone Cycle

Another version of Estrogen dominance. This explains why zinc and magnesium fall and why copper rises while on the OCP.

John R Lee's work in the 80's on Estrogen

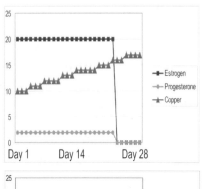

Figure 3. Oral Contraceptive Pattern.

dominance was largely ignored by the medical fraternity. The suggestion has been made that they were caught up in the glossy hype generated by pharmaceutical companies pushing Estrogen therapies.

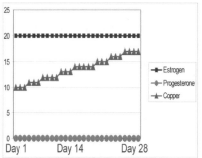

Figure 4. HRT Pattern

His premise was that even without a uterus, the women still needed progesterone. This was never really accepted despite the expanding body of evidence that Estrogen Dominance would have been directly responsible for the woman's hysterectomy! By giving Estrogen only therapy, the doctor was perpetuating the hormone imbalance. His suggestion that natural progesterone was a better treatment was shunned because progesterone was not patentable (not chic enough) and hence not lucrative enough. His work took the issue to an important level but clearly just giving progesterone creams did not always solve the clinical problems, which were quite diverse in symptoms (see list below). His original observations on women with Estrogen only HRT was expanded to include women on the oral contraceptive. (see Fig 3&4) His assumption was that the lack of progesterone in the second half of the menstrual cycle was due to pesticide exposure of the foetus in utero (while still in the womb). This observation was just the tip of the iceberg and maybe it was the lack of encompassing data that turned away many medicos.

Now despite what doctors think they may be prescribing, all HRT is unopposed Estrogen. It has the mentality of unopposed Estrogen. It has the biochemistry of unopposed Estrogen. It has the side effects of unopposed Estrogen. Some doctors have claimed that their "special" synthetic progesterone is the real thing. If you want the truth, ask them who pays for their conferences and publishing costs. The disappointing results from natural progesterone was due to the fact that the legacy of copper excess was not addressed just by giving progesterone.

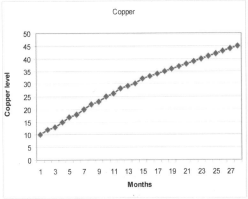

Figure 5. Slow upward shift of baseline Copper.

The effect of Xenoestrogens in the body is to shift the baseline of total Estrogen level upwards (see Fig 5). The effect on copper is that it never returns to the starting point by day 28. Hence the connection between Xenoestrogens, Estrogen only HRT and copper excess.

List of Estrogen Dominance Symptoms
Acceleration of aging
Agitation or Anxiety
Allergy (asthma, hives, rashes, sinus congestion)
Autoimmune disorders Lupus, Thyroiditis (Hashimoto's)
Breast cancer (men and women)
Breast tenderness with period
Cervical dysplasia (abnormal pap smear)
Cold hands and feet
Copper excess
Decreased sex drive

Depression with anxiety or agitation
Dry eyes
Endometriosis
Fat gain around abdomen hip & thighs
Fatigue
Fibrocystic (lumpy breasts)
Fibroids
Foggy thinking
Gall bladder disease
Hair loss
Headaches
Hypoglycaemia (low blood sugar esp. 3-4pm)
Increased blood clotting
Infertility
Irregular menstrual periods
Irritability
Insomnia
Magnesium deficiency
Memory loss
Mood swings
Osteoporosis
Ovarian cancer
Ovarian Cysts
PMS/PMT
Polycystic ovaries
Pre-menopausal bone loss
Prostate cancer (in Men)
Sluggish metabolism
Thyroid dysfunction
Uterine cancer
Water retention, bloating
Zinc deficiency

Since that time it has become clear that many chemicals behave as Estrogens. What is also clear is that we are exposed to these all of our lives, not just in the womb. This group of compounds have been called the Xenoestrogens. Xeno is the Greek word for stranger, hence the comment about strangers in the night. The list is represented below. These chemicals are cumulative in some instances and increase in quantity in the body as we get older. One of the effects of Xenoestrogens is to reduce the excretion rate of copper from the body. All estrogens cause copper accumulation, xenoestrogens *look* like estrogens to our biochemistry and hence *also cause copper retention*. These patients have very high Copper levels. These Xenoestrogens (especially the pesticides) over time have progressively been classed as carcinogens and this explains the more unpleasant problems (cancer) in this list.

List of the Xenoestrogens
Pesticides (DDT, 2,4,D 2,4,5- T, Dioxin, Dieldrin, endosulfan, methoxychlor, kepone, toxaphene, chloropicrin etc)
Petroleum products (car fumes, methlybenzene, toluene, benzene, styrene, pyrene, PCB's,)
Plastics (PVC, biphenyl, nonylphenyl, octaphenyl, lunch wraps etc)
Hormones   a.From Doctors (OCP & HRT) b.From Poultry industry & antibiotics in animal feed

How would this problem manifest? Let's take a typical example. A young girl is born. She is a difficult child. Fussy eater, poor sleep pattern, lots of colds. She loves chicken and craves chocolate. She has trouble with her periods from almost the onset of menstruation. They are irregular and painful and she suffers PMT. Her doctor puts her on the oral contraceptive to suppress ovulation and this seems to quieten things down. Eventually she comes off the pill to start a family. Her periods take 6 months to resume and they are worse than ever. She has trouble conceiving because the pill has depleted her zinc levels. She is low in progesterone and loses a few pregnancies at multiples of 4 weeks (4, 8, 12, 16). She eventually gets pregnant but her copper accumulates and she develops postnatal depression. Her baby is zinc deficient and it probably has excess copper.

She tries for another baby but this time she can't because she's developed endometriosis. Answer: the oral contraceptive. She starts to gain weight, starts to get depressed, and her skin changes. Her face and upper torso develop a reddish tinge. Then she develops anxiety symptoms. She is told that this is anxiety/panic disorder causing her depression and is put onto antidepressants, but these don't help. She can't seem to raise her iron levels with supplements. Then she's told she's got an underactive thyroid and needs thyroid replacement. But despite taking thyroid hormone, there is no real improvement in energy.

After a few years of this purgatory of health, she goes off the pill and develops heavy periods. She finds out now that she also has fibroids and consents to hysterectomy. Three months later she discovers that her Estrogen levels are low. Then the punch line. "You don't have a uterus, therefore you don't need progesterone". She starts Estrogen only HRT. Despite complaining of breast tenderness, she is told to continue. One day, one of the painful lumps in her breast is brought to her doctors' attention. She has a mammogram, then a biopsy. The pathology shows breast cancer. She has a lumpectomy with axillary node clearance. Her tumour is Estrogen receptor positive. So then it starts. Chemo then tamoxifen. Five years later she gets a terrible pain in the back. She has spinal metastases. More chemo. Then liver secondaries.

Sorry, not much more medicine can do, we've really done our best. We've followed the book; every single health recommendation. Oh, and by the way, don't go near those *natural therapists*. They have no idea of how to help you. End of story.

This case represents the full house of Xenoestrogen symptoms, and unfortunately many of the patients with breast cancer have some version of this story. Do you think that the medical profession would accept *any* blame for these events? Do you think that the Health Authorities would be interested in checking copper levels or Xenoestrogens? Recently it was found that Alcoa was burning compounds in its liquor burner that released a multitude of chemicals into the atmosphere. Guess what class of compound these were? Yep, all Xenoestrogens. Recently PCB's were found in drain water near a toxic waste plant in the Perth metropolitan area. Guess what class of compound PCB's are? Yep, xenoestrogens

again.
Do you think that the Pharmaceutical companies who make oral contraceptives, HRT or chemotherapy stand to lose or gain if doctors were aware of these problems? No, it's probably all just a conspiracy theory with *no evidence whatsoever*. Or is it....?

References:

1] Abraham G.E., Lubran MM. Serum and red cell magnesium levels in-patients with premenstrual tension. Am J Clin. Nut; 34(11) 2364-66 1981

2] Adlercreutz H., et al. Estrogen and Metabolite levels in Women at Risk for Breast Cancer. Cancer Res. 35:703, 1994

3] Arafah B.M. Increased Need for Thyroxine in Women with Hypothyroidism During Estrogen Therapy. N Engl J Med. 344(23):1743-1749, 2001

4] Asch R.H. & Greenblatt R. Steroidogenesis in the Post-menopausal Ovary. Clin Obstet Gynecol. 4(1): 85, 1977

5] Aufrere M.B., et al. Progesterone: An Overview and Recent Advances. J Pharmaceut Sci. 65:783, 1976

6] Backstrom T., et al. Estrogen and Progesterone in Plasma in Relation to Premenstrual Tension. J Steroid Biochem Mol Biol. 5:257-260, 1974

7] Baumslag, N et al Trace Mineral Content of Maternal and Neonatal Hair. Arch Environ Health 29 1974

8] Bell M. C., et al. Placebo-controlled trial of indole-3-carbinol in the treatment of CIN. Gynecol Oncol. 78(2):123-129, 2000

9] Beumont P.J.L., et al. Luteinizing Hormone and Progesterone Levels after Hysterectomy. Brit Med J. 836:363, 1972

10] Bloom T., Ojanotko-Harri A., Laine M., Huhtaniemi I. Metabolism of Progesterone and Testosterone in Human Parotid and Sub-mandibular Salivary Glands in Vitro. J Steroid Biochem Mol Biol. 44(1):69-76, 1993

11 Bourgain C., et al. Effects of Natural Progesterone on the Morphology of the Endometrium in Patients with Primary Ovarian Failure. Hum Reprod 5:537-543, 1990

12] Bradlow H. L., et al. Indole-3-carbinol. A novel approach to breast cancer prevention. Annals of the New York Academy of Sciences USA. 768:180-200, 1995

13 Bremner I Manifestations of Copper excess. Am J Clin Nutr 67 1069S-73 1998

14] Chang K.J., Lee T.T.Y., Linares-Cruz G., Fournier S. and de Lingieres B. Influences of Percutaneous Administration of Estradiol and Progesterone on Human Breast Epethial Cell Cycle in Vivo. Fertil Steril. 63:785-791, 1995

15] Christ J.E., et al. The Residual Ovary Syndrome. Obstet Gynecol. 46:551-556, 1975

16] Chuong C J & Dawson EB Zinc and copper levels in premenstrual syndrome. Fert. Steril 62:2, 313-20 1994

17] Ciampelli M., et al. Insulin and Polycystic Ovary Syndrome: A New Look at an Old Subject. Gynecol Endocrinol. 12(4):277-292, 1998

18] Clark G.M. and McQuire W.L. Progesterone Receptors and Human Breast Cells. Breast Cancer Res Treat. 3:157-163,1983

19] Colborn T., et al. Our Stolen Future. New York : Penguin Books, 1997

20] Corvol P., et al. Effect of Progesterone and Progestins on Water and Salt Metabolism. In Progesterone and Progestins (N.Y. Raven Press). 1983

21] Cover C. M., et al. Indole-3-carbinol and tamoxifen cooperate to arrest the cell cycle of MCF-7 human breast cancer cells. Cancer Research. 59:1244-1251, 1999

22] Cowan L.D., Gordis L., Tonascia J.A. and Jones G.S. Breast Cancer Incidence in Women with a History of Progesterone Deficiency. Am J Epidemiol. 114:209-217, 1981

23] Dalton K. The Aetiology of Premenstrual Syndrome is with the Progesterone Receptors. Med Hyp. 31:321-327, 1987

24] Dalton K. Premenstrual Syndrome and Progesterone Therapy. 2d ed. London: Heinemann. 1984

25] Dalton K. Progesterone Suppositories and Pessaries in the Treatment of Menstrual Migraine. Headache.12(4):151-159, 1973

26] Davis D.L., Bradlow H.L., Wolff M., Woodruff T., Hoel D.G. and Anton-Culver H. Medical Hypothesis: Xenohormones as Preventable Causes of Breast Cancer. Env Health Persoectuves. 101:372-377, 1993

27] Dannerstein L., Spencer-Gardner C., Brown J.B., Smith M.A. and Burrows G.D. Premenstrual Tension- Hormone Profiles. J Psychosomat Obstet Gynaec. 3:37-51, 1984

28] Del Giudice M.E., et al. Insulin and Related Factors in Premenopausal Breast Cancer Risk. Breast Cancer Res Treat. 47(2):111-120, 1998

29] Denouble Bnerstein L., et al. Progesterone and the Premenstrual Syndrome: A Double Blind Crossover Trial. Brit Med J. 290:1017-1021, 1985

30] Ducrey B., et al. Inhibition of 5 alpha-reductase and aromatase by the ellagitannins oenothein A and oenothein B from Epilobium species. Planta Medica. 63(2):111-114, 1997

31] Ellison P.T. Measurements of Salivary Progesterone. Ann NY Acad Sci. 694:161-176, 1993

210

32] Ellison P.T., Lipson S.F., O'Rourke M.T., Bentley G.R., Harrigan A.M., Painter-Brick C. and Vizthum V.J. Population Variation in Ovarian Function. (Letter). The Lancet. 342(8868):433-434, 1993

33] Facchinetti F et al Magnesium prophylaxis of menstrual migraine: effects on intracellular magnesium. Headache, 31:5, 298-301 1991

34] Facchinetti F et al Oral magnesium successfully relieves premenstrual mood changes. Obstet Gynecol, August; 78:2,177-81 1991

35] Foidart J.-M., et al. Estradiol and Progesterone Regulate the Proliferation of Human Breast Epithelial Cells. Fertil Steril. 69:963-969, 1998

36] Formby B. and Wiley T.S. Progesterone Inhibits Growth and Induces Apoptosis in Breast Cancer Cells: Inverse Effect on Expression of p53 and Bcl-2. Ann Clin Lab Sc. 28(6):360-9, 1998

37] Gambell R.D. Use of Progestogens in Post-menopausal Women. Int J Fertil. 34:315-321, 1989

38] Gompel A., Malet C., Spritzer P., La Lardrie J.-P., et al. Progestin Effect on Cell Proliferation and 17 -hydroxysteroid Dehydrogenase Activity in Normal Human Breast Cells in Culture. J Clin Endocrinol Metab 63:1174, 1986

39] Gompel A., Sabourin J.C., Martin A., Yaneva H., et al. Bcl-2 Expression in Normal Endometrium during the Menstrual Cycle. Am J Path. 144:1196-1202, 1994

40] Gozzo et al Xenoestrogens, pollution & health: a critical review.J Pharm Belg 1998 Jul-Aug;53(4):278-86

41] Guo D., et al. Protection by chlorophyllin and indole-3-carbinol against 2-amino-1-methyl-6-phenylimidazo[4,5-b]pyridine (PhIP)-induced DNA adducts and colonic aberrant crypts in the F344 rat. Carcinogenesis. 16(12):2931-2937, 1995

42] Hamnridge, K.M. et al Zinc Nutrtional Staus During Pregnancy: A longitudinal Study Am J Clin Nutr 37, 1983

43] Hankinson S.E. Circulating Concentrations of Insulin-like Growth Factor-I and Risk of Breast Cancer. The Lancet. 351(9113):1393-1396, 1998

44] Hess, F.M. et al Zinc Excretion in Young Women on Low Zinc Intakes and Oral Contraceptives. J Nutr 107 1977

45] Hreshchyshn M.M., et al. Effects of Natural Menopause, Hysterectomy, and Oophorectomy on Lumber Spine and Femoral Neck Bone Densities. Obstet Gynecol. 72:631-638, 1988

44] Hrushesky W.J.M. Breast Cancer, Timing of Surgery, and the Menstrual Cycle: Call for Prospective Trial. J Women's Health. 5:555-566, 1996

45] Hrushesky W.J. Menstrual Cycle Timing of Breast Cancer Resection: Prospective Study is Overdue. J Natl Cancer Inst. 87(2):143-4, 1995

46] Inoh A., Kamiya K., Fujii Y. and Yokoro K. Protective Effect of Progesterone and Tamoxifen in Estrogen-induced Mammary Carcinogenesis in Ovariectomized W/Fu Rats. Jpn J Cancer Res. 76:699-704, 1985

47] Jacobson J.L. and Jacobson S.W. Intellectual Impairment in Children Exposed to Poly-chlorinated Biphenyls in Utero. N Eng J Med. 335:783-789, 1996

48] Jellinck P.H., Michnovicz J.J. and Bradlow H.L. Influence of Indole-3-carbinol on the Hepatic Microsomal Formation of Catechol Estrogens. Steroids. 56(8):446-450, 1991

49] Kandouz M., Siromachkova M., Jacob D., Marquet B.C., et al. Antagonism between Estradiol and Progestin on Bcl-2 Expression in Breast Cancer Cells. Int J Cancer. 68:120-125, 1996

50] Katdare M., et al. Prevention of mammary preneoplastic transformation by naturally-occurring tumor inhibitors. Cancer Letters. 111(1-2):141-147, 1997

51] Kirschner M.A. The Role of Hormones in the Etiology of Human Breast Cancer. Cancer. 39(6):2716-2726, 1977

52] Krimsky S. Hormonal Chaos: The Scientific and Social Origins of the Environmental Endocrine Hypothesis. Baltimore, Md.: Johns Hopkins University Press, 2000

53] Lee, J.R. What your doctor may not tell you about premenopause. Warner Books 1999

54] Leis H.P. Endocrine Prophylaxis of Breast Cancer with Cyclic Estrogen and Progesterone. Intern Surg. 45:496-503, 1966

55] Liehr J.G. Catechol Estrogens as Mediators of Estrogen-induced Carcinogenesis. Cancer Res. 35:704, 1994

56] Liehr J.G. Genotoxic Effects of Estrogens. Mutat Res. 238(3):269-276, 1990

57] Liehr J.G. Mechanisms of Metabolic Activation and Inactivation of Catecholestrogens: A Basis of Genotoxicity. Polycyclic Aromatic Compounds. 6:229-239, 1994

58] Liehr J.G., et al. 4-Hydroxylation of Estradiol by Human Uterine Myomerium and Myoma Microsomes: Implications for the Mechanism of Uterine Turmorigenesis. Proc Nat Acad Sci. 92:1229-1233, 1995

59] Limanova Z., et al. Frequent Incidence of Thyropathies in Women with Breast Carcinoma. Vnitr Lek. 44(2):76-82, 1998

60] Lipson S.F. and Ellison P.T. Reference Value for Lutal 'Progesterone' Measured by Salivary Radioimmunoassay. Fertil Steril 61(3): 448-454, 1994

61] Lizotte L The woman with too much copper. Total health 19: 49 19997

62] Llang J., et al. Indole-3-carbinol prevents cervical cancer in human papilloma virus type 16 (HPV16) transgenic mice. Cancer Research. 59:3991-3997, 1999

63] MacLusky N.J., Naftolin F., Krey L.C. and Franks S. The Catechol Estrogens. J Steroid Biochem. 15:111-124, 1981

64] Mahesh V.B., Brann D.W. and Hendry L.G. Diverse Modes of Action of Progesterone and Its Metabolites. J Steroid Biochem Molec Biol., Dept of Cell Biology, Baylor College of Medicine, Houston, Tex. 56:67-77 , 1996

65] Malloy V. L., et al. Interaction between a semisynthetic diet and indole-3-carbinol on mammary tumor incidence in Balb/cfC3H mice. Anticancer Research. 17(6D):4333-4337, 1997

66] Matzkin H., et al. Immunohistochemical evidence of the existence and localization of aromatase in human prostatic tissues. Prostate. 21:309-314, 1992

67] Meng Q., et al. Indole-3-carbinol is a negative regulator of estrogen receptor- signaling in human tumor cells. Journal of Nutrition. 130:2927-2931, 2000

68] Mohr P.E., Wang D.Y., Gregory W.M., Richards M.A. and Fentiman I.S. Serum Progesterone and Prognosis in Operable Breast cancer. Brit J Cancer. 73:1552-1555, 1996

69] Moyer D.L., et al. Prevention of Endometrial Hyperplasia by Progesterone during Long Term Estradiol Replacement: Influence of Bleeding Pattern and Secretory Changes. Fertil Steril. 59:992-997, 1993

70] Munday M.R., et al. Correlations between Progesterone, Oestradiol and Aldosterone Levels in the Premenstrual Syndrome. Clin Endocrinol. 14:1-9,1981

72] Muneyvirci-Delale O et al Sex steroid hormones modulate serum ionized magnesium and calcium levels throughout the menstrual cycle in women. Fertil Steril, May; 69(5): 958-62 1998

73] Nagata C., et al. Relations of Insulin Resistance and Serum Concentrations of Estradiol and Sex Hormone-binding Globulin to Potential Breast Cancer Risk Factors. Jpn J Cancer Res. 91(9):948-953, 2000

74] Nolan KR Copper toxicity syndrome J Orthomol Psych 12:270-282 1983

75] O'Brien P.M.S., Selby C. and Symonds E.M. Progesterone, Fluid and Electrolytes in Premenstrual Syndrome. Brit Med J. 1:1161-1163, 1980

76] Osborne M.P., et al. Upregulation of Estradiol C16-alpha-hydroxylation in Human Breast Tissue: A Potential Biomarker of Breast Cancer Risk. J Nat Cancer Inst. 85(23):1917-1993, 1993

77] Pujol P., Hilsenbeck S.G., Chamness G.C. and Elledge R.M. Rising Levels of Estrogen Receptor in Breast Cancer over 2 Decades. Cancer. 74:1601-1606, 1994

78] Rajapakse et al Defining the impact of weakly estrogenic chemicals on the action of steroidal estrogens.Tox Sci 60(2):296-304 2001

79] Reed M.J. and Purohit A. Breast Cancer and the Role of Cytokines in Regulating Estrogen Synthesis: An Emerging Hypothesis. Endocrine Rev. 18:701-715, 1997

80] Reidel H.H., et al. Ovarian Failure Phenomena after Hysterectomy. J Reprod Med. 31:597-600, 1986

81] Rodriquez C., Calle E.E., Coates R.J., Miracle-McMahill H.L., Thun M.J. and Heath C.W. Estrogen Replacement Therapy and Fatal Ovarian Cancer. Am J Epidemiol. 141:828-834, 1995

82] Rodriguez C., Calle E.E. and Coates R.J., et al. Estrogen Replacement Therapy and Fatal Ovarian Cancer. Am J Epidemiol. 141:828-834, 1995

83] Sabourin J.C., Martin A., Baruch J., Truc J.B., et al. Bcl-2 Expression in Normal Breast Tissue during the Menstrual Cycle. Int J Cancer. 59:1-6, 1994

84] Schairer C., et al. Menopausal Estrogen and Estrogen-Progestin Replacement Therapy and Breast Cancer Risk. JAMA 283:485-491, 2000

85] Shering S.G., et al. Thyroid Disorders and Breast Cancer. Eur J Cancer Prev. 5(6):504-506, 1996

86] Sherwood RA, Rocks BF, et al. Magnesium and the premenstrual syndrome. Ann Clin Bioc 23:667-70 1986

87] Shi-Zhong Bu, De-Ling Yin, Xiu-Hai Ren, Li-Zhen Jiang, et al. Progesterone Induces Apoptosis and Up-regulation of p53 Expression in Human Ovarian Carcinoma Cell Lines. Am Cancer Soc. 1944-1950, 1997

88] Siddle N., et al The effect of Hysterectomy on the Age at Ovarian Failure: Identification of a Subgroup of Women with Premature Loss of Ovarian Function and Literature Review. Fertil Steril. 47:94-100, 1987

89] Smyth P.P. The Thyroid and Breast Cancer: A Significant Association? Ann Med. 29(3):189-191, 1997

90] Stoewsand G. S. Bioactive organosulfur phytochemicals in Brassica oleracea vegetables - a review. Food Chem Toxicol . 33(6):537-543, 1995

91] Stoll B.A. Adiposity as a Risk Determinant for Postmenopausal Breast Cancer. Int J Obes Relat Metab Disord. 24(5): 527-533, 2000

92] Stoll B.A. Dietary Supplements of Dehydroepiandrosterone in Relation to Breast Cancer Risk. Eur J Clin Nutr. 53(10):771-775, 1999

93] Stoll B.A. Western Nutrition and the Insulin Resistance Syndrome: A Link to Breast Cancer. Eur J Clin Nutr. 53(2):83-87, 1999

94] Stone S.C., et al. The Acute Effect of Hysterectomy on Ovarian Function. Am J Obstet Gynecol. 121:193-197, 1975

95] Talamini R. Selected Medical Conditions and Risk of Breast Cancer. Brit

J Cancer. 75(11):1699-1703, 1997

96] Vir, S.C. et al Serum and Hair Concentrations of Copper in Pregnancy Am J Clin Nutr 34 1981

97] Watts, D.L. Trace Elements and other Essential Nutrients Writers Block Books 1997

98] Watts, D.L. The Effects of oral contraceptive agents on Nutritional status Am Chiro March 1985

99] Watts, DL Nutritional relationships of copper J Orthomol Med 4:99-108 1989

100] Wattenburg L.W., et al. Inhibition of polycyclic aromatic hydrocarbon-induced neoplasia by naturally occurring indoles. Cancer Research. 38(5):1410-1413, 1978

101] Werbach, M. Nutritional Influences on Illness. Third Line Press. 199

102] Yuan F., et al. Anti-estrogenic activities of indole-3-carbinol in cervical cells: implications for prevention of cervical cancer. Anticancer Research. 19:1673-1680, 1999

WHAT IS HIDDEN COPPER OVERLOAD?

Many patients turn up with a mineral pattern of "hidden copper overload". This term eventuated because it is clear the patient had signs of copper overload but the level was not elevated on their hair analysis. The reason is that copper may be stored or sequestered in parts of the body for some time before it starts being excreted in the hair cells. Only when an *overflow* occurs does one detect it in the hair sample (ctually th same for mercury). Although not obvious, this type of copper overload does have clinical significance and should be treated *exactly* like overt copper excess. This involves reducing the high copper: zinc ratio foods, removing and/or blocking Xenoestrogens and giving zinc and/or molybdenum.

In the second hair analysis, one sees the copper "flushed out" and in the third analysis the copper comes back down again. The copper is hidden predominately in the digestive tract especially gullet, stomach and liver (sites of metallothionine). The patient may show excess urinary copper first. The Tessol kit from Harmonology will pick up most of these.

3 or more of the following criteria will confirm the diagnosis.

Zinc: Copper ratio less than 6
Calcium level greater than 100
Mercury level greater than 0.4
Calcium: potassium ratio greater than 10
Sodium: potassium ratio less than 2.2
Molybdenum level less than 0.003
Copper: Molybdenum ratio greater than 625
Potassium level less than 3
Barium level great than 0.26
Boron level greater than 0.91

Hidden copper overload

Copper keeps getting
delivered to the cells

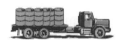
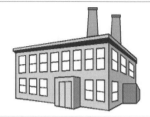

Inside, the copper
gets stored away

But there is less
room for other items

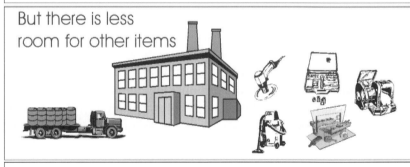

Eventually
there is no room
fo copper either

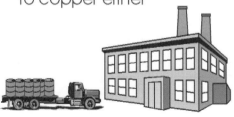
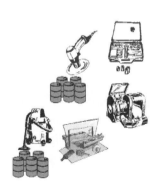

217

WHY COPPER EXCESS IS LINKED TO CANCER.

In the previous articles I have mentioned copper excess occurring in epidemic proportions. Certainly it is copper balance problems that mostly present to my clinic. What I am witnessing is not Wilson's Disease, which is a rare disorder of copper metabolism. I am witnessing an eclipse of environmental factors creating a monster nutritional imbalance. Some of my patients go back to their GP's with their hair analyses and ask for blood tests to confirm the findings. Most minerals are stored in tissues, not in the blood. In the case of *intracellular minerals*, the blood is the *least* sensitive measurement of total body stores. If you want to confirm copper overload, then a liver biopsy would be the equivalent. In fact there are studies, which have shown that hair analysis *reflects* liver copper levels. So to the armchair biologists, and medical scientists, read some texts on Tissue mineral analysis, not just biochemistry.

The University of Michigan published a paper, which showed that molybdenum supplements could alter the outcomes of cancer patients. It was called "Treatment of metastatic cancer with tetrathiomolybdate (ed molybdenum salt), an anti-copper, anti-angiogenic agent: Phase 1 study". It showed that starving tumours of copper could arrest their growth. Other studies have shown that molybdenum will affect a variety of cancers either orally or topically in humans and animal models. It begs the question of copper's involvement in the cause of cancer. Certainly copper excess is related in part to Xenoestrogen exposure. This class of compound (especially the Organochlorines) are have all been labelled as carcinogens. Hence the *cause* of the copper overload is also *the carcinogen*.

Secondly high coppers are always associated with deficiency of molybdenum, which is copper's most effective controller. This explains the mounting number of studies linking molybdenum deficiency to cancer of oesophagus, breast, stomach and colon.

Thirdly, copper has a Jekyll and Hyde personality. At normal levels it behaves itself but at high levels it blocks zinc, iron and magnesium and destroys (by oxidation) Vitamin C, Folic Acid and Vitamin E and Vitamin B1 (thiamine). Vitamin C and Folic Acid deficiency are associated with cancers like Larynx, Prostate, Breast, Cervix, Uterus, Melanoma, Bladder, Stomach and Pancreas.

Copper has another problem, which should be brought out. It has some addictive qualities and high coppers are associated with addictive behaviour patterns. Those with high coppers find themselves craving foods with high copper/low zinc ratios such as chocolate, mushrooms, avocados, grapes, almonds, crab, lobster, peanut paste and sesame seeds. This is particularly important for those who take mineral supplements long term. High copper/zinc ratio supplements will also have some "addictive" quality and may be used advantageously by Multi-level marketing companies to "hook" their customers. Most of these supplements are formulated in the USA, and they will never admit to any wrongdoing. They say that the level of copper in their supplements is simply in keeping with the RDA for copper. I have several comments about this. Firstly, they should put the RDA of *molybdenum and zinc* in the same product if they were really serious. Secondly, just following the RDA, isn't necessarily *smart* formulating. Thirdly, what suits their *laboratory rats* in Utah may not be suitable for *humans* in Western Australia where molybdenum intake is low. A simple line of research would reveal that we have been aware of our Zinc/Copper/Molybdenum problems since 1926. I would say that even a country as far away as the USA, that this information would be available to the Multimillion-dollar companies there. Fourthly, check out the Australian formulae. They are all relatively lower in copper. This reflects smart formulating. In my practice I try not to give more than 100 micrograms per day in supplements. Anyone who wished to proceed with long supplementation with copper content greater than this should have their copper status checked by hair analysis first.

References:

1] Aggett, PJ Fairweather-Tait. Adaptation to High and Low Copper Intakes:

Its relevance to Estimated Safe and adequate daily dietary intakes. Am J Clin Nut 67:1061S-63 1998

2] Beshgetoor L & Hambridge M Clinical conditions altering copper metabolism in humans. Am J Clin Nutr 67: 1017S-21S 1998

3] Bram, S., et al. Vitamin C preferential toxicity for malignant melanoma cells. Nature. 284:629-631, 1980.

4] Bremner I Manifestations of Copper excess. Am J Clin Nutr 67 1069S-73 1998

5] Brewer, G. J. Treatment of Wilson's disease with ammonium tetrathiomolybdate; Initial therapy in 17 neurologically affected patients. Archives of Neurology. 51:545-554, 1994.

6] Brewer et al. Treatment of metastatic cancer with tetrathiomolybdate, an anticopper, antiangiogenic agent. Phase I study Clin Cancer Res 6(1): 1-10 2000

7] Bruemmer, B., et al. Nutrient intake in relation to bladder cancer among middle-aged men and women. American Journal of Epidemiology. 144(5):485-495, 1996.

8] Burke, E. R. Vitamins C & E cut risk of prostate cancer cell growth. Muscular Development. 36(11):54, 1999.

9] Byers, R., et al. Epidemiologic evidence for vitamin C and vitamin E in cancer prevention. Am J Clin Nutr. 62(Supplement):1385S-1392S, 1995.

10] Cartwright et al Copper metabolism in normal subjects J Clin Nut 14: 1964

11] Cervantes C, Gutierrez-Corona F. Copper resistance mechanisms in bacteria and fungi. FEMS Microbiol Rev 1994;14:121–37.

12] Chuong et al Zinc and copper levels in premenstrual syndrome. Fertility & Sterility 62 313-20 1994

13] Daniels et al Iron and copper retention in young children J Nutr 1934

14] Dameron et al Mechanisms for protection against copper toxicity. AM J Clin Nut 67 1091S-1097S 1998

15] Eck P Insight into copper elimination. Phoenix AZ Eck Institute reference sheet 1991

16] Eck P Introduction to copper toxicity. Phoenix AZ Eck Institute reference sheet 1989

17] Epstein et al, Hair copper in primary biliary cirrhosis Am J Clin Nutr 33: 965-967.

18] Finley et al Influences of ascorbic acid supplementtion on copper stsuta in young adult men Am J Clin Nut 37 1983

19] Fitzgerald D Safety guidelines for copper in water Am J Clin Nut 67 1098S-1120S 1998

220

20] Graham, S., et al. Dietary factors in the epidemiology of cancer of the larynx. American Journal of Epidemiology. 113(6):675-680, 1981.

21] Howe, G. R., et al. Dietary factors and risk of breast cancer: Combined analysis of 12-case control studies. Journal of the National Cancer Institute. 82:561-569, 1990.

22] Jacob et al Hair as a biopsy material. V. Hair metal as an index of hepatic metal in rats: copper and zinc Am J Clin Nutr 31: 477-480

23] Karcioglu et al Zinc and copper in Medicine Springfield Charles C Thomas Pub 1980

24] Klevey LM Hair as a biopsy material II. Assesment of copper nutriture Am J Clin Nutr 23 1970

25] Klevay LM The role of copper and zinc in cholesterol metabolism. Advances in Nutritional research Draper Plenum Pub 1971

26] Komada, K., et al. Effects of dietary molybdenum on esophageal carcinogenesis in rats induced by N-methyl-N-benzylnitrosamine. Cancer Res. 50:2418-2422, 1990.

27] Levenson C Mechanisms of copper conservation in organs Am J Clin Nut 67 978S-981S 1998

28] Lizotte L The woman with too much copper. Total health 19: 49 19997

29] McKenzie, JM Alteration of the zinc anc copper concentration of hair Am J Clin Nutr 31: 470-476.

30] Luo, X. M., et al. Molybdenum and oesophageal cancer in China. Federation Proceedings. Federation of the American Society for Experimental Biology. 46:928, 1981.

31] Luo, X. M., et al. Inhibitory effects of molybdenum on esophageal and forestomach carcinogenesis in rats. J Natl. Cancer Inst. 71:75-80, 1983.

32] Malter R Copper toxicity: Psychological implications for children, adolescences and adults. Hoffman estates A Malter institute for natural development reference sheet 1984

33] Martin JM Overdosing on copper? Alive 62:43-44 1985

34] Mason KE A conspectus of research on copper metabolism and requirements of man J Nutr 109 1979

35] Maurer, K. Vitamins may prevent bladder cancer recurrence. Family Practice News. 15 December 1995:12.

36] Moss, M. A. Effects of Molybdenum on Pain and General Health: A Pilot Study J of Nutrit & Env Medicine. 5(1):56-61, 1995.

37] Nakadaira H et al Distribution of selenium and molybdenum and cancer mortality in Niigata, Japan. Arch Envir Health Sep 50:5 384-80 1995

38] Nolan KR Copper toxicity syndrome J Orthomol Psych 12:270-282 1983

39] O'Connor, H. J., et al. Effect of increased intake of vitamin C on the

221

mutagenic activity of gastric juice and intragastric concentrations of ascorbic acid. Carcinogenesis. 6(11):1675-1676, 1985

40] O'Dell BL Biochemisrty of copper The Meical Clinics of North America 60 Saunders 1960

41] Owen CA Copper deficiency and toxicity: Acquired and inherited in plants, animals and man Park Ridge NJ Noyes Pub 1981

42] Pierson, H. F., et al. Sodium ascorbate enhancement of carbidopa-levodopa methyl ester anti-tumor activity against pigmented B16 melanoma. Cancer Research. 43:2047-2051, 1983.

43] Pratt WB Elevated hair copper in idiopathic scoliosis and of normal individuals Clin Chem 24 1978

44] Schiffman, M. H. Diet and faecal genotoxicity. Cancer Surv. 6:653-672, 1987.

45] Solioz M et al Copper pumping ATPases: common concepts in bacteria and man. FEBS Lett 1994;346:44–7.

46] Turnlund et al Copper absorption, excretion and retention by young men consuming low dietary copper determined by using stable isotope 65Cu AM J Clin Nut 67: 1219-1225 1998

47] Vir et al Serum and hair concentrations of copper during pregnancy Am J Clin Nutr 34: 2382-2388 1981

48] Watts DL Nutritional relationships of copper J Orthomol Med 4:99-108 1989

49] Wei,H.J.et al. Effect of molybdenum and tungsten on mammary carcinogenesis in Sprague-Dawley (SD) rats Chung Hua Liu Tsa Chih. 9:204-207, 1987

50] Yang, C. S. Research on esophageal cancer in China: a review. Cancer Research. 40:2633-2644, 1980.

51] Zheng, W., et al. Retinol, antioxidant vitamins, and cancers of the upper digestive tract in a prospective cohort study of postmenopausal women. American Journal of Epidemiology. 142(9):955-960, 1995.

HOW COPPER OVERLOAD CAUSES IRON DEFICIENCY

There are several features of iron metabolism that can be affected by copper. Iron levels are like a bank account; they depend on how much you put in, how much you take out and how often you put in and take out.

Sources of Iron:

Food	Amount	Iron (mg)	Food	Amount	Iron (mg)
Bran flakes	1 cup	10.8	Hamburger Pattie	1 serve	2.4
Lambs Liver (Fried)	100g	8.2	Pearl Barley (Boiled)	1 cup	2.1
Spinach (Cooked)	1 cup	6.4	Cashews (Salted)	½ cup	2
Apricots (Dried)	1 cup (Halves)	6.1	Lamb	100g	2
Chickpeas (Boiled)	1 cup	4.7	Bulgur (Boiled)	1 cup	1.7
All Bran	½ cup	4.5	Raisins	½ cup	1.7
Oysters (Fried)	6 oysters	4.4	Sausages (Grilled)	2 (thick, 10cm in length)	1.3
Salmon (Canned)	1 can	3.8	Liverwurst	1 slice	1.2
Oats	½ cup	3.7	Wholegrain Bread	1 slice	1.1
Beef (Cooked)	¾ cup (Diced)	2.6	Whole wheat Pita Bread	1 (small)	0.8
Almonds	½ cup	2.6	Pate	1 tbsp	0.7
Tuna (Canned)	1 can	2.5	Baked Beans	1 cup	0.7

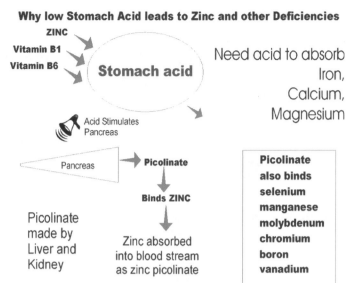

Why low Stomach Acid leads to Zinc and other Deficiencies

ZINC
Vitamin B1
Vitamin B6

Stomach acid

Need acid to absorb
Iron,
Calcium,
Magnesium

Acid Stimulates
Pancreas

Pancreas → Picolinate

Binds ZINC

Picolinate
made by
Liver and
Kidney

Zinc absorbed
into blood stream
as zinc picolinate

Picolinate
also binds
selenium
manganese
molybdenum
chromium
boron
vanadium

Input

Firstly, iron sources may not be plentiful in the diet. Above is a list of such sources with the corresponding amounts. It is believed that concurrent vitamin C will enhance iron absorption.

How Picolinate binds zinc

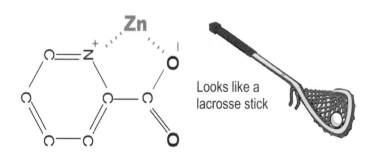

Looks like a
lacrosse stick

Also absorbed in this way are Selenium Manganese
Molybdenum Boron Chromium and Vanadium

Absorption

Secondly, iron needs to be charged with a two-plus charge to be absorbed. This requires stomach acid. Unfortuantely stomach acid requires the presence of Zinc, Vitamin B1 and vitamin B6. Calcium and magnesium also need stomach acid to absorb them. When the stomach makes acid for digestion a second message is sent to the pancreas gland to release picolinate into the intestine. This special molecule acts like a lacrosse stick to pick up ions like zinc, selenium, molybdenum, chromium, manganese and vanadium. The irony is that if you don't absorb zinc, you don't make stomach acid and if you don' make acid, you don't absorb zinc (and the iron).

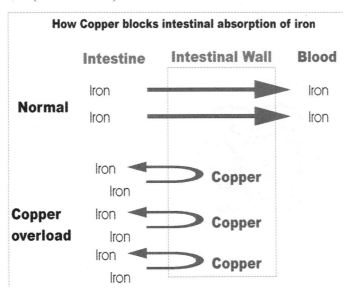

How Copper blocks intestinal absorption of iron

The next step is that iron must traverse the intestinal wall to get to the bloodstream. Copper in the intestinal wall will affect this transfer.

Loss

Iron may be lost for these reasons.

Nose bleeds

Stomach ulcers

Harmorrhoids

Menstrual loss

Liver Wastage

Storage

Lastly, the efficient of iron storage is dependent on the presence of the mineral molybdenum. If you could imagine iron as eggs in the palm of your hand, there would be a limit to how many you could hold. Molybdenum allows efficient iron storage rather like the egg cartons.

High copper levels and low molybdenum's on hair analysis are the typical findings in my patients with iron deficiency.

Iron storage

Iron storage effect of
Molybdenum

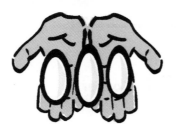

No molybdenum,
iron storage is poor

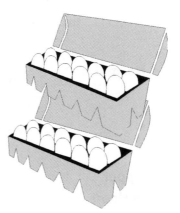

Effect of Molybdenum

WHY COPPER EXCESS CAUSES FATIGUE.

In previous articles I have mentioned the unwanted effect of having too much copper. This is a problem within the tissues and not in the blood. Naïve doctors who think that a normal blood test for copper disproves this should go back to basic cell physiology books and realise that blood tests for intracellular minerals are not representative of tissue levels as (stated earlier) blood is only a transport system.

Copper causes fatigue for several reasons.
a]   Iron deficiency and/or tissue iron blockade
b]   Magnesium deficiency and/or tissue blockade
c]   Carnitine deficiency leading to weak muscles
d]   Hypoglycaemia
e]   Poor sleep pattern
f]   Depression
g]   Tissue blockade of thyroid hormone

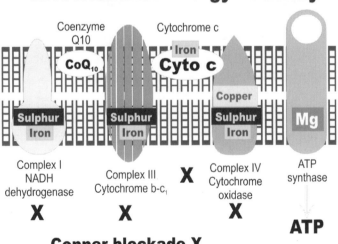

Mitochondrial Energy Pathway

Let's take iron deficiency first.

Copper excess is probably the commonest cause of *persistent* iron deficiency. It causes gastritis, hypochlorhydria (low stomach acid) and blocks the transfer of iron across the intestinal wall. See previous chapter.

Once iron is in the cells, copper blocks the effect of iron. This is most notable in the mitochondria. See the figure about Mitochondrial energy pathway and see that copper blocks most of the steps.

Muscle Metabolism, Carnitine, Iron and Vitamin C

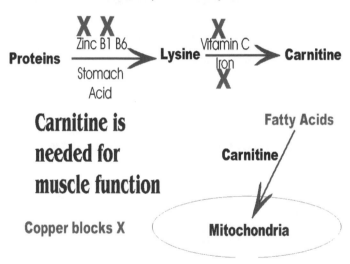

Carnitine is a vitamin, which is required for the metabolism of fatty acids. Tissues which need this type of metabolism cannot function properly. The most important tissue is muscle. Copper blocks the production of carnitine as shown in the figure above.

Copper leads to hypoglycaemia because of several mechanisms. Firstly it affects digestion and may impair the absorption of sugars. Secondly it causes an inappropriate rise in insulin, which causes the blood sugar to drop. Thirdly it affects liver function and gluconeogenesis. This is where the liver makes glucose during the fasting state.

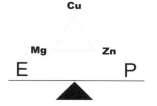

Normal Copper balance depends on Estrogen: progesterone balance

The effect on insulin is part of the Syndrome X spectrum. Its relationship to Estrogen dominance is shown below. Two hormones, Estrogen and progesterone affect normal copper metabolism and balance. If total estrogens (endogenous and foreign) are high then copper is retained. This causes the insulin level to rise and the DHEA level to fall.

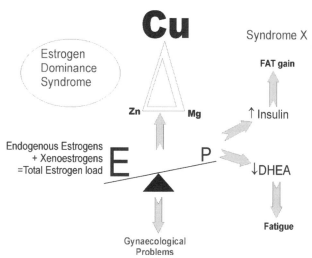

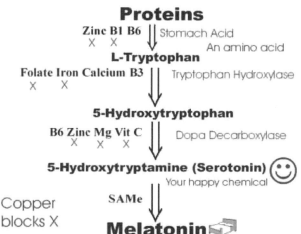

Poor sleep pattern and depression are direct results of copper blocking serotonin and melatonin production.

Lastly, the effect upon thyroid function.

Warning, after reading this section you ill know more about thyroid function than any Endocrinologist in this state.

Effect of copper upon thyroid function

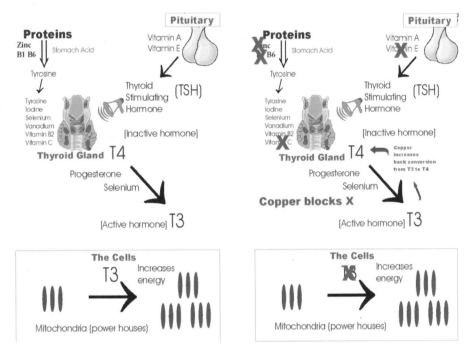

Normal thyroid function involves the release of TSH (thyroid stimulating hormone) from the pituitary. This requires Vitamin E and Vitamin A. TSH stimulates the thyroid to release T4 (thyroxine). To make T4, the thyroid needs to get tyrosine. We get this from proteins, but we need good digestion to extract this amino acid (and Zinc, B1, B6). Then the thyroid needs selenium, vanadium, Vitamin C, Vitamin B2 and iodine to make T4. To activate T4 to T3 we need progesterone and selenium. The effect by copper is to destroy Vitamin E and C, promote the back conversion from T3 to T4 and block T3 in the cells. Does this show up on a blood test? No. Do the doctors believe the blood test or the patient? You guessed it.

Those with high coppers find that they feel better taking supplements like zinc, magnesium, vitamin C and vitamin E. They are trying to match the disruptive effect of copper with the nutrients that copper blocks or destroy. The analogy is a railway bridge. The burden of copper is met by propping up the bridge with extra nutrients. Unfortunately, stress depletes zinc, magnesium and vitamin C and may sabotage this attempt to deal with copper in this manner. The best solution, of course, is to get rid of the copper.

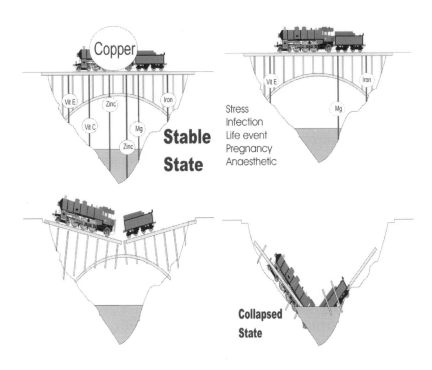

A QUICK OVERVIEW OF GLUCOSE CONTROL.

Warning: After you have read this, you will know more about diabetes than any endocrinologist in this country.

Many patients are diagnosed with hyperglycaemia. Most are started on empirical treatments without any investigation as to *why* this happened. There is much already in the literature to help define more accurately what *type* of diabetes the patients might have, but nobody bothers to check. My point is this: why not check if there is a cause that is amenable to nutritional management at the time of diagnosis? Please refer to the figure schematic on the next page.

There are two sources of glucose. Firstly from starches and sugars in the diet and secondly from the liver during fasting, especially overnight. Dietary glucose requires digestive enzymes to correctly digest carbohydrates. Carbohydrates release sugars at differing rates. This rate has been referred to as the glycaemic index. The higher the index, the faster the sugar rises. The level for pure glucose is 100.

The liver makes glucose to prop up the blood sugar level, rather like a treasury props up a country's currency. The important nutrients are zinc, magnesium and Vitamin B6.
The next phase is the production and storage of insulin. Zinc, manganese, Vitamin D and sulphur are important nutrients for this. Next comes insulin release and this is dependent upon magnesium. Think of magnesium as a valve that allows the correct and appropriate release of insulin. Glucose stimulates the release of insulin from the pancreas.
Once insulin is in the blood stream, it acts like a "front door" to let glucose into the cells, where it's used for fuel. But to get into the cell the glucose also needs an "entry ticket". This is the Glucose Tolerance Factor. It contains chromium, vanadium and Vitamin B3. In addition, chromium and vanadium need to be in balance. Alternatively, there is a "side door" entry, which can utilise selenium, arginine (an amino acid), or taurine (also an amino acid) or Vitamin E or Vitamin C.
The problem we have is that zinc and selenium are low in the soil and

magnesium levels have fallen in our diets since broad acre farming. Refining carbohydrates destroys chromium and vanadium. Overall we have increased the glycaemic index of our diets. Add these up, and you have a significant problem for glucose control.

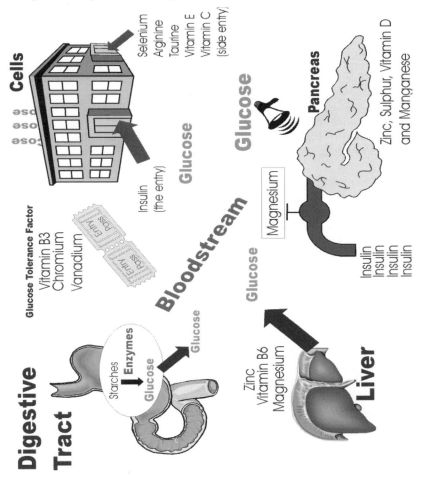

References
1] Abraham A.S., et al. The effects of chromium supplementation on serum glucose and lipids in patients with and without non-insulin dependent diabetes. Metabolism. 41:768-771, 1992.
2] Anderson R., et al. Beneficial effects of chromium for people with Type II Diabetes. Diabetes. 45(Suppl. 2):124A/454, 1996.
3] Anderson R.A., Roussel A-M, Zouari N., et al. Potential antioxidant effects of zinc and chromium supplement in people with type II diabetes mellitus. J Am Coll

Nutr. 20(3):212-218, 2001

4] Anderson R. A., et al. Chromium supplementation of human subjects: Effects on glucose, insulin and lipid variables. Metabolism. 32:894-899, 1983.

5] Anderson R. A., et al. Supplemental chromium effects on glucose, insulin, glucagon, and urinary chromium losses in subjets consuming low-chromium diets. American Journal of Clinical Nutrition. 54:909-916, 1991.

6] Anderson R.A., et al. Elevated intakes of supplemental chromium improve glucose and insulin variables in individuals with type 2 diabetes. Diabetes. 46:1786-1791, 1997.

7] Anderson R.A. Nutritional factors influencing the glucose/insulin system: chromium. J Am Coll Nutr. 16(5):404-410, 1997.

8] Baly D., et al. Effect of manganese deficiency on insulin binding, glucose transport & metabolism in rat adipocytes. J Nutr. 120:1075-1079, 1990.

9] Boden G., et al. Effects of vanadyl sulfate on carbohydrate and lipid metabolism in patients with non-insulin dependent diabetes mellitus. Metabolism. 45:1130-1135, 1996.

10] Boyd S.G., et al. Combined dietary chromium picolinate supplementation and an exercise program leads to a reduction of serum cholesterol and insulin in college-aged subjects. J Nutr Biochem. 9:471-475, 1998.

11] Cam M. C., et al. Distinct glucose lowering and beta cell protective effects of vanadium and food restriction in streptozotocin-diabetes. Eur J Endocrinol. 141(5):546-554, 1999.

12] Chan et al. the role of copper, molybdenum, selenium and zinc in nutrition and health. Clin Lab Med. 18(4):673-85, 1998.

13] Chauser A. Zinc, Insulin and Diabetes. J of American College of Nutrition 17(2):109-115, 1998.

14] Cohen N., et al. Oral vanadyl sulfate improves hepatic and peripheral insulin sensitivity in patients with non-insulin dependent diabetes mellitus. Journal of Clinical Investigations. 95(6):2501-2509, 1995.

15] Combs G.F. and Combs S.B. The Role of Selenium in Nutrition. Academic Press, Inc., Orlando, USA, 1986.

16] Corica F., Allegra A., Di Benedetto A., et al. Effects of oral magnesium supplementation on plasma lipid concentrations of patients with non-insulin dependent diabetes mellitus. Magnes res. 7:43-47, 1994.

17] Davies S., et al. Age-related decreases in chromium levels in 51,655 hair, sweat and serum samples from 40,872 patients – implications for the prevention of cardiovascular disease ad type II diabetes mellitus. Metabolism. 46(5):469-473, 1997

18] Evans G.W. The effect of chromium picolinate on insulin controlled parameters in humans. Int J Biosocial Medical research. 11:163-180, 1989

19] Evans G.W., et al. Chromium picolinate increases membrane fluidity and rate of insulin internalization. J Inorg Biochem. 46(4):243-250, 1992.

20] Fugii S., Takemura T., Wada M., et al. magnesium levels in plasma, erythrocyte, and urine in patients with diabetes mellitus. Horm Metab res. 14:161-162, 1982.

21] Haglund et al. Evidence of a relationship between childhood onset type 1 diabetes and low ground water concentration of zinc. Diabetes Care Aug. 19:8 873-5, 1996.

22] Jing M.A., Folsom A.R., Melnick S.L., et al. Associations of serum and dietary magnesium with cardiovascular disease, hypertension, diabetes, insulin, and carotid arterial wall thickness : the ARIC study. J Clin Epidemiol. 48:927-940, 1995.

23] Kelly G.S. Insulin resistance: lifestyle and nutritional interventions. Alternative medicine Review. 5(2):109-132, 2000.

24] Leach R.M., Jr. metabolism & Function of Manganese. Trace elements in Human Health & Disease. Vol. III

25] Kee N.A., et al. Beneficial effect of chromium supplementation on serum triglyceride levels in NIDDM. Diabetes Care. 17(12):1449-1452, 1994.

26] Mather H.M., et al. Hypomagnesemia in diabetes. Clin Chem Acta. 95:235-242, 1979.

27] McNeill J. Enhanced in vivo sensitivity of vanadyl-treated diabetic rats to insulin. Canadian Journal of Physiology and Pharmacology. 68(4):486-491, 1996.

28] Mechegiani E., et al. Zinc-dependent low thymic hormone level in type 1 diabetes. Diabetes. 12:932-937, 1989.

29] Mertz W., et al. Present knowledge of the role of chromium. Federation Proceedings. 33:2275-2280, 1974.

30] Nakamura t., et al. Kinetics of zinc status in children with IDDM> Diabetes Care. 14"553-557, 1991.

31] Niewoener C.B., et al. Role of zinc supplementation in type II diabetes mellitus. Am J Med. 63-68, 1988.

32] Paolisso G., et al. Improved insulin response and action by chronic magnesium administration in aged NIDDM subjects. Diabetes Care. 12(4):265-269, 1989.

33] Paolisso et al. Hypertension, diabetes and insulin resistance: the role of intracellular magnesium. Am J Hypertens. 10:3 346-55, 1997.

34] Pepato M. T., et al. effects of oral vanadyl sulfate treatment on serum enzymes and lipids of streptozotocin-diabetic young rats. Mol Cell Biochem. 198(1-2):157-161, 1999.

35] Pidduck H.G., et al. Hyperzincuria of diabetes mellitus and possible genetic implications of this observation. Diabetes. 19:240-247, 1970.

36] Preuss H.G., et al. Chromium update: examining recent literature 1997-1998. Curr Opin Clin 57] Striffler J.S., et al. Overproduction of insulin in the chromium-deficient rat. Metabolism. 48:1063-1068, 1999.

58] Toplack H., et al. Addition of chromium picolinate to a very low calorie diet improves the insulin-glucose ratio after weight reduction. International Journal of Obesity. 19(2):s057, 1995.

59] Uehara S., et al. Clinical significance of selenium level in chronic pacreatitis. J Clin Biochem Nutr. 5:201-207, 1988.

60] Wallace E. C. Diabetic epidemic. Energy times. 9(4):24-28 1999

61] Watts D.L. The nutritional relationships of manganese. J. Orthomol. Med. 5(4):219-22, 1990.

A WORD ABOUT THE EPIDEMIC OF DEPRESSION.

Depression is a common illness mostly caused by a lack of serotonin in the brain. Patients are told by their doctors that there is "an imbalance of chemicals" in the brain and that only *more chemicals* can solve this problem for them. Instead of finding out *why* the patient can't make their own serotonin, doctors give them drugs. But is it possible to fix their own innate production of this chemical? In most cases yes, but you have to know *why* it has broken down. From the previous chapters we have seen the serotonin pathway turn up several times. Let's look at it again.

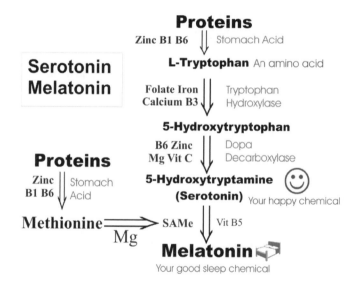

A small part of the brain called the hippocampus makes serotonin from the amino acid tryptophan. It converts tryptophan to 5-hydroxy tryptophan. In order to do this it needs Iron, Vitamin B3, Calcium and Folic acid. The next step to convert 5-hydroxy tryptophan to serotonin needs Magnesium, Zinc, Vitamin C and Vitamin B6. So there are 9 nutrients required and two enzymes.

Now, it turns out that you don't need to be deficient in any of these; you just need two borderline deficiencies in the same line or sequential lines to have a problem. In addition, the presence of a heavy metal

236

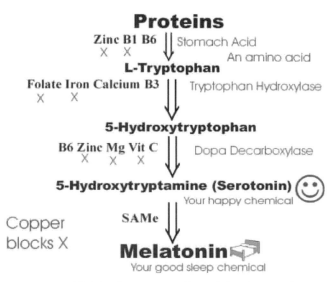

Proteins

Zinc B1 B6 ⇓ Stomach Acid
X X   An amino acid
L-Tryptophan

Folate Iron Calcium B3 ⇓ Tryptophan Hydroxylase
X   X

5-Hydroxytryptophan

B6 Zinc Mg Vit C ⇓ Dopa Decarboxylase
X   X   X

5-Hydroxytryptamine (Serotonin) ☺
Your happy chemical

Copper   SAMe ⇓
blocks X
Melatonin 🛏
Your good sleep chemical

such as copper will block Iron, Folic acid, Zinc and Magnesium. This explains the association of copper excess with depression. Mercury blocks iron and zinc. It also blocks selenium, which is also associated with depression.

So the take home message is, both deficiencies and excesses cause trouble. To solve the problems, you have to know what the abnormalities are. Giving drugs doesn't solve the reason for the serotonin deficiency and this may explain why 30% of patients don't respond to any anti-depressant.

References:
1] Baldessarini R.J. Treatment of depression by altering monamine metabolism: Precursors and metabolic inhibitor. Psychopharmacology Bulletin. 20:224-239, 1984
2] Beckmann H Kasper S Serotonin precursors as antidepressant agents: a review Fortschr Neurol Psychiatr 51:176-182 1983
3] Benton, D., et al. Selenium supplementation improves mood in a double-blind trial. Psychopharmacology. 102(4): 549- 550, 1990.
4] Benton, D., et al. The impact of selenium supplementation on mood. Biological Psychiatry. 29(11):1092-1098, 1991.

5] Birdsall TC 5-hydroxytryptophan: a clinically effective serotonin precursor Altern Med Rev 3:271-280 1998

6] Charney,D Nestler E, Bunney B eds The Neurobiological Foundation of Mental Illness. Oxford University Press. 1999.

7] Christensen L. & Burrows R. Dietary treatment of depression. Behavior Therapy. 21:183-193, 1990

8] Duman RS et al A molecular theory of depression Depression 3:187-189 1995

9] Fernstrom J.D. & Faller G.V. Neutral amino acids in the brain: Changes in response to food ingestion. Journal of Neurochemistry. 30:1531-1538, 1978

10] Gelenberg AJ et al Tyrosine for the treatment of depression Am J Psychiatry 137:622-623 1980

11] Gelenberg A.J., Gibson C.J. & Wojcik J.D. Neurotransmitter precursors for the treatment of depression. Psychopharmacology Bulletin. 18:7-8, 1982

12] Growdon J.H. & Wurtman R.J. Dietary influences on the synthesis of neurotransmitters in the brain. Nutrition Reviews. 37:129-136, 1979

13] Lieberman H.R., Caballero B. & Finer N. The composition of lunch determines afternoon plasma tryptophan ratios in humans. Journal of Neural Transmission. 65:211-217, 1986

14] Nakajima T et al Clinical evaluation of 5-hydroxy-L-tryptophan as an antidepressant drug Folia Psychiatr Neurol Jpn 32:223-230 1978

15] Shen W.W. & D'Souza T.C. Cola-induced psychotic organic brain syndrome. Rocky Mountain Medical Journal. 312-313, 1979

16] Spring B, Chiodo J. & Bowen D.J. Carbohydrates, tryptophan and behavior: A methodological review. Psychological Bulletin. 102:234-256, 1987

17] Wurtman R.J., Hefti J. & Melamed E. Precursor control of neurotransmitter synthesis. Pharmacology Reviews. 32:315-355, 1980

18] Van Praag Management of depression with serotonin precursors Biol Psychiatry 16:291-310 1981

19] Young SN Behavioral effects of dieatary neurotransmitter precursors: basic and clinical aspects. Neurosci Behaviour Rev 20:313-323 1996

IT DON'T ADD UP: THE MYTH OF ADD.

Western Australia has a high rate of Ritalin and Dexamphetamine prescribing for Attention Deficit Disorder (ADD). Despite the fuss made about this, no real progress has been made in preventing the condition or solving without using medications. The ADD problem appears to be in a part of the brain that "drives" the cerebral cortex. The best analogy would be conductor of an orchestra. If he waves softly, not much noise comes out of the orchestra pit and the audience falls asleep. If he waves wildly, the orchestra blares and wakes up all of those in the auditorium. The neurotransmitter responsible for this is noradrenaline. The defect in ADD is failure to make this chemical in sufficient quantities to "drive" the brain. Ritalin and Dexamphetamine have noradrenaline like actions and hence "prod the conductor" to work harder. The problem is that when you stop the drugs; the predicament is still there.

Perhaps just like depression (see chapter on this), we should be finding out *why* the children can't make noradrenaline. The diagram on this page shows how noradrenaline is converted from the amino acid Phenylalanine. Several familiar vitamins and minerals show their faces again. Deficiencies in these would make it more difficult to make noradrenaline. Do you thing the paediatricians and psychiatrists ever measure these?

How to make Noradrenaline

L-Phenylalanine An amino acid

Folate Iron
B3 B6 Vit C ⇓ Phenylalanine Hydroxylase

L-Tyrosine An amino acid

Folate Iron
B2 B3 Vit C ⇓ Tyrosine Hydrolase

L-Dopa

Zinc Magnesium
B6 Vit C ⇓ Dopa Decarboxylase

Dopamine

Copper Vit C ⇓ Dopamine Hydroxylase

Noradrenaline

Needed for concentration and alertness

The next scenario is to look at the effect of superimposition of the toxic minerals and copper excess in this pathway. As you can see, copper plays havoc with several of the co-factors. Mercury and cadmium also wreak havoc. But where on earth would a child get mercury? Thiomersol is the preservative in most of our vaccinations. Thiomersol *is* mercury. Where could a child get excess copper? From his/her mother via the placenta, especially if the mother had copper excess. Considering 70% of females suffer the Estrogen Dominance Dyndrome (see page 203), this is highly likely! Oh that nasty copper again.

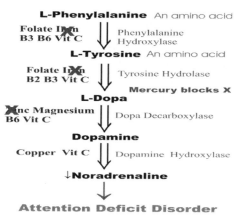

Why Mercury in the brain leads to ADD

L-Phenylalanine An amino acid

Folate Iron
B3 B6 Vit C — Phenylalanine Hydroxylase

L-Tyrosine An amino acid

Folate Iron
B2 B3 Vit C — Tyrosine Hydrolase

Mercury blocks X

L-Dopa

Zinc Magnesium
B6 Vit C — Dopa Decarboxylase

Dopamine

Copper Vit C — Dopamine Hydroxylase

↓**Noradrenaline**

Attention Deficit Disorder

So, you decide which is the better approach; give drugs or fix the noradrenaline pathway? Which is the more *logical* approach, the medical model or nutritional medicine? Which approach do you think is *encouraged* by the health authorities and governments? Which approach do you think is actively *discouraged?* Why do you think that this is the case? Yes, you guessed it; vested interests in ill health.

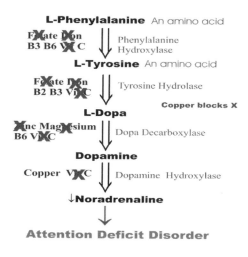

Why Copper Excess leads to ADD

L-Phenylalanine An amino acid

Folate Iron
B3 B6 Vit C — Phenylalanine Hydroxylase

L-Tyrosine An amino acid

Folate Iron
B2 B3 Vit C — Tyrosine Hydrolase

Copper blocks X

L-Dopa

Zinc Magnesium
B6 Vit C — Dopa Decarboxylase

Dopamine

Copper Vit C — Dopamine Hydroxylase

↓**Noradrenaline**

Attention Deficit Disorder

The Politics .....

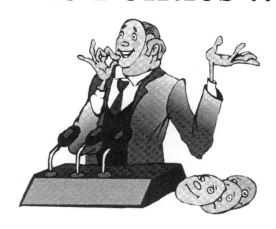

THE POLITICS OF NUTRITIONAL MEDICINE

Most of the previous chapters have concentrated on nutrients and the associated illness that result from the lack, excess or blocking of these within the body. Most agriculturists would agree that WA has significant problems with the minerals zinc, selenium and molybdenum. What about looking at the bigger picture of common illnesses and what information we have about nutrient problems in those illnesses. In 2001, Dr Brad Weeks (a Nutritional Doctor from Seattle) lectured in Perth and Mandurah about nutrition and mental illness. After a conversation with the Minister for Health he asked me to prepare some overheads for his talk on Adult Mental Health and nutrition (see table 1). He wanted me to present a very important take home message. If you do not read any further, here it is.

Systemic nutritional problems manifest in many body organs, but cause different symptoms according to the dysfunctional tissue. Mental illness is a result of these systemic processes and is part of a much larger picture of ill health in our patients.

Let's have a look at what illnesses are correlated to what nutritional problems. Below is a table (table 1) of such correlations. It tells us at least three things. Firstly, it confirms why there are such epidemics such as depression, heart disease and cancer. Secondly it suggests that preventative medicine programs should be addressing these issues now, and especially in our children. Thirdly, it is an indictment on the Medical System as a whole, which prefers to financially and professionally punish doctors who practice Nutritional Medicine, and reward doctors who practice symptom prescribing.

What is symptom prescribing? Here are some examples. Headache = Mersyndol, Asthma = Ventolin. Anxiety = Valium. Insomnia = Temazepam. Depression = Aropax. Blood pressure = Tritace. Leg cramps = quinine. Schizophrenia = Olanzapine. Dr Weeks said in his lectures that Nutritional doctors are usually "dobbed in" by other doctors. A few years ago a Perth Doctor was reported to the medical board by a colleague because he ordered a Vanadium level in a patient with thyroid problems (see table 1).

Correlations of Illness and Deficiency States

Disease	Mineral Deficiencies	Vitamin Deficiencies
Hypertension	Zinc, Selenium, Magnesium, Potassium	A, B3, B6, C, D, Coenzyme Q10
Diabetes	Zinc, Selenium, Vanadium, Magnesium, Chromium, Manganese	B3, B6, Coenzyme Q10
Asthma	Zinc, Selenium, Magnesium, Molybdenum	B6, C, E
Thyroid Disease	Selenium, Iodine, Vanadium	A, B2, B6, C, E
Heart Disease	Zinc, Selenium, Magnesium	B6, B12, Folate, C, E, Coenzyme Q10
Cancer	Zinc, Selenium, Molybdenum	A, B6, Folate, C, E, Coenzyme Q10
Depression	Zinc, Iron, Selenium, Calcium, Magnesium, Potassium	B6, B12, Folate, C
Schizophrenia	Zinc, Selenium, Magnesium, Manganese	B3, B6, Folate, C, Coenzyme Q10
Alzheimers	XS Aluminium, Magnesium	Betacarotene, B6, B12, Folate, C, Coenzyme Q10

Correlations of Illness and Deficiency States

Disease	Mineral Deficiencies	Vitamin Deficiencies
Hypertension	Zinc, Selenium, Magnesium, Potassium	A, B3, B6, C, D, Co Q10
Diabetes	Zinc, Selenium, Vanadium, Magnesium, Chromium, Manganese	B3, B6, Co Q10, Co Q10
Asthma	Zinc, Selenium, Magnesium, Molybdenum	B6, C
Thyroid Disease	Selenium, Iodine, Vanadium	A, B2, B6, C, E
Heart Disease	Zinc, Selenium, Magnesium	B6, B12, Folate, C, E
Cancer	Zinc, Selenium, Magnesium, Molybdenum	A, B6, Folate, C, E
Depression	Zinc, Selenium, Iron, Calcium, Magnesium, Potassium	B3, B6, B12, Folate, C
Schizophrenia	Zinc, Selenium, Magnesium, Manganese	B3, B6, Folate, C, Co Q10
Alzheimers	XS Aluminium, Magnesium	Betacarotene, B6, B12, Folate, C, Co Q10

Effects of Copper blocks

This is an example of where ignorance and spite manifest behind the public arena.

If doctors start ordering a lot of (say) selenium levels, they get nasty letters from the Health Insurance Commission asking for an explanation, with threats of prosecution if they continue to check for such minerals. The HIC does *not care* how many of these tests come back abnormal. Now make your own conclusion here. If selenium can help in cancer, heart disease, diabetes, depression, schizophrenia and asthma, yet the standard treatment is based on drug therapy, who has to gain by intimidating doctors?

Dr Weeks showed an interesting diagram, which tabled the deaths from prescription medicine and nutritional supplements in the USA. Now, firstly, the laws in the USA are somewhat more relaxed when it comes to things like mineral supplements compared with Australia. The statistics showed an average of 90,000 deaths per year for drug therapies and 3, yes THREE for nutritional supplements. So, if simple mineral therapies can help and have less side effects and deaths, why aren't we practicing this sort of medicine? It boils down to money and kudos. Selenium therapy might cost about $30 per year, with no kickbacks to pharmaceutical companies, prescribing physicians or regulatory bodies. The PBS (part of the HIC) subsidised drug therapies might range from $2000 to $10,000 per year for one patient. Interesting comparison don't you think?

Now, we've talked at length about the problem of copper toxicity in WA; why not add the effect of copper to our table (see table 2). Even if the sceptics did not believe the Agriculture Dept, the farmers, the vets and the nutritional doctors about the mineral deficiencies, what do they think about the blocking effect upon "normal" nutrients so plentiful from our great diets based upon our great soils and delivered by our altruistic primary producers? Now you can really see some damage occurring. Oh, that nasty copper is destroying all that **plentiful** Vitamin C in our diet. Remember the pitiful RDA of Vitamin C? What should the RDA be if the region has a problem with copper? Probably 4000mg.

Now, finally for the sceptics, who say that there is no research to back this up, I wish to draw your attention to a paper that was presented on Thursday 11th October 2001 at the University of WA. It is titled "Duty to Care" It was an 8-year study from 1990 to 1998 and included 240,000 patients. It compared death rates from various illnesses like cancer, heart disease, stroke, respiratory (lung) and suicide to the normal population.

The mentally ill death rates from cancer were 30% more than the normal population. There were 16% more deaths from heart disease, 320% more deaths from stroke, 280% more deaths from lung disease. What does this tell us? My interpretation of these findings is that these patients had nutritional problems, which were manifesting as multiorgan disease, but not being recognised as such. For example selenium deficiency could present as schizophrenia and cancer. Magnesium deficiency could present as panic disorder and asthma. Copper excess could present as depression and high blood pressure. (It may be downloaded from www. dph.uwa.edu.au).

Clearly, drug therapy and the whole current medical paradigm with all its "objective" and "non-pecuniary" resources and research have failed these people (and all of us). Even if you don't believe anything else I have written, you have to take note of this metaphorical slap-in-the-face to modern medicine.

And now for the really bad news. Nothing is going to change until the people make a fuss. There are too many vested interests in ill health, so I urge you to start making a fuss.

References
Coghlan, R et al Duty to Care. Physical Illness in people with mental illness. UWA Publishing 2001.

DO I TAKE THE RED PILL OR THE BLUE ONE? WAKING UP FROM THE MATRIX.

In the last 4 years I have been training doctors in diagnostic orthomolecular medicine (DOM). This approach uses data from several sources. These are soil science, biochemistry, dietetics, environmental science, tissue mineral biochemistry and toxicology. These are the tools needed to fully appreciate the workings and undoing of the human body today. Obviously, many of these disciplines are not taught in medical schools, and so when interacting with the bulk of the profession, certain misunderstandings occur. Another important step in the progression to embracing DOM is the need to **unlearn** some of the brainwashing that has happened during and after medical school. I call this waking up from the Matrix, from the film of that name. There are at least 11 myths to dispel. Many of these have been covered in detail in the previous articles.

Myth 1] Excess stomach acid is responsible for all dyspepsia.
Clearly from studies done in this field, most people over the age of 40 start to loose the capacity to make enough stomach acid for digestion. The process of making acid is dependent quite heavily upon the mineral zinc. Zinc is also responsible for the production of the protective mucus layer, which protects us from acid. How can we eat tripe and yet not digest ourselves? When gastroenterologists give drugs to suppress acid, the painful symptoms improve but the digestion does not. The bloating, wind, bowel actions do not improve. Despite their patients telling them this, they continue blindly on with the erroneous hypothesis the at all dyspepsia must be hyperchlorhydria.

Myth 2] Iron deficiency doesn't cause problems until anaemia occurs.
This myth is still perpetuated by teachers in medical schools all over the planet. Most of our iron is stored in places *other* than the bone marrow. When the haemoglobin falls, this means that muscle levels of iron are extremely low, because the muscles have been lending iron to the marrow for months or years before anaemia occurs. Iron

deficiency is a disease in its own right. Bodies such as the College of General Practitioners publish algorithms for investigating fatigue. These are completely useless, and this is why medicine does not deal with this symptom well. Persistent fatigue will eventually be twisted into a depressive illness. "Well Mrs Jones, you don't realise this, but you have depression. Your tiredness, poor sleep pattern, difficulty in concentrating are all symptoms of depression. See this list? You fit the college's criteria for depression. Here take these pills…they're really not addictive".

Myth 3] Calcium is the main nutrient for bone production.
There is a *team* of nutrients that is required for the product of bone. Calcium in **not** number one, has **never** been number one and will **never** be number one. No drug company or brainwashed endocrinologist can change this. Magnesium is far more important than calcium. Another myth is that without dairy, we are all on low calcium diets. Below is a list of calcium foods ranged from excellent to good to fair.

Excellent	Good	Fair
Sesame seed, kelp, collard + kale leaves, turnip greens, almonds, soya beans, hazelnuts, parsley, dandelion greens, brazil nuts, watercress, chickpeas, white beans, pinto beans, pistachio nuts, figs (dr.), sunflower seeds, beetroot green, wheat bran, mung beans, olives, broccoli, broad beans, English walnut, rhubarb, okar, spinach, prune (dr.) Swiss chard	Endive, lentils, rice, bran, cowpea, pecan nut, lima bean, wheatgerm, chive, peanut, lettuce, apricot (dr.) savoy cabbage, peas (dr.), raisings, blackcurrant, dates, snap beans, chestnut, leek, pumpkin seeds, onion-green parsnip, cabbage, peach (dr.), macadamia nut, wheat, orange, celery, turnip, cashew, rye grain, carrot, brussel sprouts, Fig (dr.) loganberry, pear (dr.), radish, barley, banana (dr.).	Blackberry, red + white current, sweet potato, brown rice, apple (dr.), black raspberry, garlic, sorghum, cauliflower, cucumber, asparagus, pumpkin, strawberry, loquat, papaya, coconut water, millet, yarn, mung bean sprouts, wild rice, apricot, pineapple, grapefruit, grapes, coconut milk, beet, blueberry, cantaloupe, melon, tomato, eggplant, mango, peach, capsicum, pear, apple, mushroom, nectarine, sweet corn.

Myth 4] Helicobacter causes stomach ulcers.

The society of Gastroenterologists say that 40% of Australians have helicobacter. Some professors say that helicobacter causes stomach ulcers. Quite clearly if 40% of Australians have helicobacter, then the majority of people with helicobacter *do not develop ulcers.* You don't need a PhD to figure that out. Then, what is different about those who develop ulcers? They have no defence against a chronic infection and they do not have enough stomach acid to kill organisms that would invade the gastric tract. Gastric physiology texts say that nothing can survive in the stomach because the acid is *too strong* for organisms to survive it. The obvious answer is that helicobacter lives in the stomach because there is *not enough acid* to kill it off. The lack of acid is due to zinc deficiency. The gastritis is due to a lack of the protective mucus, which is also due to zinc deficiency.

NUTRIENTS NEEDED FOR BONE PRODUCTION

Magnesium	Vitamin D
Calcium	Vitamin C
Phosphorus	Parathyroid Hormone
Manganese	Progesterone
Zinc	Calcitonin
Molybdenum	
Boron	
Potassium	

Myth 5] Blood tests are the best investigation for nutritional medicine.

Recently, a colleague rang me from the Gold Coast asking for advice. He was finding that some patients had normal red blood cell levels of magnesium and zinc, but had symptoms indicative of deficiency in those minerals. The answer lies in that fact that hidden inhibitors such as excess copper and the presence of cadmium will block the function of both of these minerals in the cells. Tissue mineral analysis is the best way of detecting this process. Another good example was a study by Dr Sitruk-Ware in the seventies. He found that fibrocystic breast disease could be cured by using transdermal progesterone. He published this study, but was challenged to prove it with blood tests. When he repeated the blood tests, there was no change in serum progesterone. Transdermal progesterone is transferred in the red blood cells, and so when the red cells are spun off to get a serum sample the progesterone is not detectable. Red cell progesterone will reflect the change.

Myth 6] Hair analysis is useless.

Most doctors have never been taught how to read a tissue mineral test, so their ignorance is made obvious to the patients who enquire about this test, causing them to lose face. The usual arrogant reaction is "Those things are a waste of time". This type of technology has been used for more than 40 years. A mass spectrometer is a machine that can detect single atoms. I suggest that this makes it the most accurate medical investigation available.

Myth 7] Toxic metals need to be in large amounts to cause illness.

One mercury atom antagonises 1000 zinc atoms. One cadmium atom antagonises 100 zinc atoms. You do not need to be "toxic" to manifest clinical effects from these heavy metals. Toxicity is defined by *industry*, not by medicine. Industry will use the least sensitive method of defining toxicity because legal issues are at stake.

Myth 8] Drug are more potent that natural therapies.

Those who have treated patients with magnesium deficiency have seen the cluster of symptoms like unrefreshed sleep, leg cramps, palpitations and headaches improve with monotherapy. Medicine would have prescribed an analgesic, a sleeping tablet, quinine and a beta-blocker for the same set of symptoms.

Myth 9] Natural therapies kill more patients than prescription drugs.

Biased literature regularly emerges from bodies such as the PBAC, the TGA, the medical board, the AMA, the college of general practitioners decrying the use of "dangerous herbs and supplements". The reality is that doctors kill thousands (8000 plus) of people every year with prescriptions drugs. Hundreds more than the national road toll or the number of people killed with handguns. Clearly the statistics show that it is the medical profession that should be listed as lethal.

Myth 10] Drug companies don't make natural hormones because synthetics are better.
Effective brainwashing has convinced doctors that well meaning pharmaceutical companies produce synthetic hormones because these work better with fewer side-effects that the real thing. After thousands of years of evolution to arrive at the real thing, what manner of arrogance is contained in this thinking? Natural hormones are not patentable, that's all. It's all about money, and if you brainwash enough doctors, then you can make *lots of money*. We had a 200 million dollar blow out in the PBS recently. Is that a system that's working properly?

Myth 11] Medical specialists know the biochemistry and physiology of their field well.
Best-known examples are neurologists and oncologists. Many of the patients who come with problems like Multiple Sclerosis and Motor Neurone Disease, are dismayed that the neurologist was not aware of research into heavy metal toxicity causing such conditions. They were told "These things just happen". Is this really good enough?

ALL THE WORLD'S A STAGE AND ALL THE REAL PLAYERS ARE BIG BUSINESS (A true story from the future)

Scene: The year is 2046. It is a sunny Wednesday morning and the time is 10.02 am. It is the Medi-Crime court. First Floor Megapharm Building. St George's Tce, Perth. A panel of 4 peers and one Judge sit very high above the court.

Mr Bonnet (the Medi-Crime Prosecutort) addresses the accused: Dr Yossarian, you have been charged under section 15a subsection 12 of the Medi-Crime act of 2013 with the crime of vitamin prescribing.

Dr Yossarian: I don't recognize that act or this court. You are all employees of Megapharm. This is a joke.

Mr Bonnet: Your career is on the line here Doctor, so I suggest you humour us.

The trial of the Nutritional Doctor Continues......

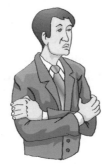 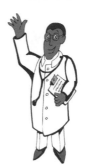

Mr Bonnet
Inquisitor for the Medical Board

Dr Yossarian
Nutritional Medicine Practitioner

Dr Yossarian: What actually did I do again?

Mr Bonnet: You were reported by a Dr Pita for prescribing zinc and magnesium to one of your patients. This type of prescribing was abolished in 2014 to protect the world from unscrupulous vitamin companies selling dangerous products to innocent NHS victims.

Dr Yossarian: This patient had documented zinc and magnesium
252

deficiency.

Mr Bonnet: That brings me to charge number 2. "Illegal use of a pathology laboratory for the misdirection of science".

Dr Yossarian: That was an accredited laboratory in South Africa. One of the few countries, which did not subscribe to this bullshit.

Mr Bonnet: Never-the-less, its use lead to a felony crime in this country. The obsolete belief that you ascribe to has been extinct for 32 years. Why do you continue to follow the "wizards" that led the Nutritional Medicine cults in the early century?

Dr Yossarian: They are extinct because most of them were killed at a conference in 2014. Probably, by the very company which employs you.

Mr Bonnet: I come from a long line of Medical Board representatives. We can sniff a heretic a mile away. These people committed mass suicide by drinking concentrated selenium and zinc. I have the newspaper article here. Do you wish to see it? (Hands it to Dr Yossarian).

Dr Yossarian: This is not the original article. I clearly remember the Australian reporting this differently.

Mr Bonnet: Do you have that article now?

Dr Yossarian: No.

Mr Bonnet: Then you have no proof really do you?

Dr Yossarian (mumbling): He who controls the past controls the future.

Mr Bonnet: What did you say?

Dr Yossarian: Its from Orwell's 1984.

Mr Bonnet: Oh, the comedy "When I'm 64". Most amusing. Yes, Orwell wrote a comedy called "When I'm 64". I believe that I have a copy of that somewhere too. Shall I produce it?

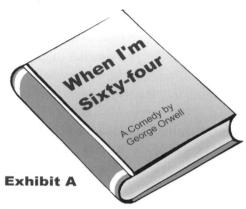

Exhibit A

Dr Yossarian: Probably no point now is there?

Mr Bonnet: Anyway, back to business. This crime is serious one.

Dr Yossarian: Because the patient got better?

Mr Bonnet: But she did not get better. She complained to Dr Pita that the tablets were too expensive and asked him was there something she could have on the NHS which was cheaper?

Dr Yossarian: The patient *did* get better, that's why Dr Pita dobbed me in. He did it out of spite.

Mr Bonnet: Whatever the reason, you're still in trouble.

Dr Yossarian: I acted in the interest of the patient and within a scientific framework. Test, treat and retest.

Mr Bonnet: What you did was illegal. Measuring minerals is illegal.
254

Prescribing minerals is illegal. These laws are in place to protect the public.

Dr Yossarian: These laws are in place to protect vested interest in ill health. Megapharm bought out all the supplement companies and then stopped production. In order to combat underground producers they forced the governments to outlaw vitamin sales and production. They were responsible for wiping out the best minds in Nutritional Medicine by murdering them and covering their tracks with assistance of people like you.

Mr Bonnet: Your attitude is quite belligerent: you obviously didn't train at our local Medical School. We filter out people like you in the first year. Only conservative line-toers ever leave *our* Medical School.

Dr Yossarian: I did train here, but I kept an open mind. They didn't have thought police then, so I was lucky.

Mr Bonnet: Your peers….

Dr Yossarian: These are not my peers. What have you get here? A neurosurgeon, a gynaecologist, a psychiatrist and a GP registrar. All of you work in medical centres owned by Megapharm. All of you are on their payroll. This is a Kangaroo Court , not an enquiry. None of them know anything about nutrition anyway, so don't call them my peers!

Mr Bonnet: These doctors practice conventional medicine. Medicine as written in books like Harrison's textbook of medicine. Your medicine is not in these books, so how, why do you practice it?

Dr Yossarian: All of the contributors to Harrison's are on the payroll of Megapharm. This is not objective information anymore. The chapter on depression basically deals with the various characteristics of the Drugs available. It does not discuss causes at all. Same with diabetes. These "peers" are just part of the *retail arm* of the

Pharmaceutical companies. They have been for *50 years!* The authors of DSM-IV were all on the payroll of Pharmaceutical Companies too. Pharmaceutical companies control medical school curricula now, but they started in the 80's when they realised that early brainwashing paid big dividends.

Mr Bonnet? You're quite a heretic aren't you? The panel has decided to jail you for 30 years.

Dr Yossarian: I'll appeal.

Mr Bonnet? This is the highest court for Medi-Crimes, sorry. By the way we have a questionnaire that we'd like you to fill out about your experience. We'd like your feedback, so we can improve the way we deal with doctors. Would you mind filling it in before you go to prison?

THE LAST WORD.

Well, what have we learned?

Point 1. Important nutritional information is not getting through to the people who could really benefit from it: the medical profession.

Point 2. Deficiency states can occur even with normal blood tests or even hair analysis.

Point 3. Digestive disturbances such as Helicobacter stomach infection can severely reduce absorption of nutrients, even with those on "good" diets.

Point 4. Environmental toxicity is occurring everyday in our children and ourselves. Generally the symptoms are not recognised for what they are.

Point 5. An ignorant medical profession bedazzled by clever marketing from Drug companies has dismissed important nutritional information out of hand.

Point 6. Health Authorities do not wish to public to "band together" and pool the large number of "anecdotes" into a huge chronicle. The Health Authorities (you can probably guess who we are talking about here) and other businesses with vested interests threaten (financially and professionally) anyone discovering such patterns. We actually have an "ill health" industry.